Natural Products in Clinical Trials

(Volume 2)

Edited by

Atta-ur-Rahman, *FRS*
Kings College, University of Cambridge, Cambridge, UK

Shazia Anjum
Department of Chemistry,
The Islamia University of Bahawalpur, Pakistan

&

Hesham R. El-Seedi
Department of Medicinal Chemistry, Uppsala University,
Biomedical Centre, Sweden

Natural Products in Clinical Trials

Volume # 2

Editor(s): Atta-ur-Rahman, *FRS*, Shazia Anjum and Hesham R. El-Seedi

ISSN (Online): 2468-0702

ISSN (Print): 2468-0699

ISBN (Online): 978-981-14-2576-9

ISBN (Print): 978-981-14-2575-2

need for a court order if at any point you breach any terms of this License Agreement. In no event will any delay or failure by Bentham Science Publishers in enforcing your compliance with this License Agreement constitute a waiver of any of its rights.

3. You acknowledge that you have read this License Agreement, and agree to be bound by its terms and conditions. To the extent that any other terms and conditions presented on any website of Bentham Science Publishers conflict with, or are inconsistent with, the terms and conditions set out in this License Agreement, you acknowledge that the terms and conditions set out in this License Agreement shall prevail.

Bentham Science Publishers Pte. Ltd.
80 Robinson Road #02-00
Singapore 068898
Singapore
Email: subscriptions@benthamscience.net

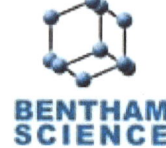

BENTHAM SCIENCE

CONTENTS

PREFACE

Nature provides mankind with an amazing diversity of chemical structures, which is accompanied with corresponding variety of biological activities. This volume presents the discovery of new bioactive natural products that have been clinically tested for use as drugs.

Silva *et al.* in chapter 1 cover all recent patents on natural products in clinical trial to treat schistosomiasis- a neglected tropical diseases found in about 70 tropical and subtropical countries

Salem *et al.* in two separate chapters 2 and 4 of this volume describe natural products used to treat metabolic disorders and cardiovascular diseases. A brief outline of the pathophysiology of metabolic disorders is provided in chapter 2. The chapter includes all natural products based drug therapies that are currently applied in clinical trials attributed to metabolic disorders. In chapter 4 those natural products that are specifically used to cure cardiovascular diseases have been discussed with special emphasis on their efficacy and safety under preclinical studies and clinical trials.

Fluorine-containing natural products possess remarkable bioactivities. Statistical data regarding the role of fluorine in medicinal chemistry and drug design is very well established. Zhuang *et al.* in chapter 3 summarize the use of fluorinated natural products in drug development in a comprehensive way.

Prevalence of various ocular diseases is high, but few remedies are available. Interestingly, natural compounds are also used for the prevention of ocular diseases. Johar *et al.* describe several avenues for the application of natural compounds in the prevention and treatment of various ocular diseases in chapter 5. The chapter also covers probable mechanisms responsible for the disease formation, identification of targets, and the evaluation of candidate molecules by *in silico*, *in vitro* and *in vivo* assays. It is hoped that the readers will enjoy reading the wide-ranging and comprehensive reviews contributed by eminent scholars.

We would like to thank the editorial staff of Bentham Science Publishers, particularly Ms. Asma Ahmed, Mr. Obaid Sadiq and Mr. Mahmood Alam for their constant support.

Prof. Atta-ur-Rahman, *FRS*
Kings College
University of Cambridge
Cambridge
UK

Shazia Anjum
Department of Chemistry
The Islamia University of Bahawalpur
Pakistan

&

Hesham R. El-Seedi
Division of Pharmacognosy, Department of Medicinal Chemistry
Uppsala University, Biomedical Centre
Sweden

List of Contributors

Ahmed Elissawy — Department of Pharmacognosy, Ain Shams University, Abbassia, Cairo 11566, Egypt

Assem M. El-Shazly — Department of Pharmacognosy, Zagazig University, Zagazig 44519, Egypt

Ahmed Zayed — Department of Pharmacognosy, Tanta University, Tanta, Egypt

Amr A. Mahrous — Department of Pharmacology and Toxicology, Cairo University, Cairo 11562, Egypt
Department of Neuroscience, Cell Biology, and Physiology, Wright State University, Dayton, Ohio 45435, USA

A.R Vasavada — Iladevi Cataract and IOL Research Centre, Ahmedabad, India

Ademar Alves da Silva Filho — Department of Pharmaceutical Sciences, Federal University of Juiz de Fora, R. José Lourenço Kelmer s/n, Juiz de Fora, Brazil

Chunlin Zhuang — School of Pharmacy, Second Military Medical University, Shanghai, China

Dalia I. Hamdan — Department of Pharmacognosy, Menoufia University, Shibin Elkom, Egypt

Everton Allan Ferreira — Department of Pharmaceutical Sciences, Federal University of Juiz de Fora, R. José Lourenço Kelmer s/n, Juiz de Fora, Brazil

Islam Mostafa — Department of Pharmacognosy, Zagazig University, Zagazig 44519, Egypt

Josué de Moraes — Núcleo de Pesquisa em Doenças Negligenciadas, Universidade Guarulhos, Guarulhos, São Paulo, Brazil

Kaid Johar SR — Department of Zoology, Biomedical Technology and Human Genetics, Gujarat University, Ahmedabad , India

Lívia Mara Silva — Department of Pharmaceutical Sciences, Federal University of Juiz de Fora, R. José Lourenço Kelmer s/n, Juiz de Fora, Brazil

Lara Soares Aleixo de Carvalho — Department of Pharmaceutical Sciences, Faculty of Pharmacy, Federal University of Juiz de Fora, R. José Lourenço Kelmer s/n, Campus Universitário, 36036-900, Juiz de Fora, Minas Gerais, Brazil

Lucas Sales Queiroz — Department of Pharmaceutical Sciences, Federal University of Juiz de Fora, R. José Lourenço Kelmer s/n, Juiz de Fora, Brazil

Mahitab H. El Bishbishy — Department of Pharmacognosy, October University for Modern Sciences and Arts (MSA), Giza, Egypt

Maha M. Salama — Department of Pharmacognosy, Cairo University, Cairo 11562, Egypt
Department of Pharmacognosy, British University in Egypt, Cairo 11837, Egypt

Mohamed A. Salem — Department of Pharmacognosy, Menoufia University, Shibin Elkom, Egypt

Ohana Zuza — Department of Pharmaceutical Sciences, Faculty of Pharmacy, Federal University of Juiz de Fora, R. José Lourenço Kelmer s/n, Campus Universitário, 36036-900, Juiz de Fora, Minas, Gerais, Brazil

Priscila de Faria Pinto — Department of Biochemistry, Institute of Biological Sciences, Federal University of Juiz de Fora, Juiz de Fora, MG, Brazil

Pooja Rathaur — Department of Life Science, Gujarat University, Ahmedabad, India

Rasha Adel — Department of Pharmacognosy, Zagazig University, Zagazig 44519, Egypt

Shraddha Bhadada Institute of Pharmacy, Nirma University, Ahmedabad, India

Shahira M. Ezzat Department of Pharmacognosy, October University for Modern Sciences and Arts (MSA), Giza 12451, Egypt
Department of Pharmacognosy, Cairo University, Kasr El-Aini Street, Cairo 11562, Egypt

Wannian Zhang School of Pharmacy, Second Military Medical University, Shanghai, China
School of Pharmacy, Ningxia Medical University, Yinchuan , China

Yuelin Wu School of Chemical and Environmental Engineering, Shanghai Institute of Technology, Shanghai, China

Zhenyuan Miao School of Pharmacy, Second Military Medical University, Shanghai, China

A Review of Recent Patents and Natural Products in Clinical Trial to Treat Schistosomiasis

Lívia Mara Silva[1], Lara Soares Aleixo de Carvalho[1], Ohana Zuza[1], Lucas Sales Queiroz[1], Everton Allan Ferreira[1], Josué de Moraes[2], Priscila de Faria Pinto[3] and Ademar Alves da Silva Filho[1,*]

[1] *Department of Pharmaceutical Sciences, Faculty of Pharmacy, Federal University of Juiz de Fora, R. José Lourenço Kelmer s/n, Campus Universitário, 36036-900, Juiz de Fora, Minas Gerais, Brazil*

[2] *Núcleo de Pesquisa em Doenças Negligenciadas, Universidade Guarulhos, Guarulhos, São Paulo, Brazil*

[3] *Department of Biochemistry, Institute of Biological Sciences, Federal University of Juiz de Fora, Juiz de Fora, MG, Brazil*

Abstract: Schistosomiasis, caused by trematode flatworms of the genus *Schistosoma*, is one of the most significant neglected tropical diseases in about 70 tropical and subtropical countries. It is estimated that over 200 million people are infected and more than 770 million are at risk of infection. *S. mansoni*, *S. haematobium* and *S. japonicum* are the major etiological agents of human schistosomiasis, whose treatment is dependent on a single drug, praziquantel (PZQ). In the light of the exclusive dependency on PZQ, there is an urgent and unmet need to discover novel therapeutic agents against this pathogen. In this chapter, we comprehensively addressed chemical and pharmacological aspects of the schistosomicidal patented compounds in the early 20th century, beginning with antimonials as the first compounds in the schistosomiasis treatment, passing over the next years with many chemical derivatives, such as imidazoline, acridone and carbazoles, and, after, with PZQ and artemisinin, in the 1980s. Also, recent patents have been described covering other drugs, such as *N*-phosphorylate amino acids, peroxide derivatives, and cysteine protease inhibitors along with new patents based on natural compounds, such as alkaloids, terpenes, and anthraquinones.

Keywords: Alkaloids, Antimonials, Artemisin, Bilharzia, Natural Products, Patent, Piperazine, Praziquantel, Schistosomiasis, *Schistosoma*, Terpenes.

* **Corresponding Author Ademar Alves da Silva Filho:** Department of Pharmaceutical Sciences, Faculty of Pharmacy, Federal University of Juiz de Fora, R. José Lourenço Kelmer s/n, Campus Universitário, 36036-900, Juiz de Fora, Minas Gerais, Brazil; E-mail: ademar.alves@ufjf.edu.br

Atta-ur-Rahman, Shazia Anjum and Hesham Al-Seedi (Eds.)

INTRODUCTION

Schistosomiasis, also known as bilharzia, is one of the most significant neglected diseases, affecting more than 207 million people worldwide and exposing about 700 million to the risk of infection in more than 70 countries [1 - 3]. Schistosomiasis, which was described in 1852 by Theodor Bilharz, is a disease caused by trematodes worms of the genus *Schistosoma*. The main species that reach man are *Schistosoma mansoni, S. guineans, S. japonicum, S. mekongi, S. intercalatum* and *S. haematobium* [2]. Of these species, *S. haematobium* causes urinary schistosomiasis, classically manifested as inflammation and deformation of the bladder, ureters or kidneys, while *S. mansoni, S. japonicum, S. intercalatum, S. guineans* and *S. mekongi* are associated with intestinal inflammation and hepatosplenic schistosomiasis [4 - 6].

Schistosoma is a parasite that presents a high sexual dimorphism, having separated and easily distinguishable sexes. Male adult worms are shorter than female, which in turn are larger and thinner. Usually, the couple is found together due to the gynecophore channel (opening on the back of the male worm that houses the female) and the intercourse between them is constant [7].

Adult worms of *S. mansoni* live in the mesenteric veins, mainly in the inferior mesenteric vein, migrating against the circulatory current. Each female puts about 400 eggs *per day* on the walls of capillaries and venules. Some eggs are transported to the liver, where they cause fibromatous inflammation and chronic problems [7 - 9]. In the gut, the eggs are released along with the faecal cake.

The eggs produced by adult worms are released by feces or urine in the water, where the mature eggs release the miracidium, which are the infective forms for the snails and can penetrate into various molluscs, mainly into snails of *Biomphalaria, Bulinus* and *Oncomelania* genus. After penetrating, the miracidium undergoes a sequence of transformations, originating the cercariae that are released in the water and, after contacting with the skin, penetrate into definitive host (human or other host) [7 - 9]. The cercariae are bifurcated larvae that actively penetrate the skin and mucous of the definitive hosts, through their suckers, intense movement and histolytic secretions [9]. Inside of the definitive host, the cercariae lose their bifurcated tail and transform into schistosomula, which migrate to the hepatoportal circulation, where they mature into male and female adult worms. After the coupling, pairs of adult worms migrate to their final niche in the mesenteric circulation where they begin egg production, which is responsible for the resulting immunopathological lesions [8 - 10].

The pathology that characterizes schistosomiasis is caused mainly by deposition of eggs in tissues, including the urinary tract, intestine and liver. Also, parasite eggs may trigger more serious health problems such as bladder cancer, hepatic cirrhosis, hydronephrosis, and reproductive complications [4].

The control of schistosomiasis is based on large-scale treatment of at-risk population groups, access to safe water, improved sanitation, hygiene education, and snail control. Current schistosomiasis control programs rely on one drug, praziquantel (PZQ). Chemotherapy with this drug, that was developed in the 1970s, has emerged as the major tool, because its safe and low-cost intervention produces a rapid impact [11]. However, the reliance on a single drug for the treatment of a disease as severe as schistosomiasis raises major concerns for health agencies and it is necessary to research and discover new drugs to act against the disease. In this context, this chapter attempts to summarize the schistosomicidal compounds patented in the early 20th century, and the main aspects related to the new patented schistosomicidal drugs, as well as clinical trials with some of them to treat schistosomiasis.

1. DRUGS DISCOVERY AND PATENTED UNTIL 2000

The period prior to 2000 was remarkable for the treatment of schistosomiasis, since it was a period of discovery of important drugs, such as PZQ, until now used as a pillar for the treatment of schistosomiasis.

1.1. Antimonials and Piperazine Derivatives

In 1917, emetic tartar (**1**) was first used in the treatment of schistosomiasis [12]. Antimony derivatives (Fig. **1**) have been used for the treatment of leishmaniasis in humans and dogs for decades [13, 14]. However, the use of antimony derivatives has been abandoned due to its undesirable toxic effects and the appearance of less toxic drugs such as oxamniquine and praziquantel. In order to develop alternatives to these drugs, the antimonial derivatives (patent WO2006000069 A1) were improved with the aid of liposomes and cyclodextrins aiming to inhibit the toxic effects and to deliver the drug exactly to its site of action. As a result, this present invention found that both promote cutaneous and transdermal drug absorption. Antimony derivatives include preferentially the pentavalent antimonial, meglumine antimoniate (**2**) and sodium stibogluconate (**3**), and antimony complexes [15]. In agreement with the present invention, it has been demonstrated that the association of an antimonial to cyclodextrin results in increased oral, cutaneous and percutaneous absorption of antimony. In this way, this invention presents a potential drug for use by oral and topical routes, for the treatment of schistosomiasis [15].

The patent DE2901350 A1 (1980) provided a novel agent for the treatment of schistosomiasis, with the administration of alkali metal salts of 2,3-dimercaptopropane-1-sulfonic acid together with the known antimony compounds. The association enhances the effect of the compounds but also, at the same time, significantly reduce their toxicity [16].

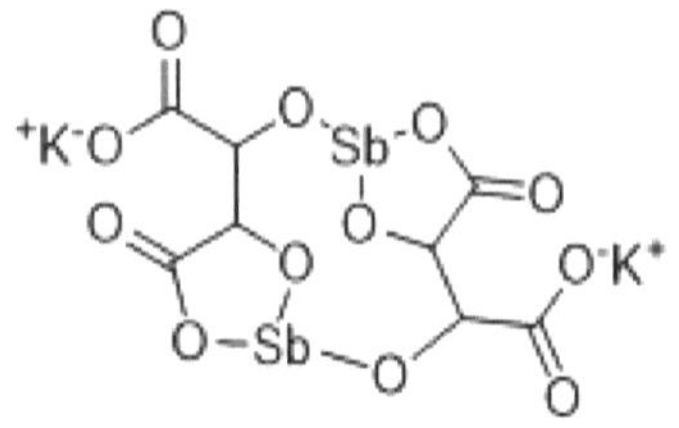

1

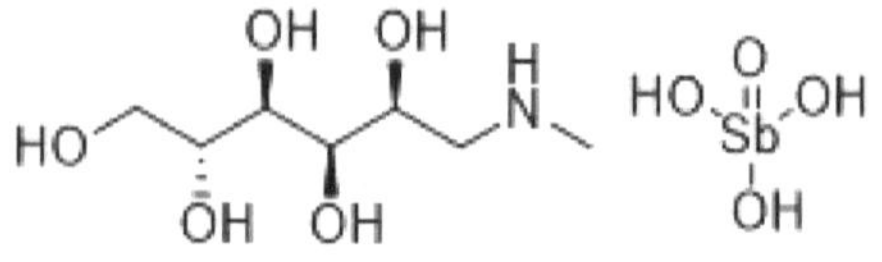

2

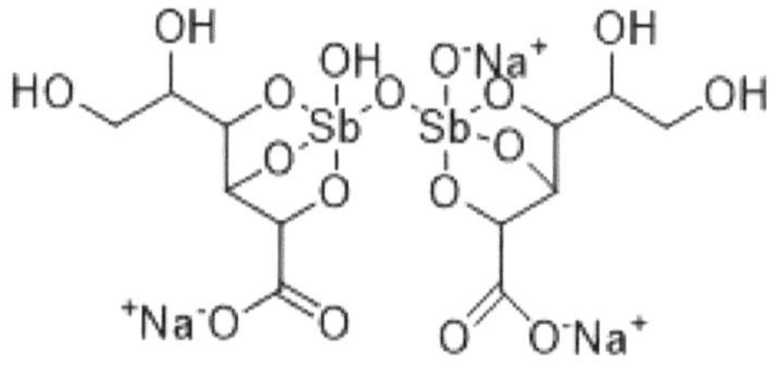

3

Fig. (1). Antimony derivatives. Tartar emetic (**1**), meglumine antimoniate (**2**) and sodium stibogluconate (**3**)

Other compounds used were the piperazine derivatives. Among potential drugs, piperazine compounds (Fig. **2**) possess a six membered heterocyclic ring containing nitrogen, which is present in several drugs with important medicinal potentials [17]. In 1964, Abbott Laboratories patented the use of piperazine derivatives, for the treatment of schistosomiasis. One of these derivatives, named as A-16612 (**4**), showed high schistosomicidal activity in mice. However, in monkeys and humans, A-16612 (**4**) caused serious adverse effects, such as hallucinations and asthenia [18]. Following, in 1965, the Patent US 3203858 A described arylpiperazine sulfones, such as (**5**), as effective agents against *S. mansoni* in some animals and, especially, in humans by oral or parenteral routes of administration [19]. In 1971, Tomcufcik *et al.* deposited a patent describing the synthesis of various schistosomicidal aminoalkylene piperazines 1,4-substituted, such as (dimethylamino-3-propyl)-1-piperazine (**6**) and benzoyl-1 (dimethylamino-3-propyl)-4-piperazine (**7**), which inhibited the development of the *S. mansoni* cycle in mice [20]. Also, in 1972, the patent US3639602 A reported the use of 2,4-di-4-arylpiperazine compounds, such as (**8**), and their acid salts as effective *in vivo* agents for treating schistosomiasis, when orally or parenterally administered at the doses of 50 to 500 mg/kg [21]. Similarly, the patent US4515793 described the use of phenylpiperazines derivatives, such as (**9**), as *in vivo* antischistosomial compounds. Results showed that after 120 days of treatment, when mice were treated with two oral doses of 40 or 125 mg/kg, a 100% of worm's reduction was observed [22].

Fig. (**2**). Some schistosomicidal piperazine derivatives: A-16612 (**4**), bis-[4-(3-chloro-4-methylphenyl)piperazine] ethyl sulfones (**5**), (dimethylamino-3-propyl)-1-piperazine (**6**), benzoyl-1 (dimethylamino-3-propyl)-4-piperazine (**7**), 2,4-di-(4-arylpiperazino) (**8**) and 2-[4-[3-Chloro-4-(hydroxymethyl)phenyl-l-piperazinyl]-l-phenylethanone (**9**).

At that time, other compounds were developed and researched (Fig. **3**). The patent GB908986 A in 1962 comprised racemic and optically active compounds, such as (**10**), which are particularly useful in reacting with trivalent antimony compounds to yield complexes that could be used in the treatment of *S. mansoni* infections [23]. In 1976, the patent CH 571475 A5 described interesting chemotherapeutic properties, as well as low toxicity for diethylaminobenzaldehydes, such as (**11**), with was active against helminths, especially against *Schistosoma sp* [24]. Likewise, nitrofuranepropenamides, such as (**12**), was patented in 1986 with the number JO 1360 B. The invention described their parasiticidal activity against certain types of infective worms, including *Schistosoma* species [25].

Fig. (3). Some schistosomicidal compounds. 2,3-dimercapto-succinic acid (**10**), 4-(2-diethylami-o-ethylamino)-benzaldehydes (**11**) and N-(4-methoxy-2-methyl phenyl)-3-(5-nitro-2-furanyl) propenamide (**12**).

1.2. Imidazolidine Derivatives

The use of imidazolidine compounds (such as **13**) was introduced as an alternative to treat schistosomiasis in 1964. Since that, new derivative compounds have emerged to improve the treatment. It is known that the imidazolidine core is an extremely important pharmacophore group, known in the literature by its large spectrum of biological activities, including the schistosomicidal activity. The following patent, GB1278272 A (1972) described the use of the new hexahydro-imidazoquinoline compound (**13**) (Fig. **4**) in the treatment of schistosomiasis [26].

The new hexahydro-imidazoquinoline compound (**13**) was orally and intraperitoneally administered in mice. The dosages were 25mg/Kg daily, during 4 days, or 50 mg/kg in a single dose. The efficacy was checked 24 hours after the last treatment, showing that all compounds were only slightly less active than the parent compound. However, the derived compounds demonstrated a longer-acting than their parent compounds and their therapeutic effectiveness seems to be as good as or even better than the parent compounds [26].

13

Fig. (4). Example of imidazolidine compounds (**13**).

1.3. Acridanone Derivatives

Some acridanone derivatives, developed by Hoffmann-La Roche in 1985, have demonstrated schistosomicidal activities through distinct mechanisms of action. The main compound appointed to have powerful antischistosomal activity, is Ro 15-5458 (**14**) (Fig. **5**), which was patented (US4711889). This compound exhibited significant action in comparison with standard antischistosomal drugs against the three principal human species of the parasite [27, 28]. Firstly, it was demonstrated, by Sturrock *et al.*, (1985), that doses of 25 mg/kg were fully effective against *S. mansoni* [27, 28]. Moreover, the association of PZQ with Ro 15-5458 (**14**) was high effective on reducing *S. mansoni* infection [29]. Other researches have demonstrated the effectiveness of this compound on different phases of the parasite development, and different *Schistosoma* species [30 - 32].

14

Fig. (5). Chemical structure of the Ro 15-5458 (**14**).

1.4. Carbazoles

The Patent WO 8911480 A1 (1989) described the schistosomicidal and antitumor effects of the 6H-pyrido(4,3-b)carbazoles derivatives, which are synthetic compounds related to ellipticine (**15**) and olivacine (**16**) (Fig. **6**) [33, 34]. It was found that the compound *cis*-octahydro-6H-pyrido[4,3-b]carbazole (**17**) presented schistosomicidal activity in both hycanthone-sensitive and hycanthone-resistant worms. Hycanthone is a drug with known schistosomicidal activity [33].

15   **16**   **17**

Fig. (6). Carbazoles and its derivatives. Ellipticine (**15**), olivacine and (**16**) 5-hydroxymethyl-11-methy--6H-pyrido [4,3-b] carbazole N-methylcarbamate carbazole (**17**).

1.5. Aminoacyl Adenylate Mimics

Aminoacyl-tRNA synthetases (AARS) are a family of essential enzymes that may be found in every biological cell that are responsible for maintaining the fidelity of protein synthesis, by catalyzing the aminoacylation of tRNA [35]. The disruption of protein translation in some organisms may be caused by inhibition of tRNA synthetases. According to the patent US5726195 A (1998) new tRNA synthetases inhibitors have emerged, such as aminoacyl adenylate mimics, which inhibit isoleucyltRNA synthetases and have efficacy against a broad spectrum of bacteria, fungi, and parasites [35]. It was found that the compound (**18**) (Fig. **7**) were active against parasites, including *Entamoeba*, *Leishmania*, and *Schistosoma* [35].

18

Fig. (7). Aminoacyl adenylate mimic compound (**18**).

1.6. Praziquantel, Its Derivatives and Recent Studies

In the late 1970s, PZQ (**19**), an isoquinoline-pyrazine derivative, was introduced and immediately proved to be superior to any other schistosomicidal drug, quickly becoming the drug of choice in most endemic areas. PZQ is effective against all human adult worms of *Schistosoma* species, but has poor activity against juvenile worms. It has very low toxicity, and no important long-term safety difficulties have been documented in people so far. PZQ has several advantages, such as low cost, single administration with high efficacy, broad therapeutic profile, high tolerability, and few and transient side effects [36]. The mechanism of PZQ action is not clearly understood; calcium alterations appear to be the primary effects of this drug [37].

Considering that more than 218 million people need treatment for the disease each year and that the drug is the only one indicated by WHO to treat the disease, the emergence of praziquantel-resistant parasites is a concern [11, 38]. Currently, there are several patents involving this drug, its derivatives, medicinal associations and pharmaceutical formulations in order to improve its pharmacokinetic and pharmacokinetic characteristics. In addition, because it is a drug worldwide and extensively used, there are many clinical trials with PZQ.

The patent EP0024868B1 (1981), also published as DE3063894 D1, EP0024868 B1 and US4303659, reported the association of PZQ and oxamniquine [39]. Oxamniquine, a tetrahydroquinoline derivative, is described as one of the most promising schistosomicides [40]. In the last thirty years this drug has been widely used on the American continent, in particular in Brazil, where *S. mansoni* is the only endemic species. Oxamniquine is relatively safe, with limited side effects, but has some disadvantages, such as be effective only against *S. mansoni*. Oxamniquine is being withdrawn from the market and replaced by PZQ [41]. The finding involved in this patent is that the concomitant use of oxamniquine and PZQ is particularly valuable in the treatment of schistosomiasis, due to a synergism. Different concentrations of the associated compounds were tested, the oxamniquine to PZQ ratio being 1: 0.5 to 1.0: 5.0, in dosage forms for oral administration (syrup, tablets, capsules and the like). The reported dose is dependent on the individual's body weight, but is generally 1-20 mg/kg of oxamniquine and 2.5-40 mg/kg of PZQ, when administered orally or parenterally. The assay was performed on Charles River (UK) CD-1 mice, infected with the Puerto Rican strain of *S. mansoni*. Formulations were orally administered by gavage and after 14 days the animals were euthanized. Then, worms were recovered by portal hepatic perfusion and the liver was histologically evaluated. Comparing the association with the isolated compounds, the total dose required for the combination to promote the same efficacy of the individual compounds is the half dose of using oxamniquine alone and 1/7 of the dose using PZQ alone [42].

Regarding the improvement of PZQ activity by new formulations, the Patent CN102138890 A (2011) describes the preparation of a transdermal formulation of PZQ to 35%, adjuvant 206 of 40% to 60% and aqueous solution [43]. The transdermal formulation may enhance the bioavailability of pharmaceutical preparations, provided it ensures the penetration of the drug. Therefore, a transdermal penetration enhancer was used in the formulation, consisting of a mixture of isopropyl myristate, nitrione, propylethylglycol, oleic acid, and the like. The formulation was tested on New Zealand white rabbits infected with *S. japonicum*, 28 days post infection. The rabbits were divided into groups and group I received formulation with a concentration of the drug equal to 24%, given once. Group II also received the concentration of 24%, but 2-fold. After 45 days of treatment, the rabbits were sacrificed, worms were collected after portal hepatic perfusion and the eggs present in the liver were collected for counting under an optical microscope. The results show a reduction of 80% of adult worms in group I and 96.23% in group II [43].

Among PZQ derivatives (Fig. **8**), the patent CN102285985 B (2011), also published as CN 201110142534 [44] related the used of the hydroxylated praziquantel derivative (10-hydroxyl PZQ, **20**). This compound has some advantages over PZQ. While PZQ is active only against the adult forms of *S. japonicum*, 10-hydroxyl praziquantel (**20**) demonstrated activity against adult and larval forms, in addition to better solubility. Previous work modified the aromatic ring with the addition of nitro groups or amides, but derivatives with nitro grouping showed no activity against *S. japonicum* and amides were less effective than PZQ [44, 45]. The schistosomicidal activity of 10-hydroxyl praziquantel (**20**) was also compared with other compounds, such as artemisinin derivatives, as reported by Duan *et al.* [46]. *In vitro* and *in vivo* results demonstrated that 10-hydroxy praziquantel (**20**) is a promising schistosomicidal compound, since it was very active against larval and adult forms of the parasite [46].

The patent CN105037354 A (2015), also published as CN102432607 A, related the use of other pyrazine isoquinoline derivatives (**21** and **22**) similar to PZQ and their application for the treatment of schistosomiasis, with a focus on the elimination of adult worms and larvae [47]. The compounds of this invention and the mechanism of action are not well understood. However, the activity is similar to PZQ, being related to calcium channels, contraction of the muscles and damages in tegument, with affect the absorption of nutrients [47]. These compounds show rapid absorption after oral administration, and highest plasma concentration of the drug in the plasma is reached after 1 to 2 hours. Metabolization occurs in the liver and its main product is a hydroxylated metabolite. The compound does not cross the placenta, does not accumulate in tissues, and binds to serum proteins by up to 80%. The compounds (**21** and **22**) were tested in pharmaceutical formulations for oral or parenteral administration and satisfactory results were obtained at 10 to 25 mg/kg. The *in vitro* assay was performed with *S. japonicum* and compounds were tested at concentrations of 5-50 mol/mL. Results showed that the new compounds are more active than PZQ, causing the death of both larvae and adult worms [47]. Other active PZQ derivatives were also matter of invention in the patent CN104327076 A (2015), which related the use of the racemic compounds **23**, **24** and **25** for the treatment of schistosomiasis [48].

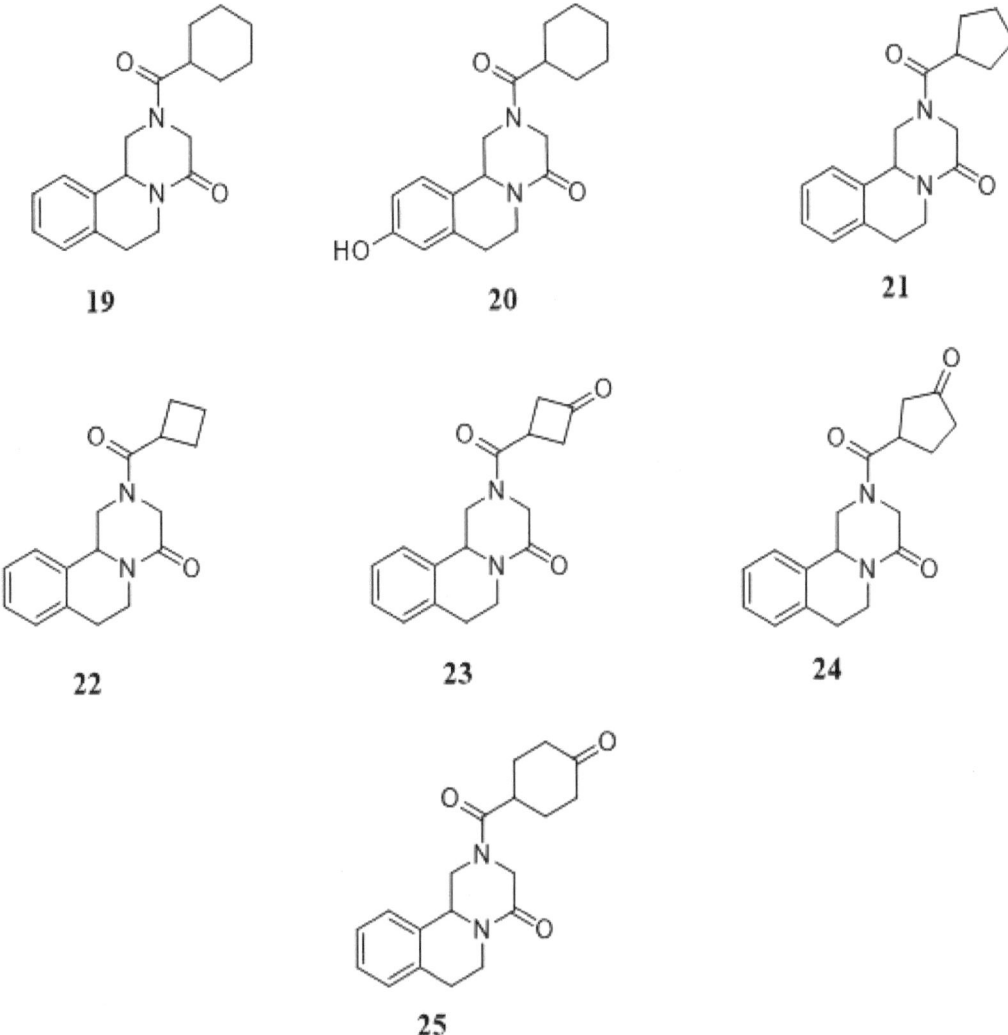

Fig. (8). Praziquantel and related compounds. Praziquantel (**19**), 10-hydroxyl praziquantel (**20**), pyrazine isoquinoline derivatives (**21** and **22**), Rac-1 (**23**), Rac-2 (**24**) and Rac-3 (**25**).

2. ARTEMISIN, ITS DERIVATIVES AND RECENT STUDIES

The schistosomicidal activity of artemisinin (**26**) was first reported by Chen *et al.*, 1980 [49]. Since then, laboratory-based studies have revealed that some artemisinin derivatives, best known for their antimalarial properties, also have potential effects against the juvenile forms of *S. mansoni* [12, 50]. In 2003, Li *et al.* patented (WO2003022855 A1) the new tert-butoxy dihydro-artemisinin derivative (**27**) (Fig. **9**) against *Schistosoma*. Comparing with other artemisinin derivatives, the tert-butoxy dihydro-artemisinin (**27**) has a highest therapeutical index (> 1700), as well as it may reduce the toxicity and side effects [50 - 52].

In 2004, according to the patent CN102276632 B, it was introduced the idea of using the combination of the artemisinin derivatives artesunate (**28**) and artemether (**29**) with PZQ against *S. japonicum* [53]. In this regard, a new compound DW-3-15 (**30**) was synthesized, bonding covalently a PZQ molecule with an artemisinin derivative. This new compound DW-3-15 (**30**) was tested against young and adult schistosomes of *S. japonicum*, showing 100% of dead against both phases in 24 hours at 25 μM concentration. When tested in mice, the oral administration of DW-3-15 (**30**) (200 mg/kg, for 5 days) was able to reduce in 55.3% the worm burden, while the rate of reduction of PZQ was 50.3% [54].

Fig. (9). Artemisinin and its derivatives. Artemisinin (**26**), tert-butoxy dihydro artimisinin (**27**), artesunate (**28**), artemether (**29**) and DW-3-15 (**30**).

More recently, in 2013, another patent has been filed in respect of artesunate (**28**) derivatives. This invention (CN103405779 A) disclosed a long-acting artesunate drug for preventing schistosome infection. According to this invention, artesunate was coupled to the GST-NSP protein, producing an artesunate *n*-GST-NSP conjugate, with low immunogenicity. This conjugate is able not only to maintain the activity in juvenile schistosome, but also to prolong the half-life period of the artesunate in the host, being active in the early phases, as well as in preventing schistosome infection [55].

3. RECENT PATENTS AND CLINICAL TRIAL OF SYNTHETIC DRUGS

3.1. N-phosphorylated Amino Acid

The invention, described in the patent CN1262929 A in 2000, reported some phosphorylated amino acids for the reduction of the hepatic granulomas caused by schistosomiasis, possessing reduced toxicity [56]. *N*-(O, O- diethyl) - phosphoryl tyrosine (**31**) were tested in mice infected with *S. japonicum*, intraperitoneally administered at doses of 6 mg/day for 10 days. After 3 weeks of treatment, mice were sacrificed and the number of *S. japonicum* eggs was quantified. Results demonstrated that after ten days treatment, the new compound (**31**) (Fig. **10**) showed remarkable therapeutic effect, reducing in 49.33% the adult worms and 72.29% the number of eggs. Results of the trial demonstrated that the novel compounds have significant effect for the treatment of schistosomiasis [56].

31

Fig. (10). *N*-phosphorylated amino acid. *N*-(O, O- diethyl) - phosphoryl tyrosine (**31**).

3.2. Peroxide Derivatives

The patent CN101909627 A (2010) also known as WO2009071553, described the new therapeutic use of peroxide derivatives to treat schistosomiasis [57]. Similar molecules were described in the patent applications US 6486199 B1 and US 20040039008 A1 [58]. In this patent (CN101909627) it was shown the *in vitro* schistosomicidal activity of PA1259 (**32**) (Fig. **11**). PA1259 (**32**) was tested at 300, 100, 10, and 5 µg/mL on schistosomules and adult worms. PA 1259 (at 5 µg/mL) was able to kill 100% of schistosomules in 3 hours of incubation, as well as 100% of adult schistosomes in 1 hour when tested at 100 µg/mL [57, 59].

Another peroxide derivative useful for the prophylaxis and treatment of schistosomiasis was patented in 2013 (US2013245108). This peroxide derivative (**33**) (Fig. **11**) was capable of killing *S. mansoni* at the immature stage, *in vivo* inhibiting the growth of the schistosomes and preventing the development of liver dysfunction [60]. *In vivo* experiments showed a reduction of about 86% in the number of recuperated worms and a reduction of 98% in the number of eggs produced by adult female schistosomes [60].

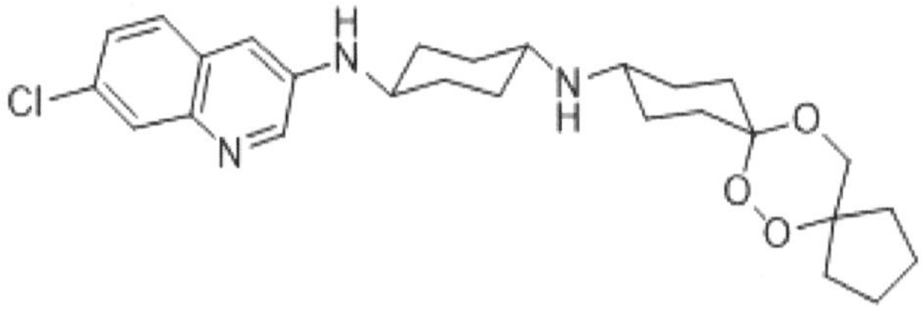

32

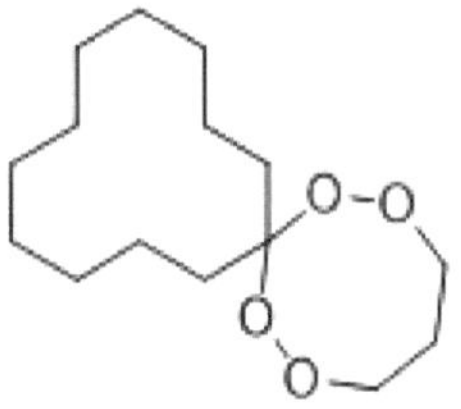

33

Fig. (11). Peroxide derivatives PA1259 (**32**) and (**33**).

3.3. Oxadiazole N-oxide Derivatives

As *S. mansoni* worms lives in an aerobic environment, they have to minimize damages caused by oxygen radicals, such as superoxide, H_2O_2, and hydroxyl radical. In this regard, an option in the development of new compounds is new drugs that will target the parasite's redox system, which depends on thioredoxin-glutathione reductase (TGR), an enzyme that replaces both glutathione reductase and thioredoxin reductase in the parasite. Based on that, it is described in the patent WO2009076265 A1 (2009) the inhibition of TGR and the schistosomicidal activity of selected oxadiazoles *N*-oxide derivatives. *In vitro* assays showed that the oxadiazol 2-oxide (**34**) (Fig. **12**) was able to kill adult worms and to inhibit TGR in schistosome [61]. As furoxan (**35**) (Fig. **12**) shares with another member of its family 1,2,5-oxadiazole ring, it was tested to check its ability to inhibit TGR in the parasite [61]. *In vivo* experiments indicated furoxan (**35**) was significantly active against all intra-mammalian lifecycle stages of *S. mansoni*, with at least an 89% of reduction in worm burdens [61].

Also, the patent US2011207784 A1 (2011) worked in the same field, assessing the schistosomicidal activity of oxadiazoles compounds, specifically oxadiazole-2-oxides [62]. Results showed that the oxadiazole-2-oxides derivatives (**36**) were able to inhibit TGR at concentrations of 0.11 µM and 11.2 µM, as well as to kill 100% of treated *S. mansoni* worms after 48h of incubation [62].

34 **35** **36**

Fig. (12). Oxadiazoles compounds. Oxadiazole 2- oxide (**34**), Furoxan (**35**) and Oxadiazole derivative (**36**).

3.4. Trioxolanes

The invention of 1,2,4-trioxolanes, with their prodrugs and analogues (Patent EP2599779, 2013), comprises novel compounds able to treat malaria and schistosomiasis. The trioxolanes analogues of 1,2,4-trioxolane (**37**) (Fig. **13**) have been found to be effective in the treatment of schistosomiasis with a low degree of neurotoxicity, being suitable for both oral and non-oral administration. Trioxolanes are active against both cercaria and adult *S. mansoni* and *S. japonicum* when administered at 100-200 mg/kg/day orally. It is also believed that these trioxolanes will be active against *S. haematobium* [63, 64].

Fig. (13). Structure of 1,2,4-trioxolanes analogues (**37**).

3.5. Cysteine Protease Inhibitors

Cysteine proteases are a class of proteolytic enzymes that help schistosomes to degrade the ingested blood proteins. The cysteine proteases play an important role in the life cycle of parasite organisms [65, 66]. *In vivo* experimental studies with cysteine protease inhibitors (Fig. **14**), such as the phenyl vinyl sulfone (K11777) (**38**) and valproic acid (**39**) was performed in mice infected with *S. mansoni*. The inhibition of these schistosome enzymes resulted in a significant reduction in parasite burden in experimentally infected mice. Using cysteine protease-specific substrates and active site labelling, they identified cathepsin B1 as the molecular target of K11777 (**38**) and the major cysteine protease associated with the schistosome gut. However, as disadvantage, K11777 (**38**) should be administered intraperitoneally, during long-course treatment. On the other hand, experiments using valproic acid (**39**) as the protease inhibitor resulted in moderate worm burden reduction (41%), but a considerable decrease in the faecal egg counts (84%) [67]. Similarly, the Patent US 2012101053 (2012) is an invention related to inhibition of the papain cysteine proteases, which can be useful in the treatment of parasitic diseases. Two cysteine proteases (SmCL1 and SmCL2) are present in the human blood fluke *S. mansoni*. SmCL1 may play a role in the degradation of host hemoglobin, while SmCL2 may be important to the reproductive system of the parasite [68]. Inhibition of one or both proteases may provide an effective treatment for human schistosomiasis. Then, this patent is related to the use of compounds (general formula **40** and **41**) as cysteine proteases inhibitors, being capable of inhibiting and/or decreasing the cathepsins activities, including, but not limited to, cathepsins and papain-like cysteine proteases [68]. Likewise, the patent WO 2009067797 A1 (2009) described some cysteine protease inhibitors for the treatment of parasitic diseases [10]. This invention reported the use of compounds (**42** and **43**) for inhibiting or decreasing the activity of cruzipain, a cysteine protease necessary for some parasites life-cycle. Compounds of this present invention are capable of treating and/or preventing parasitic diseases, including malaria, trypanosomiasis, and schistosomiasis [69].

Fig. (14). Cysteine Protease Inhibitors. Phenyl vinyl sulfone (K11777) (**38**) and valproic acid (**39**) and related compounds (**40, 41, 42** and **43**).

3.6. Decoquinate Analogues

The recent invention in 2016 (Patent CN105330602 A) disclosed decoquinate analogues (Fig. **15**) and their application in pharmaceutical chemistry. Decoquinate analogues are active compounds that kill schistosomes and can open up a new way for finding new lead schistosomicidal compounds. This patent described decoquinate analogues which have relevant activity against *S. japonicum*, especially JD487 (**44**) and JD458 (**45**), which are able to cause 100% of dead worms of *S. japonicum* at 25 µM [70].

44   **45**

Fig. (15). Decoquinate analogue. JD487 (**44**) and JD458 (**45**).

3.7. Platinum Complexes

Patent US 2005080131 A1 (2005) described the use of platinum to treat oncological, viral, bacterial, and parasitic disease, such as schistosomiasis. It has been suggested that cellular cytotoxicity of platinum compounds is a result of platinum compounds being reduced to platinum in the cell. Surprisingly, platinum complexes of the present invention may not require this type of reduction in the cells to have a cytotoxic effect. Therefore, platinum complexes of the present invention are distinct from platinum compounds in the art by maintaining their correct oxidative conformation as platinum compounds which are more effective than the existing platinum compounds. In addition, platinum complexes of the invention can also form nitric oxide in the cells as radicals thereby killing the cells through the formation of oxide radicals [71].

3.8. Other Compounds

In the patent BR 1020130279226 A2 (2015) it was described the schistosomicidal potential of 3,7-dimethyl-1-octanol (**46**) (Fig. **16**) against adults worms of *S. mansoni* and its use in the pharmaceutical formulations for prevention and treatment of schistosomiasis. *In vitro* studies with adult schistosomes showed that this compound caused dead of worms after 24 h of incubation with 3,7-dimethy-

-1-octanol (**46**) (50 μg/mL) [72].

The compounds, in the patent CN103622977 A in 2014, were developed aiming to inhibit the 3-oxoacyl-ACP reductase (OAR), a key rate-limiting enzyme of the fatty acid synthesis pathway of *Schistosoma* [43, 52]. Based on that, compound (**47**), and its analogues, act inhibiting the OAR (Fig. **16**). According to Liu *et al.* (2013) the compounds OAR 22 (**48**) and OAR 27 (**49**) exhibited strong antischistosomal activity and inhibitory effects on the enzymatic activity of OAR, as well as low toxicity against the host cells [73, 74].

46   **47**   **48**

49

Fig. (16). Other compounds with schistosomicidal activity. 3,7-dimethyl-1-octanol (**46**), 2- [2- (4-chloro-2-nitrophenyl) amine-1-hexene] -4,6-difluoro (2 - [2- (4-chloro-2-nitrophenyl) diaz-1-enyl] -4,- -difluorophenol) (**47**), OAR 22 (**48**) and OAR 27 (**49**).

4. RECENT PATENTS AND CLINICAL TRIAL OF NATURAL COMPOUNDS

4.1. Polyunsaturated Fatty Acids

Fatty acids are termed saturated fatty acids, when no double bonds are present between the carbon atoms, and are termed unsaturated fatty acids, when double bonds are present [75]. Polyunsaturated fatty acids (PUFAs) are classified based on the position of the first double bond from the methyl end of the fatty acid. An example of PUFA is the arachidonic acid (ARA) (**50**), an all-*cis* 5,8,11,14-eicosatetreanoic acid, called an omega-6 fatty acid: 20:4(ω-6), which is present in the phospholipids of membranes and has been hypothesized to act to kill juvenile and adult male and female worms of *S. mansoni* and *S. haematobium* [75].

In 2009, the patent GB2460056 reported a formulation containing an omega-6 unsaturated fatty acid, preferably arachidonic acid (**50**), together with an omega-3 unsaturated fatty acid, such as docosahexaenoic acid (**51**) for use in the treatment of schistosomiasis (Fig. **17**) [75]. More recently, Hadley and Rashika (2015), in the patent WO2015123480 A2, described the application of arachidonic acid (**50**) for the treatment of schistosomiasis [76]. Also, authors have performed a randomized controlled trial, assessing the effect of dietary supplementation with arachidonic acid (**50**) on the cure rates of children (with clinically confirmed schistosomiasis) with or without concomitant treatment with PZQ. In this clinical trial described in patent (WO2015123480A2), children were randomly divided into groups, where the first group received a single oral dose of PZQ (40 mg/kg) on the first day of treatment, while the second group received ARA (10 mg/kg b.w./day) for 15 days over three weeks [76], and the third group received PZQ and ARA. The ARA treatment resulted in a 77% of cure rate for children having low infection and 50% of cure rate for children having moderate and high infection. Also, the PZQ-ARA treatment showed 94% of cure rate for children having low infection and 71% cure rate children having moderate and high infection [76].

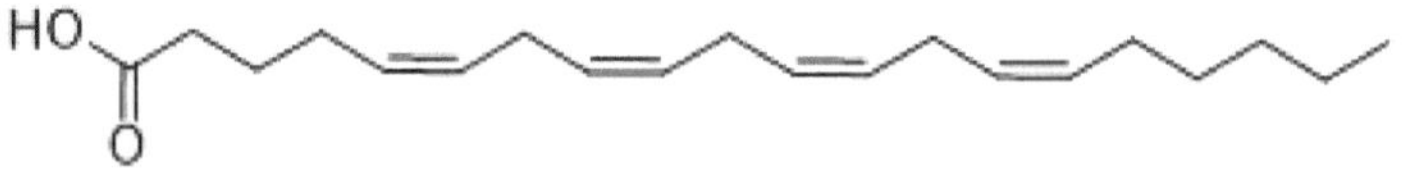

50

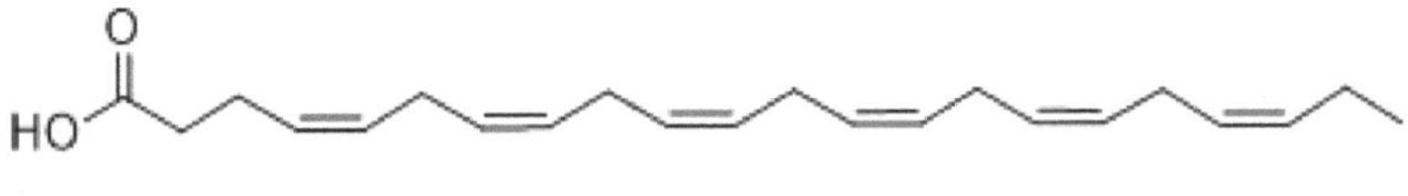

51

Fig. (17). Structure chemical of Arachidonic acid (**50**) and Docosahexaenoic acid (**51**).

4.2. Alkaloids

Epiisopiloturine (**52**) (Fig. **18**) is an imidazole alkaloid with activity against some parasitic infections, such as schistosomiasis and leishmaniasis. This alkaloid was found in the leaves of *Pilocarpus microphyllus*, known as "Jaborandi" [77]. Lima *et al.* (2011) described the application of this compound in the patent PI09041109 A2 for the treatment of leishmaniasis and schistosomiasis [78]. Cytotoxicity was evaluated in peritoneal cells of Swiss female mice at different concentrations, showing that at concentrations of 4 to 128 µg/mL this alkaloid did not interfere with macrophage functions. Also, in the *in vitro* schistosomicidal assay epiisopiloturine (**52**) (50, 100, 150 and 200 µg/mL) caused damage in schistosome tubercle and parasite death [79]. *In vivo* assays, using single doses of 40 and 300 mg/kg, decreased in about 50% the worm burden, as well as reduced in 80% the number of excreted eggs [80].

4.3. Natural Oils and Peptides

Mirazid is an antischistosomal drug available in the local Egyptian market since 2001 (Mirazid®). It originates from Myrrh, a medicinal herb that has been used for thousands of years. Myrrh (Arabian or Somali Myrrh) is an oleo-gum resin, obtained from the stem of various species of *Commiphora* (Burseraceae) growing in northeast Africa and Arabia [81]. From this plant, it is possible to extract oils, specifically the oleo-gum resin that is very useful as an antischistosomal agent [81]. The pharmaceutical composition, described in patent US 6077513 (2011) for treating *S. mansoni*, consisting of isolated myrrh oil and myrrh resin, contains 7-17% of volatile oil, 25-40% of resin, and 57-61% of gum [81]. A combination of resin and volatile oil from *Commiphora* resulted in a marked reduction in worm load, reaching 100% after two weeks of treatment [81]. Mirazid is under investigation in clinical trial (phase III) in an open-label randomized non-placeb--controlled study in which the investigators will compare the efficacy and safety of Mirazid to PZQ for the treatment of schistosomiasis.

Within the structural class of natural peptide active compounds, the so-called cephaibols are distinguished, containing many amino acids. They are synthesized from *Acremonium tubakii* FH 1685 DSM 12774 during fermentation and released into the culture medium. The cephaibols, according to patent US 2003203848 A1, are suitable to control human and animal pathogens, including *S. mansoni* [82].

4.4. Terpenes

Nerolidol (**53**) (Fig. **18**) is a sesquiterpene used as flavor enhancer and can be found in many essential oils. It can currently be purchased in the form of an isolated or synthetic product. The patent BR 1020120063310 refers to the schistosomicidal activity of this compound [83]. *In vivo* experiments showed that the treatment with nerolidol did not provoke any acute toxicity in animals, as well as a low mortality rate was observed among the groups that received doses ranging from 1000 to 5000 mg/kg of this compound [83]. Also, when *in vitro* tested against S. *mansoni*, nerolidol (**53**) (12.5 µg/mL) killed all adult worms in a dose dependent rate [83]. According to authors, a single dose of nerolidol (100, 200 or 400 mg/kg) administered orally to mice infected with adult schistosomes resulted in a reduction in the worm burden and egg production [83, 84].

(+)- epoxy-limonene (**54**) (Fig. **18**) is a secondary metabolite of (+) limonene epoxidation. It consists of a mixture of *cis* and *trans* isomers that posses antimicrobial activity against *S. aureus* ATCC 25923 and *C. albicans* ATCC 76645 reported and proven [4]. This compound was described in the patent BR102012006336 (2013), which reported the *in vitro* schistosomicidal activity of (**54**) [85]. (+)-epoxy-limonene (**54**) reduced motility and killed all adults [86].

Carvacrol (**55**) (Fig. **18**) (patent BR 10 2012 007004 9 A2, 2013) is a monoterpene present in essential oils of many species of medicinal and aromatic plants. It has been widely used both as a food or food additive in the food industry for a long time. In recent years, its multiple functions have been well studied in different fields. Carvacrol has shown several biological activities, such as antioxidant, antiviral, antibacterial, fungicidal, insecticidal and acaricidal properties. Moreover, this monoterpene has been shown to have antiprotozoal activities against *Giardia lamblia*, *Leishmania chagasi* and *Trypanosoma cruzi* parasites. Although the carvacrol is widely used and well known for its medicinal properties, this natural product has been poorly investigated for its anthelmintic potential. It was demonstrated that carvacryl acetate, at 6.25 µg/mL, has antischistosomal activity, affecting parasite motility and viability [87].

4.5. Other Triterpene Derivatives, Diterpenes and Saponins

The patent RU20130151703 20131120 reported a method of production and the schistosomicidal potential of triphenylphosphonium salts of lupane and ursane triterpenoids (**56**) (Fig. **19**) [88].

Pulsatilla herbs are derived from the dry roots of *Pulsatilla chinensis* (Bunge). In the Traditional Chinese Medicine, this plant is used for stomach diseases and amoeba dysentery. It was found that *Pulsatilla* decoction had great effect on killing some parasites. Pentacyclic triterpenoid saponins, mainly oleanolic and lupane-type, especially the oleanolic saponin: 3(1 → 2) -α-L-arabinose-oleanolic acid-28-O-β-D-glucose- (1 → 3) -α-L-rhamnose- (1 → 6) -β-D-glucose ester (**57**) (Fig. **19**), are one of the major classes of secondary metabolites found in this plant [89]. The patent (CN102631361 A) reported the used of these saponins, including (**57**) for the treatment and/or prevention of schistosomiasis [89].

52   53

54   55

Fig. (18). Natural compounds with schistosomicidal activity. Epiisopiloturine (**52**), Nerolidol (**53**), (+) - epoxy-limonene (**54**) and Cavacrol (**55**).

The WO2016097759 A1 patent related the schistosomicidal activity of diterpenes derivatives from sempervirol (**58**) (Fig. **19**), particularly 7-keto-sempervirol (**59**) (Fig. **19**), which is a phenol diterpene isolated from *Lycium chinense* [90]. According to authors, 7-keto-sempervirol (**59**), selectively kills schistosomula, inducing tegumental damage and motility disruption. Furthermore, 7-ket- -sempervirol (**59**) dramatically inhibits the developmental maturation and oviposition of phenotypically normal *S. mansoni* eggs. Collectively these findings suggest that diterpenoids, such as 7-keto-sempervirol, have broad activities against related trematodes [90, 91].

4.6. Tocopherols, Naphthoquinones and Anthraquinones

Tocopherols arc methylated phenols with antioxidant activity [92]. Alpha-tocopherol (**60**) (Fig. **19**) is the most biologically active preventing peroxidation of polyunsaturated fatty acids from cellular and subcellular membranes [92]. Zhiyue *et al.* (2015) reported the application of alpha-tocopherol (**60**) in preparation of a drug for treating schistosomiasis (patent CN105078963 A) [93]. According to authors, alpha-tocopherol has *in vitro* schistosomicidal activity, inhibiting the development of the reproductive organ of schistosome, and then, the eggs laid by schistosome in a host are reduced [93]. *In vivo* experiments showed that the administration of alpha-tocopherol (**60**) (1, 15 and 20 mg/Kg/day, per gavage) is able to reduce the number of testicles and cause testicular atrophy in male worms, while in female worms it was observed immature ovary, uterus and vitellarium, causing a significant reduction in eggs laid [93].

Fig. (19). Other natural compounds with schistosomicidal activity. Triterpene derivative (**56**), saponin (**57**), diterpenes (**58** and **59**), alpha-tocopherol (**60**), anthraquinones (**61** and **62**), and naphthoquinone derivatives (**63** and **64**).

The patent WO 03089577 (A2) described the anthelminthic activity of anthraquinones, which is an important class of natural compounds with a wide range of applications. Besides their utilization as colorants, anthraquinone derivatives have been used since centuries for medical applications, such as laxatives and anti-inflammatory agents [94]. This invention related to *in vitro* and *in vivo* activities of anthraquinones against *Schistosoma sp* [95]. Anthraquinones extracted from *Hemerocallis fulva* 'Kwanzo' were *in vitro* tested for their activity against multiple life-stages (cercariae, schistosomula, and adult) of *S. mansoni* [95]. Anthraquinones (**61**) and (**62**) (Fig. **19**), at 25 µg/mL, were found to rapidly immobilize *Schistosoma* cercariae to kill 50% of them by 24 hours post-exposure [96].

The use of some naphtoquinones as schistosomicidal compounds, such as the menadione derivatives LJ83K (**63**) and LJ81K (**64**) (Fig. **19**), was object of the patent application US9409879 B2 (2016) [97]. This work described the *in vitro* activity of LJ83K (**63**) and LJ81K (**64**) against *S. mansoni* worms in culture. Both compounds cause dead of parasites after 4 hours of treatment, when parasites showed "hairy phenotype" with the appearance of spicula on the tegument, suggesting that occurs an important perturbation in metabolism. *In vivo* assays were also performed, showing a large reduction in worm burden [97]. Other antiparasitic studies with some synthetics naphtoquinones have already shown that these naphthoquinones are also able to block the cercarial skin penetration. It was not shown the mechanism by which naphthoquinones work, but it is generally recognized that their antiparasitic activity involves modulation of parasite redox cycling, as well as production of reactive oxygen species, which provides a variety of oxidative stress in proteins, lipids and DNA and others macromolecules [98].

CONCLUDING REMARKS AND FUTURE PERSPECTIVES

In this chapter, the schistosomicidal compounds patented in the early 20th century, as well as the main aspects related to the new patented schistosomicidal drugs and natural products were addressed, some of which are in clinical trials to treat schistosomiasis. In comparison with other drugs, only a few synthetic or natural compounds have been studied and recently patented against *Schistosoma* and, unfortunately, only a few have been subjected to clinical trials. Although schistosomiasis is an important infectious disease that afflicts millions of people worldwide, it is still largely neglected and underappreciated. Schistosomiasis is a neglected disease, affecting people mainly in developing countries, which can not yet afford to pay for the high costs of research and drug development.

After 1917, when tartar emetic was first used in the treatment of schistosomiasis, little advance was made in the development of antischistosomal drugs. Antimonial compounds were previously used but are now obsolete due to their toxicity. Oxamniquine was used on a large scale in Brazil, but it was also discontinued. In the late 1970s, praziquantel was introduced and became the drug of choice. After discovery of praziquantel in the 1970s, neither the pharmaceutical industry nor international donor agencies thought much about the possible need for alternative drugs for schistosomiasis. Currently, schistosomiasis control programs still rely on one drug, PZQ, which is the drug submitted to the most new clinical trials, mainly in association with another antiparasitic drug. However, in addition to the dependence on the praziquantel, its drug resistance is an imminent threat, particularly by means of its large-scale use. In this sense, researches into new antischistosomal drugs, as well as their clinical trials are imperative and urgent matters. In recent years, there has been an increase in the number of studies and publications using experimental models with *Schistosoma*. Currently, a number of natural and synthetic compounds have been *in vitro* and *in vivo* evaluated against *Schistosoma* species, but only a few compounds are effectively promising in order to be submitted to clinical trials.

Unfortunately, it seems that no innovative schistosomicidal drug has been approved or submitted to relevant clinical trials in the last few years, and the investigations have been limited to combinations of repurposed compounds, with some exceptions for artemisinin derivatives, arachidonic acid, phytocomplexs (such as mirazid), and other natural products. In view of this alarming situation, many efforts should be made in order to find new effective and safe drugs that could be clinically evaluated and made a successful against schistosomiasis.

CONSENT FOR PUBLICATION

Not applicable.

CONFLICT OF INTEREST

The author confirms that this chapter contents have no conflict of interest.

ACKNOWLEDGEMENTS

The authors are grateful to FAPEMIG (Grant numbers # APQ 0171/11; APQ 02015/14; PPM-00296-16; BPD 00284-14) and CNPq (Grant number # 487221/2012-5) for financial support, as well as to CAPES, PIBIC/CNPq/UFJF and CNPq for fellowships.

REFERENCES

[1]   de Moraes J. Natural products with antischistosomal activity. Future Med Chem 2015; 7(6): 801-20.
        [http://dx.doi.org/10.4155/fmc.15.23] [PMID: 25996071]

[2]   Utzinger J, N'goran EK, Caffrey CR, Keiser J. From innovation to application: social-ecological context, diagnostics, drugs and integrated control of schistosomiasis. Acta Trop 2011; 120(0) (Suppl. 1): S121-37.
        [http://dx.doi.org/10.1016/j.actatropica.2010.08.020] [PMID: 20831855]

[3]   Sustaining the drive to overcome the global impact of neglected tropical diseases: second WHO report on neglected diseases. Geneva: World Health Organization 2013.

[4]   Colley DG, Bustinduy AL, Secor WE, King CH. Human schistosomiasis. Lancet 2014; 383(9936): 2253-64.
[http://dx.doi.org/10.1016/S0140-6736(13)61949-2] [PMID: 24698483]

[5]   Schistosomiasis: progress report 2001 - 2011, strategic plan 2012 - 2020. Geneva: World Health Organization 2013.

[6]   Schistosomiasis. Geneva: World Health Organization 2016.

[7]   Gryseels B, Strickland GT. Schistosomiasis.Hunter's Tropical Medicine and Emerging Infectious Disease. 9th ed. Saunders 2012; pp. 867-83.

[8]   Ross AG, Bartley PB, Sleigh AC, *et al.* Schistosomiasis. N Engl J Med 2002; 346(16): 1212-20.
[http://dx.doi.org/10.1056/NEJMra012396] [PMID: 11961151]

[9]   Souza FPC, Gomes AP, Faria Júnior FC, Costa AP, Santana LA, Vitorino RR. *Schistosomiasis mansoni*: general aspects, immunology, pathogenesis and natural. Rev Bras Clin Med 2011; 9(4): 300-7.

[10]   De Castro CCB, Dias MM, Rezende TP, Magalhães LG, Da Silva Filho AA. Natural products with activity against schistosoma species. Fighting multidrug resistance with herbal extracts, essential oils and their components. 1st ed. San Diego: Academic Press 2013; pp. 109-34.
[http://dx.doi.org/10.1016/B978-0-12-398539-2.00008-2]

[11]   Summary of global update on preventive chemotherapy implementation in 2015. Wkly Epidemiol Rec 2016; 91(39): 456-9.
[PMID: 27758092]

[12]   Leow CY, Willis C, Hofmann A, Jones MK. Structure-function analysis of apical membrane-associated molecules of the tegument of schistosome parasites of humans: prospects for identification of novel targets for parasite control. Br J Pharmacol 2015; 172(7): 1653-63.
[http://dx.doi.org/10.1111/bph.12898] [PMID: 25176442]

[13]   Berman JD. Chemotherapy for leishmaniasis: biochemical mechanisms, clinical efficacy, and future strategies. Rev Infect Dis 1988; 10(3): 560-86.
[http://dx.doi.org/10.1093/clinids/10.3.560] [PMID: 3293160]

[14]   Christopherson JB. The successful use of Antimony in Bilharziosis administered as intravenous injections of antimonium tartaratum (tartar emetic). Lancet 1918; 192(4958): 325-7.
[http://dx.doi.org/10.1016/S0140-6736(01)02807-0]

[15]   Millan RDS, De Michele CP, Frezard FJG, De Melo AL, Ferreira LAM, Bejarano RO. Pharmaceutical compositions consisting of cyclodextrin and an antimony derivative, their preparation as well as their use. WO Patent 2006000069 2006 Jan 05.

[16]   Bertram HP, Kemper HF, Khayyal MT. inventors; Heyl & CO Chemisch - Pharmazeutische Fabrik, assignee. Schistosomiasis treatment with antimony cpds. *e.g.* tartar emetic - in combination with alkali 2,3 di:mercapto-propane-1-sulphonate to increase activity and reduce toxicity. DE Patent 2,901,350 A1 1980 Jul 31.

[17]   Rathi AK, Syed R, Shin HS, Patel RV. Piperazine derivatives for therapeutic use: a patent review (2010-present). Expert Opin Ther Pat 2016; 26(7): 777-97.
[http://dx.doi.org/10.1080/13543776.2016.1189902] [PMID: 27177234]

[18]   Katz N, Pellegrino J, Oliveira CA, Cunha AS. Experimental chemotherapy of schistosomiasis. II. Laboratory and clinical trials with A-16612, a piperazine derivative. J Parasitol 1967; 53(6): 1229-32.
[http://dx.doi.org/10.2307/3276685] [PMID: 4965716]

[19]   Buting WE. inventor; Eli Lilly and Company, assignee. Bis-beta-(4-arylpiperazino) ethyl sulfones for treating schistosomiasis. US Patent 3,203,858 1965 Aug 31.

[20]   Tomcufcik AS, Fabio PF, Hoffman AM. inventors; American Cyanamid Company, assignee. Anti-protozoal piperazine derivs. CH Patent 514,608 A 1971 Oct 31.

[21]   Porter HD. inventor; Eli Lilly and Company, assignee. 2,4-Di-(4-arylpiperazino)-3-pentanones for treating schistosomiasis. US Patent 3,639,602 1972 Feb 1.

[22]   Werbel LM, Colbry N, Turner W, Worth DF. inventors; Edna McConnell Clark Foundation, assignee. Phenylpiperazines which are useful in the treatment of schistosomiasis. US Patent 4,515,793 1985 May 7.

[23]   La Roche H. inventor; La Roche H, assignee. Sulphur-containing dicarboxylic acids and derivatives thereof and a process for the manufacture of same. GB Patent 908,986 1962 Oct 24.

[24]   Sandoz AG. inventor; Sandoz AG, assignee. 2-Substd. 4-(2-diethylamino-ethylamino)-benzaldehydes - with anthelmintic activity, from 4-aminobenzaldehyde acetals. CH Patent 571,475 A5 1976 Jan 15.

[25]   Rossignol JF. assignee. n-(4-methoxy-2- methyl phenyl)- 3-(5- nitro-2-furanyl) propenamide and antiparasitic use thereof, from 4-aminobenzaldehyde acetals. JO Patent 1,360 B 1986 Nov 30.

[26]   Baxter CAR. inventor. Pfizer, assignee. Substituted hexahydro-imidazoquinolines. GB Patent 1,278,272 A 1972 Jun 21.

[27]   Sturrock RF, Otieno M, James ER, Webbe G. A note on the efficacy of a new class of compounds, 9-acridanone-hydrazones, against *Schistosoma mansoni* in a primate--the baboon. Trans R Soc Trop Med Hyg 1985; 79(1): 129-31.
         [http://dx.doi.org/10.1016/0035-9203(85)90256-1] [PMID: 3992631]

[28]   Sturrock RF, Bain J, Webbe G, Doenhoff MJ, Stohler H. Parasitological evaluation of curative and subcurative doses of 9-acridanone-hydrazone drugs against *Schistosoma mansoni* in baboons, and observations on changes in serum levels of anti-egg antibodies detected by ELISA. Trans R Soc Trop Med Hyg 1987; 81(2): 188-92.
         [http://dx.doi.org/10.1016/0035-9203(87)90210-0] [PMID: 3113001]

[29]   Kamel G, Metwally A, Guirguis F, Nessim NG, Noseir M. Effect of a combination of the new antischistosomal drug Ro 15-5458 and praziquantel on different strains of *Schistosoma mansoni* infected mice. Arzneimittelforschung 2000; 50(4): 391-4.
         [PMID: 10800639]

[30]   Bombacher URS, Link H, Montavon M. inventors; F Hoffmann-La Roche AG, assignee. Acridanone derivatives. CA Patent 1,258,854 1989 Aug 29.

[31]   Guirguis FR. Efficacy of praziquantel and Ro 15-5458, a 9-acridanone-hydrazone derivative, against *Schistosoma haematobium*. Arzneimittelforschung 2003; 53(1): 57-61.
         [PMID: 12608016]

[32]   Pereira LH, Coelho PM, Costa JO, de Mello RT. Activity of 9-acridanone-hydrazone drugs detected at the pre-postural phase, in the experimental schistosomiasis *mansoni*. Mem Inst Oswaldo Cruz 1995; 90(3): 425-8.
         [http://dx.doi.org/10.1590/S0074-02761995000300021] [PMID: 8544746]

[33]   Archer S. inventor. Rensselaer Polytechnic Institute, assignee. Substituted 6h-pyrido (4,3-b) carbazoles. WO Patent 8,911,480 A1 1989 Nov 30.

[34]   Archer S, Ross BS, Pica-Mattoccia L, Cioli D. Synthesis and biological properties of some 6H-pyrido[4,3-b]carbazoles. J Med Chem 1987; 30(7): 1204-10.
         [http://dx.doi.org/10.1021/jm00390a014] [PMID: 3599025]

[35]   Hill JM, Yu G, Shue YK, Zydowsky TM, Rebek J. inventors. Cubist Pharmaceuticals, assignee. Aminoacyl adenylate mimics as novel antimicrobial and antiparasitic agents. US Patent 5,726,195 1998 Mar 10.

[36]   Cioli D, Pica-Mattoccia L, Basso A, Guidi A. Schistosomiasis control: praziquantel forever? Mol Biochem Parasitol 2014; 195(1): 23-9.
         [http://dx.doi.org/10.1016/j.molbiopara.2014.06.002] [PMID: 24955523]

[37]   Abdul-Ghani R, Loutfy N, el-Sahn A, Hassan A. Current chemotherapy arsenal for schistosomiasis

mansoni: alternatives and challenges. Parasitol Res 2009; 104(5): 955-65.
[http://dx.doi.org/10.1007/s00436-009-1371-7] [PMID: 19255786]

[38]   Wang W, Wang L, Liang YS. Susceptibility or resistance of praziquantel in human schistosomiasis: a review. Parasitol Res 2012; 111(5): 1871-7.
[http://dx.doi.org/10.1007/s00436-012-3151-z] [PMID: 23052781]

[39]   Bramemer KW, Shaw JR. inventors; Pfizer, assignee. Schistosomicidal composition comprising oxamniquine and praziquantel. EP Patent 0,024,868 B1 1983 Mar 11.

[40]   Richards HC, Foster R. A new series of 2-aminomethyltetrahydroquinoline derivatives displaying schistosomicidal activity in rodents and primates. Nature 1969; 222(5193): 581-2.
[http://dx.doi.org/10.1038/222581a0] [PMID: 4977703]

[41]   De Moraes J. Antischistosomal natural compounds: Present challenges for new drug screens.Current topics in tropical medicine. 1st ed. Rijeka: InTech 2012; pp. 333-58.

[42]   Shaw JR, Brammer KW. The treatment of experimental schistosomiasis with a combination of oxamniquine and praziquantel. Trans R Soc Trop Med Hyg 1983; 77(1): 39-40.
[http://dx.doi.org/10.1016/0035-9203(83)90008-1] [PMID: 6679362]

[43]   Zhu C, Lin J, Lu K, Li H, Shi Y, Jiang Y. inventors; Shangai Veterinary Research Institute, assignee. Praziquantel transdermal preparation and applications thereof. CN Patent 102,138,890 2011 Aug 3.

[44]   Qiao C, Xia C, Duan W, Qiu S, Zhao Y. inventors; Soochow University, assignee. Preparation method of 10-hydroxyl praziquantel and application thereof as antischistosomiasis medicine. CN Patent 102,285,985 B 2011 Aug 8.

[45]   Ronketti F, Ramana AV, Chao-Ming X, Pica-Mattoccia L, Cioli D, Todd MH. Praziquantel derivatives I: Modification of the aromatic ring. Bioorg Med Chem Lett 2007; 17(15): 4154-7.
[http://dx.doi.org/10.1016/j.bmcl.2007.05.063] [PMID: 17555960]

[46]   Duan WW, Qiu SJ, Zhao Y, Sun H, Qiao C, Xia CM. Praziquantel derivatives exhibit activity against both juvenile and adult *Schistosoma* japonicum. Bioorg Med Chem Lett 2012; 22(4): 1587-90.
[http://dx.doi.org/10.1016/j.bmcl.2011.12.133] [PMID: 22264473]

[47]   Yue Y, Dequn S, Chunhua Y. inventors; Weihai Xiushui Pharmaceutical, assignee. Application of pyrazine isoquinoline derivatives in preparing drugs for treating schistosomes. CN Patent 105,037,354 2015 Nov 11.

[48]   Dequn S, Yue Y, Yang Z, Yi Z, Yanchen Q. invetors; Shandong Jingpeng Bio Pesticide, assignee. Compound. CN Patent 104,327,076 2015 Feb 4.

[49]   Chen DJ, Fu LF, Shao PP, Wu FZ, Shu H, Ren CS, *et al.* Experimental studies on antischistosomal activity of qinghaosu. Zhonghua Yi Xue Za Zhi 1980; 60: 422-5.

[50]   Alencar AC, Santos TdaS, Neves RH, Lopes Torres EJ, Nogueira-Neto JF, Machado-Silva JR. Simvastatin and artesunate impact the structural organization of adult *Schistosoma mansoni* in hypercholesterolemic mice. Exp Parasitol 2016; 167: 115-23.
[http://dx.doi.org/10.1016/j.exppara.2016.05.007] [PMID: 27228897]

[51]   Li HJ, Wang W, Li YZ, *et al.* Effects of artemether, artesunate and dihydroartemisinin administered orally at multiple doses or combination in treatment of mice infected with *Schistosoma japonicum*. Parasitol Res 2011; 109(2): 515-9.
[http://dx.doi.org/10.1007/s00436-011-2474-5] [PMID: 21626153]

[52]   Li Y, Wang F, Zhang Y, Sui Y, Xiao S. inventors; Shangai Institute Materia Medica, assignee. Tert-butoxy dihydro artemisinin, its production and pharmaceutical composition. WO Patent 03,022,855 2003 Mar 20.

[53]   Xia C, Qiao C. inventors; Soochow University, assignee. Praziquantel derivative as well as preparation and application thereof. CN Patent 102,276,632 2014 Dec 14.

[54]   Dong L, Duan W, Chen J, Sun H, Qiao C, Xia CM. An artemisinin derivative of praziquantel as an

orally active antischistosomal agent. PLoS One 2014; 9(11)e112163
[http://dx.doi.org/10.1371/journal.pone.0112163] [PMID: 25386745]

[55]   Chuanxin Y, Yi J, Lijun S, Jie W, Xuren Y, Shuang S. inventors; Jiangsu institute Parasitic Diseases, assignee. Long-acting artesunate drug for preventing schistosome infection and preparation method thereof. CN Patent 103,405,779 2013 Nov 27.

[56]   Yufen Z, Shengli C, Yanmei L. inventors; Qinghua University, assignee. Medicine for curing schistosomiasis and its preparation method. CN Patent 1,262,929 A 2000 Aug 16.

[57]   Meunier B, Cosledan F. inventors; Palumed, assignee. New therapeutic uses of dual molecules containing a peroxide derivative. CN Patent 101,909,627 A 2010 Dec 8.

[58]   Vennerstrom JL, Dong Y, Chollet J, *et al.* inventors; Medicines for Malaria Venture MMV, assignee. Spiro and dispiro 1,2,4-trioxolane antimalarials. US Patent 2004/0,039,008 A1 2004 Feb 26.

[59]   Vennerstrom JL, Dong Y, Chollet J, Matile H. inventors; Medicines for Malaria Venture MMV, assignee. Spiro and dispiro 1,2,4-trioxolane antimalarials. US Patent 6,486,199 B1 2002 Nov 26.

[60]   Wataya Y, Kim HS, Hiramoto A, *et al.* inventors; Okayama University, assignee. Novel Antischistosomal Agent. US Patent 2013/245,108 A1 2013 Sep 19.

[61]   Williams DL, Sayed A. inventors; Illinois State University, assignee. Treatments for the control of schistosomiasis. WO Patent 2009/076,265 A1 2009 Jun 18.

[62]   Thomas CJ, Maloney DJ, Bantukallu GR, Sayed AA, Simeonov A, Williams DL. inventors; Illinois State University, assignee. Oxadiazol-2-oxides as antischistosomal agents. US Patent 2011/207,784 A1 2011 Aug 25.

[63]   Vennerstrom JL, Tang Y, Dong Y, *et al.* inventors; Medicines for Malaria Venture MMV, assignee. Dispiro 1,2,4 - trioxolane antimalarials. EP Patent 2,599,779 2013 Jun 5.

[64]   Xiao SH, Keiser J, Chollet J, *et al. In vitro* and *in vivo* activities of synthetic trioxolanes against major human schistosome species. Antimicrob Agents Chemother 2007; 51(4): 1440-5.
[http://dx.doi.org/10.1128/AAC.01537-06] [PMID: 17283188]

[65]   Brady CP, Brinkworth RI, Dalton JP, Dowd AJ, Verity CK, Brindley PJ. Molecular modeling and substrate specificity of discrete cruzipain-like and cathepsin L-like cysteine proteinases of the human blood fluke *Schistosoma mansoni.* Arch Biochem Biophys 2000; 380(1): 46-55.
[http://dx.doi.org/10.1006/abbi.2000.1905] [PMID: 10900131]

[66]   Doenhoff MJ, Curtis RH, Ngaiza J, Modha J. Proteases in the schistosome life cycle: a paradigm for tumour metastasis. Cancer Metastasis Rev 1990; 9(4): 381-92.
[http://dx.doi.org/10.1007/BF00049526] [PMID: 2097086]

[67]   Abaza SM, El-Moamly AA, Ismail OA, Alabbassy MM. Cysteine proteases inhibitors (phenyl vinyl sulfone and valproic acid) in treatment of schistosomiasis *mansoni*-infected mice: an experimental study to evaluate their role in comparison to praziquantel. Parasitol United J 2013; 6(1): 99-108.

[68]   Black C, Beaulieu C. inventors; Black C, Beaulieu C, assignee. Cathepsin cysteine protease inhibitors for the treatment of various diseases. US Patent 2012/101,053 A1 2012 Apr 26.

[69]   Isabel E, Mellon C, Beaulieu C. nventors; Merck Frosst Canada, assignee. Cysteine protease inhibitors for the treatment of parasitic diseases. WO Patent 2009/067,797 A1 2009 Jun 4.

[70]   Wang W, Yu C, Feng B, *et al.* inventors; Jiangnam University, Jiangsu institute of Parasitic Diseases, assignee. Decoquinate analogue and application thereof. CN Patent 105,330,602 A 2016 Feb 17.

[71]   Kay H, Palmer J, Stanko J. inventors; University of South Florida, assignee. Platinum complexes and methods of use. US Patent 2005/080,131 A1 2005 Apr 14.

[72]   Costa JP, Oliveira GZS, Araujo AJF, *et al.* inventors; Federal University of Piaui, assignee. Use of 3,7-dimethyl-1-octanol in pharmaceutical formulations for the treatment of schistosomiasis. BR Patent 102,013,027,922-6 A2 2015 Sep 8.

[73]   Wei H, Jian L, Jipeng W, *et al.* inventors; National institute of Parasitic Diseases, Chineses Center for Disease Control and Prevention, assignee. Application of compound in preparation of drug used for resisting Schistosomiasis *japonicum*. CN Patent 103,622,977 A 2014 Mar 12.

[74]   Liu J, Dyer D, Wang J, *et al.* 3-oxoacyl-ACP reductase from *Schistosoma japonicum*: integrated in silico-*in vitro* strategy for discovering antischistosomal lead compounds. PLoS One 2013; 8(6)e64984 [http://dx.doi.org/10.1371/journal.pone.0064984] [PMID: 23762275]

[75]   Rashika ER, Hatem T, Mohamed S. inventors; Arab Science & Technology Foundation, assignee. Compositions comprising omega-6 fatty acids for use in treating schistosomiasis. GB Patent 2,460,056A 2009 Nov 18.

[76]   Hadley K, Rashika ER. inventors; DSM IP Assets BV, assignee. Compositions and methods for the prevention and/or treatment of schistosomiasis. WO Patent 2015/123,480 2015 Aug 20;

[77]   Pinheiro CUB. Jaborandi (*Pilocarpus spp.*, Rutaceae): A Wild Species and Its Rapid Transformation into a Crop. Econ Bot 1997; 51(1): 49-58. [http://dx.doi.org/10.1007/BF02910403]

[78]   Miura LMCV, De Moraes J, Lima DF, *et al.* inventors; Federal University of Piaui, assignee. Process for obtaining epiisopiloturin and its application in the fight against parasitic infections. BR Patent 0,904,110-9 A2 2011 May 31.

[79]   Veras LM, Guimarães MA, Campelo YD, *et al.* Activity of epiisopiloturine against *Schistosoma mansoni*. Curr Med Chem 2012; 19(13): 2051-8. [http://dx.doi.org/10.2174/092986712800167347] [PMID: 22420337]

[80]   Guimarães MA, de Oliveira RN, Véras LMC, *et al.* Anthelmintic activity *in vivo* of epiisopiloturine against juvenile and adult worms of *Schistosoma mansoni*. PLoS Negl Trop Dis 2015; 9(3)e0003656 [http://dx.doi.org/10.1371/journal.pntd.0003656] [PMID: 25816129]

[81]   Massoud AMA. inventor; Massoud AMA, assignee. Drug for treatment of bilharziasis (Schistosomiasis). US Patent 6,077,513 2011 Jun 20.

[82]   Vertesy L, Kurz M, Schiell M, Hofmann J. inventors; Aventis Pharma, Sanofi-Aventis Deuschland, assignee. Cephaibols: novel antiparasitics from Acremonium tubakii, process for their production, and use thereof. US Patent 2003/203,848 2003 Oct 30.

[83]   Freitas RM, Costa JP, Santos PS, Moraes J, Nakano E, Souza DP. inventors; Costa JP, assignee. Applications in pharmaceutical formulations of nerolidol for the treatment of schistosomiasis. BR Patent 102,012,006,331-0 2015 Oct 6.

[84]   Silva MP, de Oliveira RN, Mengarda AC, *et al.* Antiparasitic activity of nerolidol in a mouse model of schistosomiasis. Int J Antimicrob Agents 2017; 50(3): 467-72. [http://dx.doi.org/10.1016/j.ijantimicag.2017.06.005] [PMID: 28666754]

[85]   Nunes LCC, Almeida AAC, Carvalho RBF, *et al.* inventors; Nunes LCC, assignee. Pharmaceutical application of (+) epoxy-limonene in the treatment of schistosomiasis. BR Patent 102012/006336-0 A2 2013 Nov 26.

[86]   Moraes Jd, Almeida AAC, Brito MRM, *et al.* Anthelmintic activity of the natural compound (+)-limonene epoxide against *Schistosoma mansoni*. Planta Med 2013; 79(3-4): 253-8. [http://dx.doi.org/10.1055/s-0032-1328173] [PMID: 23408270]

[87]   Fortes AC, Andrade LN, De Moraes J, Nakano E, Sousa DP, Freitas RM. inventors; Fortes AC assignee. Applications of carvacrol acetate in pharmaceutical formulations for the treatment of schistosomiasis. BR Patent 102,012,007,004-9 A2 2013 Nov 19.

[88]   Kajzer D, Julevna SA, Aleksandrovna ND, Ravilevich GR, Nikolaevich OV, Memetovich DU. inventors; Institute of Petrochemistry and Catalysis of the Russian Academy of Sciences, assignee. Triphenylphosphonium salts of lupine and ursane triperpenoids, method of production and use for treating bilharzias. RU Patent 2013/0151703 2013 May 27.

[89]   Xu Q, Liu Y, He W, Chen Z, Li X, Yang S. inventors; Soochow University, assignee. Application of oleanane glycoside in preparation of drugs for treating and/or preventing schistosomiasis. CN Patent 102,631,361 A 2012 Aug 12.

[90]   Edwards J, Brown M, Peak E, Bartholomew B, Nash RJ, Hoffmann KF. The diterpenoid 7-ket--sempervirol, derived from *Lycium chinense*, displays anthelmintic activity against both *Schistosoma mansoni* and *Fasciola hepatica*. PLoS Negl Trop Dis 2015; 9(3)e0003604
[http://dx.doi.org/10.1371/journal.pntd.0003604] [PMID: 25768432]

[91]   Hoffmann KF, Nash RJ, Peak E. inventors; University Aberystwyth, assignee. Anthelmintic compounds. WO Patent 2016/097759 2016 Jun 23.

[92]   Cayuela JA, García JF. Sorting olive oil based on alpha-tocopherol and total tocopherol content using near-infra-red spectroscopy (NIRS) analysis. J Food Eng 2017; 202: 79-88.
[http://dx.doi.org/10.1016/j.jfoodeng.2017.01.015]

[93]   Zhiyue L, Zhongdao W, Limei Z, *et al.* inventors; University Sun Yat Sen, assignee. Application of alpha-tocopherol in preparation of drug for treating schistosomiasis. CN Patent 105,078,963 2015 Nov 25.

[94]   Malik EM, Müller CE. Anthraquinones as pharmacological tools and drugs. Med Res Rev 2016; 36(4): 705-48.
[http://dx.doi.org/10.1002/med.21391] [PMID: 27111664]

[95]   Cichewicz RH, Lim K-C, McKerrow JH, Nair MG. Kwanzoquinones A–G and other constituents of *Hemerocallis fulva* 'Kwanzo'roots and their activity against the human pathogenic trematode *Schistosoma* mansoni. Tetrahedron 2002; 58(42): 8597-606.
[http://dx.doi.org/10.1016/S0040-4020(02)00802-5]

[96]   Cichewicz RH, Nair MGN, Mckerrow JH. inventors; Board of Trustees of Michigan State University, assignee. Antihelminthic anthraquinones and method of use thereof. US Patent 03,092,690 A2 2005 Jul 5.

[97]   Davioud-Charvet E, Lanfranchi DA, Johann L, Williams DL, Rodo EC. inventors; Davioud-Charvet E, Lanfranchi DA, Johann L, Williams DL, Rodo EC, assignee. Total synthesis of redox-active 1.4-naphthoquinones and their metabolites and their therapeutic use as antimalarial and schistomicidal agents. US Patent 9,409,879 2016 Aug 09.

[98]   Magalhães LG, Rao S, Soares IAO, Badocco FR, Cunha WR, Rodrigues V, *et al.* Chemoprevention of Schistosomiasis: *In vitro* Antiparasitic Activity of Nineteen Plant-derived and Synthetic Simple Naphthoquinones and Naphthols against *Schistosoma Mansoni* Adult Worms. J Trop Dis Public Health 2014; 2(4): 1-7.

CHAPTER 2

Natural Products, the New Intervention Regime of Metabolic Disorders

Mohamed A. Salem[1], Dalia I. Hamdan[1], Islam Mostafa[2], Rasha Adel[2], Ahmed Elissawy[3] and Assem M. El-Shazly[2,*]

[1] Department of Pharmacognosy, Faculty of Pharmacy, Menoufia University, Shibin Elkom 32511, Egypt

[2] Department of Pharmacognosy, Faculty of Pharmacy, Zagazig University, Zagazig 44519, Egypt

[3] Department of Pharmacognosy, Faculty of Pharmacy, Ain Shams University, Abbassia, Cairo 11566, Egypt

Abstract: Nature is considered an indispensable source of natural products and natural products-derived drug leads. Over the last decade, the use of natural products-based medicine (herbal medicine or phytomedicine) has increased tremendously worldwide especially with the exceeding prevalence of metabolic disorders. Metabolic disorders are the major worldwide epidemic associated with obesity, diabetes mellitus, cardiovascular diseases associated with hyperlipidemia, and many other endocrine and nutrition-related issues. Since metabolic disorders are multi-factorial in their pathophysiology, they can be targeted by natural products that have synergy between diverse metabolites. Therefore, it is important to find the proper formulas not only for the treatment but also for reduction of associated risks and for prophylaxis and prevention of long-term complications. At the present work, a brief outline of the pathophysiology of metabolic disorders is provided. Additionally, natural product-based drug therapies that are currently applied in clinical trials attributed to metabolic-related diseases are critically discussed.

Keywords: Cardiovascular diseases, Clinical trials, Diabetes, Dyslipidemia, Metabolic disorders, Natural products, Obesity, Osteoporosis, Pathophysiology.

1. INTRODUCTION

Our body is a complex factory that is made up of several machines represented by different systems. Each complex machinery system requires energy to be fully functional. Additionally, each unit, the cell, requires energy to perform its unique function. Energy is utilized in our body through a complex process, metabolism,

* **Corresponding author Assem M. El-Shazly**: Department of Pharmacognosy, Faculty of Pharmacy, Zagazig University, Zagazig 44519, Egypt; E-mail: assemels2002@yahoo.co.uk

Atta-ur-Rahman, Shazia Anjum and Hesham Al-Seedi (Eds.)

which occurs within the living organism in order to maintain life. The word "metabolism" is derived, since late 19th century, from the Greek metabolē "a change" (from metaballein "to change") with the English suffix -ism. Through metabolism, chemical transformations are performed within the cells of organisms for the conversion of food to energy [1]. Metabolic system is among the most fundamental essentials for survival. The major organs that constitute our metabolic system include the gastro-intestinal tract, pancreas, liver, gall bladder, thyroid, cardiovascular system and hypothalamus. All these units must work harmoniously to achieve the proper rate of metabolism. Inappropriate connections between these units or disturbed function in any of these units lead to a metabolic disorder.

Disturbance of metabolism leads to the development of several disorders such as obesity, diabetes mellitus, dyslipidemia and osteoporosis (Fig. **1**) [2]. Such disorders constitute the greatest current threat to the human population worldwide [3]. The incidence of metabolic disorders worldwide has increased drastically during the last years. Consequently, obesity, diabetes mellitus, dyslipidemia, osteoporosis and associated disorders are considered among the most serious threats to the current and future health of human population worldwide. The World Health Organization (WHO) estimates that about 1.6 million deaths in 2016 were caused by diabetes [4]. Additionally, diabetes is considered one of the four main non-communicable diseases (NCDs) accounting for serious threats next to cardiovascular diseases, cancer and chronic respiratory diseases [4]. Intriguingly, in 2016, there was more than 10-fold increase in the number of obese children and adolescents from 11 million in 1975 to 124 million globally [4].

The most common pathophysiologies of these disorders include changes in miRNA expression, oxidative stress and nuclear factor erythroid 2 related factor 2 (Nrf2) pathways [2]. Lack of safety, serious side effects and high cost of chemically-synthesized drugs are considered challenges in the treatment and prevention of metabolic disorders. An alternative therapy that is sufficiently accessed by all the population worldwide, even in less-developed countries, is phytotherapy. Plant-derived therapy has raised more attention in the last decades, owing to more safety, lower cost and less side effects. In this chapter, we will briefly discuss the pathophysiology of the most prevalent metabolic disorders and the role of natural products in the prevention and treatment of such disorders.

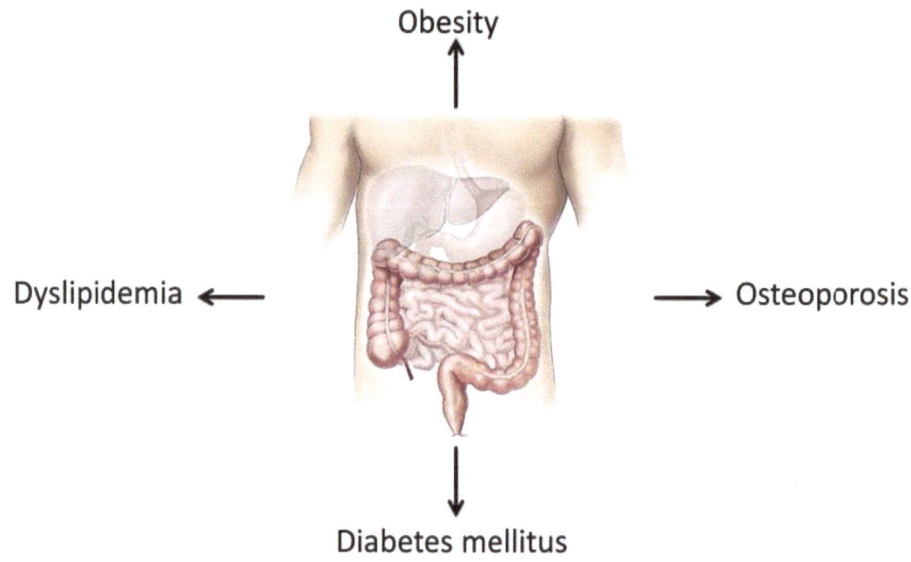

Fig. (1). Metabolism and associated metabolic disorders.

2. OBESITY

Obesity derived from the Latin word obesity as, (stout, fat, or plump) or ob-esum, (fatness with moderately abusive overtones). Ēsus is the past participle of edere (to eat), with ob (over) added to it [5, 6]. Obesity and overweight are defined as excessive fat deposition in adipose tissue which normally represents 15-20% of body weight in men and 20-25% in women and constitutes one of the largest body organs and includes lipid-filled adipocytes, endothelial cells that form vasculature, fibroblasts for structural support, pericytes which are changed to adipocytes, preadipocytes, mast cells and immune cells. In addition, fat tissue is a special form of connective tissue consisting of fat cells which are the largest cells in the body embedded in stroma and originates from more rudimentary cells associated with the capillary network. Obesity and overweight are measured using body mass index (BMI) which is calculated by dividing person's weight (in kilograms) over the square of person's height (in meters). Additionally, BMI equal to or greater than 25 means overweight, while, a body mass index 30 or more indicates that a person is obese [7].

Below 40 years of age, obesity is associated with few symptoms such as tiredness, breathlessness, back pain, arthritis, sweatiness, poor sleeping, depression and menstrual disorders. On the other hand, overweight and obesity that resulted from disturbance in metabolism have been associated with several chronic diseases such as type-2 diabetes mellitus, dyslipidemia, cancer, hypertension, cardiovascular diseases and endothelial dysfunction [8]. Obesity represents a health burden that threatens the population worldwide particularly children (in low- and middle-income countries, predominantly in urban era). This indicates that strong preventive measures are required [9].

2.1. Pathophysiology of Obesity

Adiposity, in humans, is developed when there is an imbalance between excessive caloric intake and energy expenditure as our body is endowed to keep homeostasis between fat available, fat storage and fat utilized [10]. Food with high calories more than the body requirements is stored within adipocytes as triglycerides which protects against the toxicity of fatty acids, in other respects, free fatty acids produce oxidative stress because they circulate in the vasculature and disseminate throughout the body [11]. Additionally, the deposited fat is released gradually and not converted into carbohydrates, but the liver utilizes them in ketones production through normal process of lipolysis. Moreover, reduction of appetite and maintaining energy balance occurred *via* physiological mechanisms derived from afferent signals from the periphery as the gastrointestinal tract (pancreas and liver). Also, nutrient digestion, absorption and the vagus satiety feeling are regulated by hormones released from the gut as cholecystokinine (CCK), peptide YY (PYY) and glucagon-like peptide 1 (GLP1). Finally, carbohydrates metabolism and hypothalamus stimulating satiety are regulated by pancreatic hormones as insulin, glucagon and amylin. An imbalance in the regulation of adipose tissue remodeling results in obesity [12, 13].

In the recent studies, it was found that obesity, premature aging, cancer, cardiovascular diseases, cognitive impairment and mood disorders are circadian disruption (CD) comorbidities. CD is defined as a breakdown of the normal phase relationship between the internal circadian rhythms and 24-h environmental cycles [14]. The mechanisms that linking CD with obesity are unknown, but it was found that, reduction of daily sleep, high snacking frequency and more exposure to night light reduce brain feeling for internal and external rhythms which lead to disturbance of metabolism, involve obesity [8]. Additionally, weight gain could be addressed through different strategies including, but not limited to, modulation of energy balance either by increasing energy output, increasing lipolysis or decreasing energy intake by appetite suppression, modulation of signal transduction, stimulation of anorexigenic or inhibition of orexigenic pathways, modulation of lipid metabolism and adipogenesis, regulation of adipocytes differentiation, modulation of lipid digestion and absorption through lipase inhibition.

Table 1. Phytoconstituents used in treatment of obesity.

Phytoconstituents	Source	Mechanism
Capsaicin	*Capsicum annuum*	Suppressing 3T3-L1 differentiation, promote lipolysis and thermogenesis.
Catechins	*Camellia sinensis*	Energy expenditure and fat oxidation in humans
Copteroside B	*Acanthopanax senticosus*	Pancreatic lipase inhibitor
Curcumin	*Curcuma longa*	suppressing 3T3-L1 differentiation, inhibits preadipocyte proliferation, lipogenesis and fat accumulation in liver
Damulin-A and B	*Gynostemma pentaphyllum*	Activation of the AMPK pathway.
Epigallocatechin gallate	*Camellia sinensis*	Appetite supression through interaction with a component of leptin-independent pathway
Foenumoside B	*Lysimachia foenum-graecum*	Suppressing 3T3-L1 differentiation and exhibits potent activation of the AMPK pathway.
Fucosterol	*Ecklonia stolonifera*	inhibits adipocyte differentiation *via* suppression of adipocyte marker proteins PPAR and CCAAT/enhancer-binding protein
Gordonosides	*Hoodia gordonii*	Suppress hunger and thirst
Hederagenin 3-*O*-β-D-glucuronopyranoside 6-*O*-methyl ester	*Acanthopanax senticosus*	Pancreatic lipase inhibitor
5-Hydroxytryptophan (5-HT)	*Griffonia simplicifolia*	Direct precursor for serotonin which exhibits appetite suppression effects
1H-indole-2-carbaldhyde, 1H-indole-6-carbaldhyde	*Sargassum thunbergii*	Inhibition of adipogenesis through the suppression of 3T3-L1 differentiation *via* AMPK pathway activation.
Meridianin C	Macroalgae *Aplidium*	Inhibition of adipogenesis by down-regulation of C/EBPα and PPARγ.
Methyl xestospongic ester	*Xestospongia testudinaria*	Pancreatic lipase inhibitory activity with a decrease in circulating TAG.
Phlorotannins	*Ecklonia stolonifera*	Inhibition of adipocyte differentiation
Piperine alkaloid	*Piper nigrum*	Enhances lipolysis through sympathetic activation and inhibits the differentiation of 3T3-L1 cells.
Protopanaxadiol saponins	*Panax ginseng*	Increase the levels of cholecystokinin (anorexigenic mediator)

(Table 1) cont.....

Quercetin and isoquerctin	*Nelumbo nucifera*	Both compounds enhance lipolysis mediated by β-adrenergic pathways.
Synephrine alkaloid	*Citrus aurantium*	Lipolytic effects in human fat cells.
Sulphorafane	*Brassica oleracea*	Suppression of 3T3-L1 adipocyte differentiation and stimulates lipolysis in adipocytes.

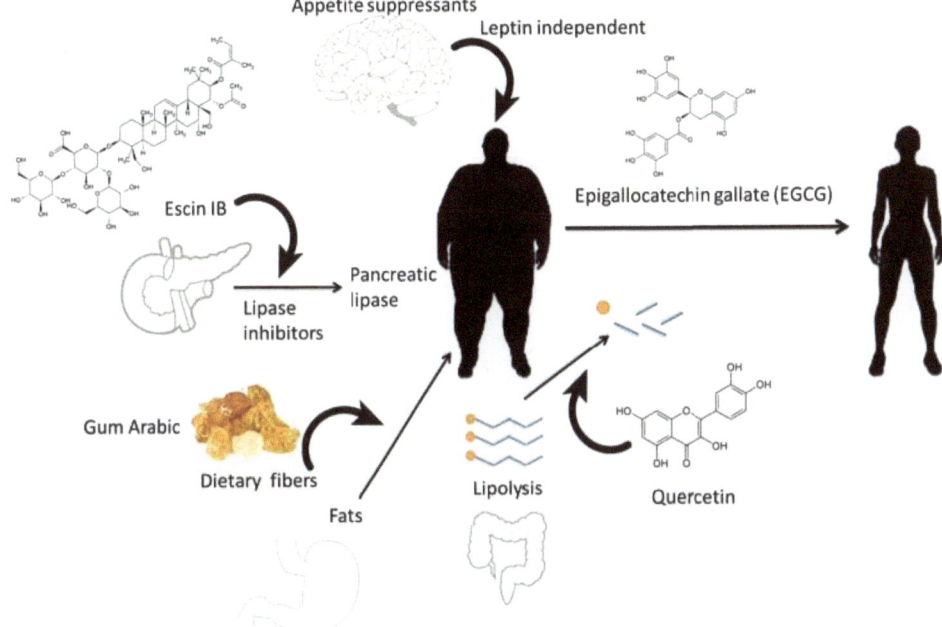

Fig. (2). Role of some active ingredients in obesity control.

2.2. Natural Products and Obesity

As usual, nature offers an unlimited source for confronting any health problem, whereas, natural sources provide a solution for problems developed with obesity management regarding the development of serious side effects, cost/benefit ratio and maintaining a healthy status (Figs. **2** and **3**). Additionally, there is a continuous increasing demand for the development of new anti-obesity products from natural sources either in the form of plant extracts, isolated bioactive compounds or functional foods (Table **1**). This demand arises from the fact that many synthetic products as sibutramine, rimonabant, fenfluramine, among others had been withdrawn from the market due to development of serious side effects including stroke, hypertension and anxiety [15, 16]. Other strategies for obesity treatment, for example surgical interventions may also show economic limitations beside the common post-operative side effects. The best strategy for controlling obesity represents the non-medical, non-surgical weight loss through life-style modulation by increasing the physical activity and healthy controlled diet, however, this strategy is very difficult to follow due to the busy schedule and sedentary life style, beside the slow rate of weight loss following this strategy [17].

Fig. (3). Representative natural secondary metabolites used to treat obesity.

2.2.1. Natural Products as Appetite Suppressants

Appetite suppression represents one of the major strategies in weight loss, through creating a sensation of fullness and satiety. Serotonin, leptin, ghrelin, among others, are important metabolic signals that mediate appetite control. The molecular basis behind appetite suppression and satiety could be regarded as multifactorial combining both central and peripheral effects and involving the interaction between vast group of neurotransmitters, peptides and hormones. The hypothalamic arcuate nucleus (ARC) plays the major role in controlling the appetite through the interaction between orexigenic neuropeptides Y (NPY) and agouti-related peptide (AgRP) and anorexigenic proopiomelanocortin (POMC) and cocaine- and amphetamine-regulated transcript (CART) [18, 19].

Epigallocatechin gallate (EGCG) isolated from green tea controls appetite *via* interaction with a component of leptin-independent pathway [20]. Additionally, it was previously reported that, EGCG attenuated body fat deposition in a dose-dependent manner by reducing leptin and stearoyl-CoA desaturase-1 (SCD1) gene expression in white fat, while, uncoupling proteins (UCP1) expression was not changed in brown fat [21]. Also, energy expenditure and fat oxidation in humans was increased by catechins (polyphenols) from green tea [22].

The stem of leafless spiny plant of *Hoodia gordonii* (bushman's hat) is considered one of the promising medicinal plants for the development of new anti-obesity products that is used in South Africa and Namibia mainly to suppress hunger and thirst [23]. Clinical data regarding this use are not sufficient mainly due to the narrow geographical distribution of the plant [23]. The major constituents as pregnane, steroidal glycosides (hoodigosides and gordonosides) and compound P57 (an oxypregane derivative) are considered the marker compounds of Hoodia and exhibited promising *in vivo* results [24 - 27]. Reports by Phytopharm showed that double-blind, placebo-controlled studies performed on 20 obese free-feeding subjects indicated a reduction in caloric intake by approximately 1000 calories per day [28]. Moreover, other reports revealed that Hoodia extract (400 mg/capsule) twice daily for one month resulted in weight loss (2-15 pounds) and intake reduction of about 1000 calorie/day [28]. The active constituent P57 revealed possible central action, as it increases hypothalamic ATP resulting in reduction in food intake by 40–60% with a dose-dependent effect [29].

Griffonia simplicifolia seed, which is indigenous to Central Africa, is another promising source for appetite suppression. It is rich in 5-hydroxytryptophan (5-HT) a direct precursor for serotonin, a neurotransmitter that is directly linked to anorexigenic pathways in the hypothalamus. Serotonin was evaluated clinically for its appetite suppression effects showing maximum effects at a dose of 900 mg/day. *In vivo* evaluation of 5-HT showed a significant increase in the circulating levels of leptin, an important mediator of food intake and body weight regulation secreted by adipocytes [30 - 32].

The rhizomes of *Panax ginseng* (Korean red ginseng), are one of the most popular medicinal herbs and among the most famous constituents in traditional Chinese medicine (TCM). It is well known for its adaptogenic properties, increasing stamina, physical activities and immune response. Recently, *P. ginseng* was studied as anti-obesity agent *via* significant reduction in neuropeptide Y (NPY) in the hypothalamus [33]. Moreover, protopanaxadiol and protopanaxatriol saponins showed significant increase in the levels of the anorexigenic mediator cholecystokinin coupled with decreased expression of neuropeptide Y [34].

2.2.2. Natural Products as Lipase Inhibitors

Pancreatic lipase (PL) is the major enzyme involved in the digestion of dietary fats, secreted in the duodenum catalyzing the hydrolysis of triacylglycerols (TAG) into monoacylglycerols and free fatty acids, the later are then incorporated with bile acid-phospholipid micelles and absorbed in the small intestine entering the circulation as chylomicrons [35]. Through inhibition of PL, a considerable fraction of the ingested TAG will not be converted to free fatty acids and hence neither absorbed nor utilized in the synthesis of new fats, this in turn allows the body to utilize stored fats to obtain its requirements from the fatty acids.

Orlistat is considered as one of the most famous products used in anti-obesity regimens, exerts its action mainly through inhibition of PL, however, unpleasant side effects are usually associated with its use [36]. So, hundreds of medicinal plant extracts, and/or secondary metabolites were screened for their PL inhibitory activity among which saponin rich medicinal plants showed a remarkable activity [37]. Additionally, silphioside F, copteroside B, hederagenin-3-*O*-β-D-glucuronopyranoside-6'-*O*-methyl ester isolated from *Acanthopanax senticosus* herb (Siberian ginseng) [38], and chiisanoside, 11-deoxyisochiisanoside, isochiisanoside, and sessiloside identified in *A. sessiliflorus* [39], exhibited weight reduction activity through potent PL inhibitory activity comparable with those of orlistat. Moreover, saponin rich fractions and purified saponins from the closely related Panax sp. showed potent inhibition of PL [40], total Chikusetsu saponins, isolated from *P. japonicus* and *P. quinquefolium* (American ginseng) leaves showed significant dose-dependent weight reduction with less side effects mainly the absence of severe diarrhea coupled with orlistat administration [41 - 43]. Japanese Horsechestnut showed weight reduction capability with the inhibition of PL and increase in the fecal fat content with lowering of circulating TAG [44 - 46].

Polyphenolics (flavonoids, tannins and phenolic acids) are another class of compounds exhibiting significant PL inhibitory effect, demonstrating protein binding and aggregating capabilities through hydrophobic and hydrogen bonding interactions. Grape seed and green tea extracts are rich sources of polyphenolics which exert potent PL inhibitory activity leading to limited dietary fat absorption and fat accumulation in adipose tissue. This action is mainly attributed to the synergistic action between flavonoids and procyanidins, rather than by a single compound [47 - 49]. Furthermore, roots and stems of *Salacia reticulate* (marking nut tree) are traditionally used in preventing obesity *via* PL inhibition which is attributed to polyphenolic compounds [50].

2.2.3. Natural Products Modulating Adipocyte Differentiation

Adipose tissue consists of two main types, white adipose tissue (WAT) that represents the most prevalent type and the major storing site for excess fats acting as an energy depot. The other less prevalent one is brown adipose tissue (BAT) restricted in the cervical, supraclavicular and may extend to the front of the neck and thoracic regions. BAT is mainly linked to thermogenesis through energy dissipation in the form of heat by breakdown of the stored fat mediated *via* β-adrenergic receptors. A third type is beige adipose tissue which formed mainly from WAT in a process called WAT browning expressing UCP-1 on their mitochondria. Therefore, the increase in BAT mass, browning of WAT through formation of beige adipocytes and increasing UCP expression represent promising target for the search of new anti-obesity candidates [51 - 53].

Curcumin isolated from the rhizome of *Curcuma longa* (turmeric) and sulphorafane (SFN), a glucosinolate from *Brassica oleracea* (broccoli), showed significant reduction in body weight in mice with high fat diet due to suppression of 3T3-L1 adipocyte differentiation. Moreover, curcumin significantly decreased the expression of PPARγ and CCAAT enhancer binding protein α (C/EBPα), which are two key transcription factors in adipogenesis, and this effect modified lipid metabolism in adipocytes and inhibited white adipogenesis [54 - 56]. Also, *Artemisia iwayomogi*, *Codonopsis lanceolata* (deodeok), *Populus balsamifera* (balsam poplar) and its active component (salicortin), in addition, *β*-glucan-rich extract from *Pleurotus sajor-caju* (Oyster mushroom) are used as anti-obesity *via* modulation of PPARγ [57].

Capsaicin, isolated from *Capsicum annuum* (Chili Pepper), revealed thermogenic activity through stimulating the browning of WAT and increasing the mitochondrial population in BAT with over expression of UCP-2 and UCP-3. Additionally, capsaicin significantly suppresses 3T3-L1 differentiation into WAT causing significant decrease in WAT biomass [58, 59].

2.2.4. Natural Products Modulating Lipid Metabolism

Inhibition of fatty acid synthesis through targeting key enzymes such as acetyl

Co-A carboxylase, malonyl Co-A, HMG-Co-A reductase or increasing the rate of lipid breakdown through lipolysis represents an important strategy in the management of obesity. *Nelumbo nucifera* (Indian Lotus or sacred Lotus), a well-known aquatic plant which is traditionally used in India, China and southwest Asia, showed enhanced lipolysis mediated by β-adrenergic pathways using ethanolic leaf extract and isolated phenolic compounds such as quercetin, isoquercitin and catechin [60, 61]. Moreover, administration of the phenolic-rich extract of *N. nucifera* leaves and the ethanolic extract of *Gynostemma pentaphyllum* herb (Asian creeping herb commonly found in Japan, China, Korea and Philippines) showed significant ability to reduce body weight through lipid synthesis suppression, potent activation of AMPK in the liver with subsequent increase in β-oxidation and glucose uptake in skeletal muscles and suppression of hepatic fat synthesis [60, 62].

Moreover, dammarane type saponins damulin-A and B, isolated from *G. pentaphyllum*, foenumoside B saponin isolated from *Lysimachia foenum-graecum* (loosestrife) and momordicoside S and karaviloside XI (cucurbitane glycosides) isolated from the fruit of *Mormordica charantia* (bitter melon) exhibited potent activation of the AMPK pathway [62 - 66]. Furthermore, foenumoside B and *M. charantia* dried juice showed significant weight reduction in obese mice through inhibition of 3T3-L1 adipocyte differentiation and epinephrine stimulating lipolysis, respectively [66]. Also, Sulphorafane (SFN) isolated from *B. oleracea* (cabbage) showed ability to stimulate lipolysis in adipocytes and this effect was regulated by hormone-sensitive lipase [59].

The pungent alkaloid piperine isolated from the unripe fruits *Piper nigrum* (Black pepper) was found to promote lipolysis through sympathetic activation, with increase in catecholamine secretion from the adrenal gland in addition to inhibiting the differentiation of 3T3-L1 cells [67, 68]. Similarly, capsaicin from *Capsicum annuum* (red chilies) promotes lipolysis and thermogenesis by similar mechanism [69].

In addition, the aqueous extract of *Hibiscus sabdariffa* (roselle), as well as curcumin isolated from turmeric rhizome and resveratrol found in grapes act as initiators of insulin resistance. Moreover, curcumins and resveratrol as polyphenols showed significant inhibition in preadipocyte proliferation, lipogenesis and fat accumulation in liver [70]. Additionally, curcumin as anti-obesity, affected insulin resistance and improved adipokine imbalances [71]. Supplementation of curcuminoid showed significant reduction in the concentrations of serum triglycerides but there is no significant influence on body mass index, body fat and other lipid parameters [72].

One of the dietary supplements that exhibited an effect on body mass index (BMI), deposition of body fat and lipid metabolism through different mechanisms is Gum Arabic (GA). Additionally, it showed a reduction in glucose level, fat absorption and visceral adipose tissue associated with downregulation of 11β-hydroxysteroid dehydrogenase type I in liver, triglyceride and low-density lipoprotein. Moreover, GA supplementation as dietary fiber could regulate adipose triglyceride lipase, hormone sensitive lipase. Moreover, it reduced total cholesterol in plasma by lowering HMG-CoA reductase which is the rate-limiting enzyme in mRNA expression that is required for cholesterol biosynthesis [73, 74].

In recent years, different ephedra species as *Ephedra sinica*, *E. intermedia* and *E. equisetina* have been used as dietary supplements to treat obesity [75, 76]. Where, *E. sinica* with acarbose 0.5-5% modulated gut microbiota, reduced weight gain, improved lipid profiles, epididymal fat accumulation, decreased fasting blood glucose and glucose intolerance when administered by oral gavage for 6 weeks in high fat diet-fed mice through increasing peroxisome proliferator-activated receptor alpha (PPAR-β), adiponectin activity and reducing tumor necrosis factor alpha (TNF-β) activity [77, 78]. Additionally, clinical trials carried out on obese korean women and the clinical data measured before and after intake of 4g water extract of *E. sinica* (equivalent of 24g of crude herb), revealed that body weight, body mass index and body fat percentage were reduced *via* alteration of gut microbiota that was confirmed during subject analysis using 16S rRNA gene-based pyrosequencing [79].

Although, Ephedra has been marketed to reduce obesity as dietary supplements, Food and Drug Administration (FDA) banned the sale of dietary supplements containing ephedrine alkaloids in the US market due to adverse effects [80, 81]. However, extracts of *Citrus aurantium* (Bitter orange) containing similar alkaloid synephrine are weight-loss products [81]. In contrast, Bent, *et al.*, 2004 [80] built a systematic review and found that *C. aurantium* containing herbal products for weight loss, exhibited no significant benefit compared with placebo-controlled group containing 20 patients which followed for 6 weeks in a clinical study. Additionally, clinical trials were applied using animals to ensure the safety and efficacy of *C. aurantium* and synephrine alkaloid due to safety information of these products are not adequate and warrants rigorous clinical study to draw adequate conclusions regarding the safety of this plant and its constituents [81]. Fugh-Berman and Myers revealed that *C. aurantium* contains the sympathomimetic synephrine which has lipolytic effects in human fat cells only at high doses, but it increases blood pressure, pulse, and cardiovascular problems [82]. Additionally, *C. aurantium* contains 6′,7′-dihydroxybergamottin and bergapten, both inhibit cytochrome P450-3A, and may increase the serum levels of many drugs [82]. Moreover, *C. aurantium* extract and synephrine were investigated in rats to ensure safety and efficacy *via* monitoring weight gain, arterial blood pressure, electrocardiogram (ECG) and mortality [83]. Calapai *et al.* observed that administration of *C. aurantium* decreased food intake and weight gain but with mortality in treated groups compared to control ones [83]. In addition, there were ventricular arhythmias with enlargement of QRS complex in ECG. All the previous data concluded that *C. aurantium* containing products are associated with cardiovascular toxicity [83].

2.2.5. Marine Products as Potential Anti-obesity

Marine organisms provide a relatively new source of bioactive metabolites, representing unique products with potent bioactivities. Generally, they are classified as plants or seaweeds exemplified by the algae and animals or invertebrates exemplified by sponges, corals, tunicates, *etc.*

Phlorotannins isolated from polar fractions of different species of brown algae *Ecklonia stolonifera* were evaluated for their anti-obesity activity and showed potent inhibition of adipocyte differentiation. The activity was linked to the suppression of C/EBPα and PPAR expression [84]. Also, fucosterol, isolated from the same algae inhibited adipocyte differentiation *via* suppression of adipocyte marker proteins PPAR and CCAAT/enhancer-binding protein in a concentration-dependent manner [85, 86]. Additionally, indole alkaloids *e.g.* 1H-indole-2-carbaldhyde and 1H-indole-6-carbaldhyde isolated from the brown algae *Sargassum thunbergii*, showed inhibition of adipogenesis through the suppression of 3T3-L1 differentiation *via* AMPK pathway activation [87]. In addition, meridianin C, another indole alkaloid isolated from the macroalgae *Aplidium* showed inhibition of adipogenesis by down-regulation of C/EBPα and PPARγ [88].

It was found that methyl xestospongic ester, a brominated fatty acid isolated from the marine sponge *Xestospongia testudinaria* demonstrated potent PL inhibitory activity with a decrease in circulating TAG [89]. Moreover, chitosan, a glucosamine polymer obtained by N-deacetylation of chitin from the shells of crustaceans as crabs and shrimps, is a well-known anti-obesity agent. Mixture of chitin (20%) and chitosan (80%) enhance fat excretion and inhibiting lipid absorption [90]. Alginates, other polysaccharides obtained from different brown algae species, are commonly used to reduce body weight through the physical sensation of fullness as they expand in the GIT resulting in low food intake [91].

3. DIABETES MELLITUS

3.1. Pathophysiology of Diabetes Mellitus

Diabetes mellitus is considered to be one of the most common diseases worldwide [2]. Diabetes is mainly divided into two main categories based on the cause of its development; type 1 diabetes (T1D) with deficiency in insulin secretion due to autoimmune disease that destroys β-cells of pancreas and type 2 diabetes (T2D) in which insulin resistance with subsequent alteration in carbohydrates, lipids and protein metabolism is the main cause [92]. Pregnancy can be a cause of special type of diabetes called gestational diabetes that may persist after delivery and become a T2D, external factors like utilization of certain drugs can cause T2D also [92]. Genetic defect can be a reason for diabetes development [92]. Symptoms and complications of diabetes include hyperglycemia, polyuria, ketoacidosis, cardiovascular disorders and renal failure [92, 93]. Several tests have been developed to diagnose diabetes including fasting blood glucose, postprandial blood glucose and hemoglobin A1c with values over 126 mg/dl, 200 mg/dl and 6.5%, respectively, to be considered as a diabetic case [92]. Diabetes treatment strategy depends on its virulence and etiology, it ranges from life style changes like exercise and diet control in mild cases to drug treatment (either synthetic or natural) or a combination of drugs in case of T2D moderate cases and to insulin therapy in severe cases of T2D and T1D [92, 94, 95].

Table 2. Antidiabetic activity of some phytoconstituents.

Phytoconstituent	Source	Mechanism
Amorfrutins	*Amorpha fruticosa*	Target peroxisome proliferator-activated receptor γ
Anthocyanins	Strawberry, raspberry, blueberry, and blackcurrant	Inhibit α-glucosidase and α-amylase
Berberine	Barberry	Stimulates insulin secretion and glycolysis and prevent adipogenesis
Curcumin	*Curcuma longa*	Increases insulin secretion, decrease insulin resistance and increase glycogen synthesis
Eremanthin	*Costus speciosus*	Increases insulin level
Genistein	Soybean	Enhances insulin secretion and protect β-cells
Glucosinolates	Brassicaceae family	Activate Nrf2
Guggulsterone	*Commiphora mukul*	Increases plasma insulin, hepatic and muscle glycogen
Gum Arabic	*Acacia senegal* and *A. seyal*	Inhibits glucose absorption
Iridoid glucoside	*Vitex negundo*	Increases in insulin
Kaempferitrin	*Bauhinia forficate*	Action may be attributed to its anti-oxidant activity

(Table 2) cont.....

Phytoconstituent	Source	Mechanism
Mangiferin	*Mangifera indica*	Activates glucokinase enzyme
Oleanolic acid	Apple peel	Stimulates glucose uptake
Peonidin	*Ipomoea batatas*	Inhibits α-glucosidase and α-amylase
Quercetin	Apple, onion, citrus and tea	Activates AMPK
Salicylates	Salix species	Activate AMPK
Sulfated flavonoids	*Potentilla discolor*	Inhibit aldose reductase
Tannins	Strawberry, raspberry, blueberry, and blackcurrant	Inhibit α-glucosidase and α-amylase
Ursolic acid	Apple peel	Stimulates glucose uptake
Vitamin E	Sunflower, olive oil and nuts	Reduces BGL and glycated hemoglobin A1c and elevate insulin level

3.2. Natural Products and Diabetes Mellitus

Multiple reviews had dealt with collecting data of natural products (herbal form, extracts or pure compounds) used as antidiabetic [2, 96 - 105]. Based on the mode of action, they can be classified into herbs that possess antidiabetic action that may be attributed to their antioxidant properties [2, 102], enhance insulin secretion [102, 105], increase insulin sensitivity [97], act as α-glucosidase and α-amylase inhibitor [102, 105], target glucose uptake and transport [102] and herbs with several modes of action [105]. Many Chinese herbs and herbal formulas were prepared to target treatment of diabetes with some of them were tested clinically; a review summarizing these herbs was performed by Tao *et al.* [96]. Indian antidiabetic plants were collected in a review by Grover *et al.* [106]. The use of molecular docking and drug modeling for discovery of natural hypoglycemics and their mode of action was reviewed by Ye *et al.* [107]. As to pure natural compounds, numerous flavonoids exhibited antidiabetic action, compounds from this class can act by several mechanisms like aldose reductase inhibition, increasing glucose transporter GLUT-4 level, increasing insulin release, inhibition of protein tyrosine phosphatase 1B, inhibition of α-glucosidase enzyme, increasing glucose uptake and insulin like action [98]. Terpenoids represent another class that showed hypoglycemic activity *via* increasing glucose transporter GLUT-4 level, AMPK activation, decreasing glycosylated hemoglobin A1c, decreasing LDL, triglyceride and total cholesterol and increasing insulin and HDL levels [98]. Some terpenoids can activate protein kinase B, extracellular-signal-regulated kinases and glycogen synthase kinase 3b and inhibit α-glucosidase activity [98]. Triterpenoids may act as antidiabetic agents *via* Nr2f activation [2]. Cinnamic aldehyde, scopoletin, as well as some phenolics like anthraquinones, phenyl propanoyl esters, lignans and acylated anthocyanins showed also antidiabetic action; generally, cinnamic aldehyde and phenolics activity can be attributed to Nr2F activation [2, 98, 108, 109]. Other natural products with hypoglycemic action as alkaloids, glycosides and polysaccharides were also reported [110]. Nutraceuticals including amino acids, fatty acids, vitamins and minerals are good sources for treatment of diabetes (Table **2**) [111]. In this part, we will focus on summarizing studies dealt with investigating antidiabetic action of natural products *via* clinical trials or even in animal models and *in vitro* as well, but with promising results that should be recommended to be tested clinically (Fig. **4A-D**).

Fig. (4A). Representative natural secondary metabolites used to treat diabetes.

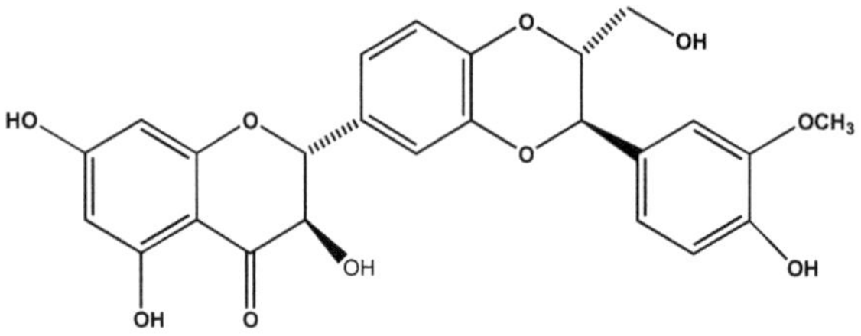

Silymarin

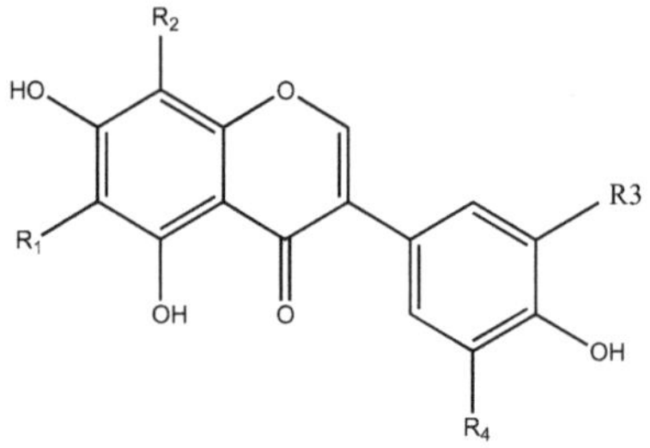

R1 = H, R2 = H, R3 = H, R4 = H; Genistein
R1 = H, R2 = H, R3 = prenyl, R4 = prenyl; 3',5'-diprenylgenistein
R1 = prenyl, R2 = prenyl, R3 = H, R4 = H; 6,8-diprenylgenistein

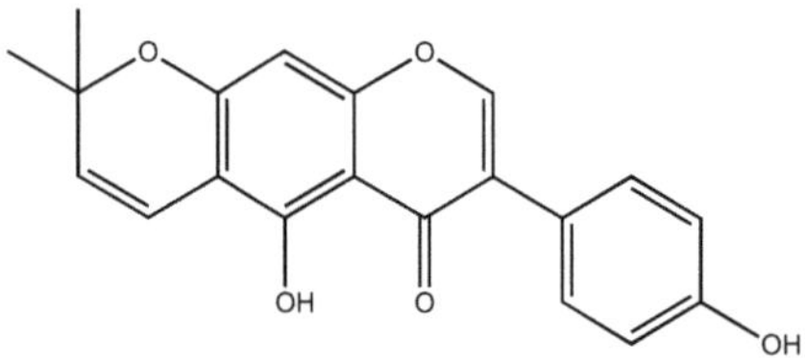

Alpinumisoflavone

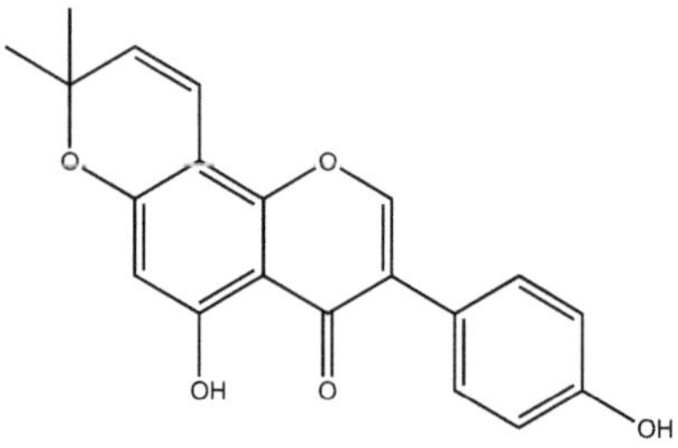

Derrone

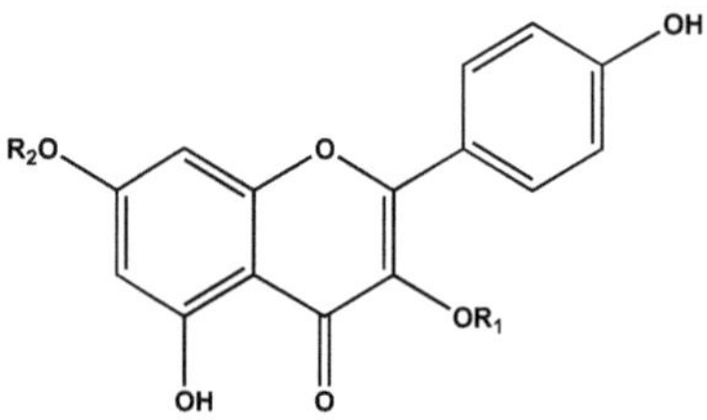

R1 = rhamnose, R2 = rhamnose; Kaempferitrin

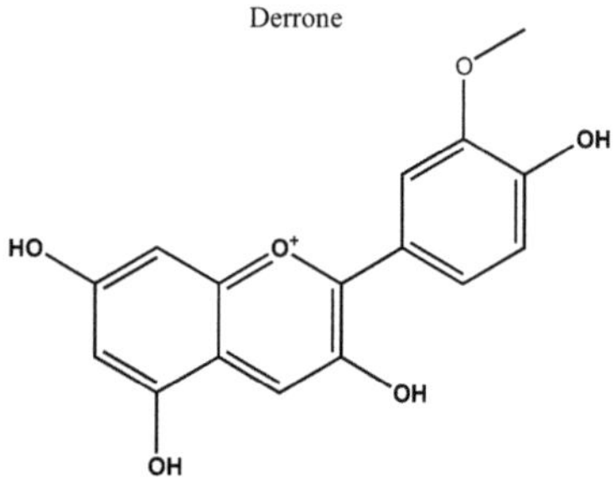

Peonidin

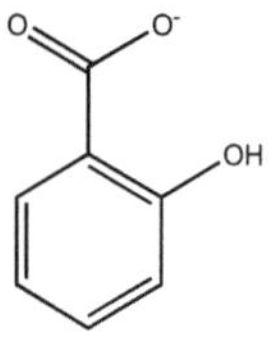

Salicylate

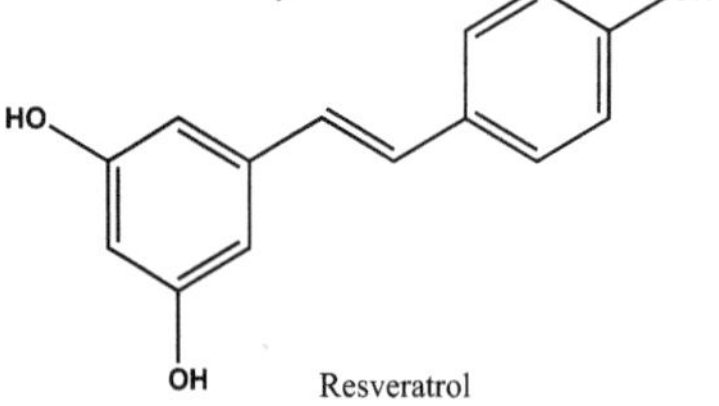

Resveratrol

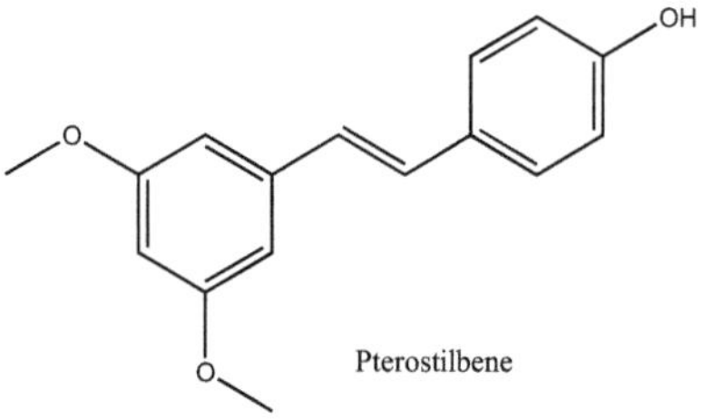

Pterostilbene

Fig. (4B). Representative natural secondary metabolites used to treat diabetes.

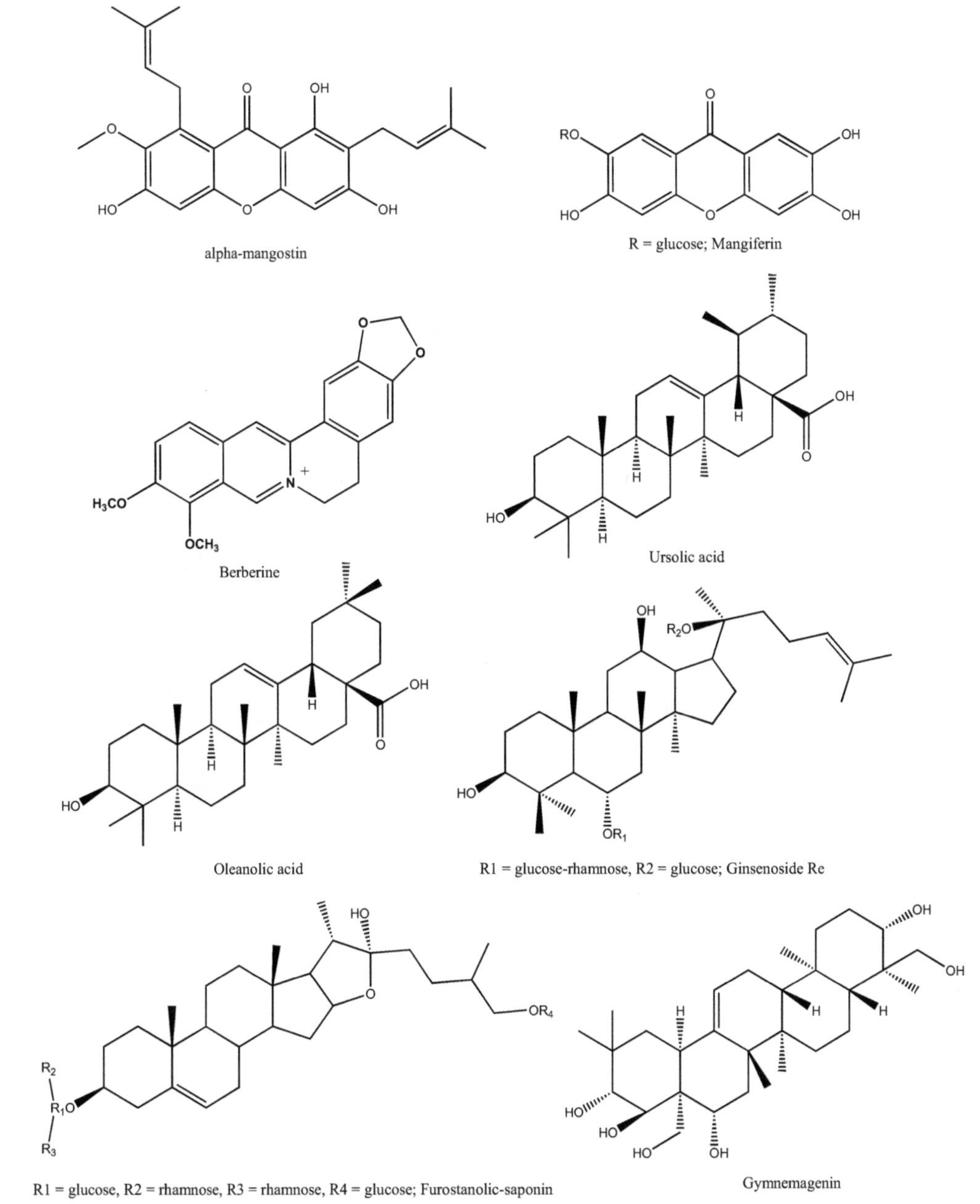

alpha-mangostin

R = glucose; Mangiferin

Berberine

Ursolic acid

Oleanolic acid

R1 = glucose-rhamnose, R2 = glucose; Ginsenoside Re

R1 = glucose, R2 = rhamnose, R3 = rhamnose, R4 = glucose; Furostanolic-saponin

Gymnemagenin

Fig. (4C). Representative natural secondary metabolites used to treat diabetes.

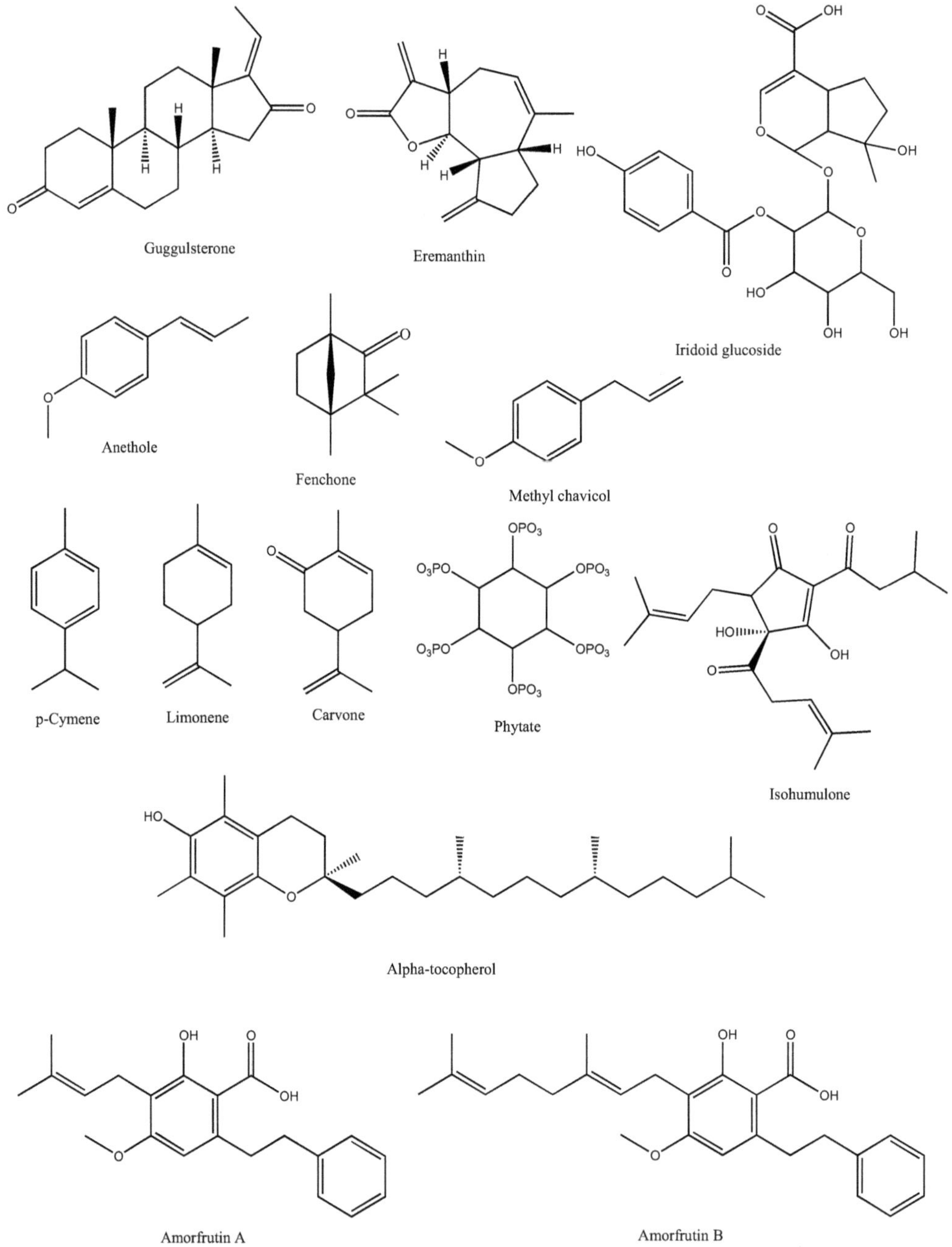

Guggulsterone

Eremanthin

Iridoid glucoside

Anethole

Fenchone

Methyl chavicol

p-Cymene

Limonene

Carvone

Phytate

Isohumulone

Alpha-tocopherol

Amorfrutin A

Amorfrutin B

Fig. (4D). Representative natural secondary metabolites used to treat diabetes.

3.2.1. Flavonoids

Flavonoids represent a major class that possesses hypoglycemic action, several studies had been performed to investigate the mode of action of such compounds, luteolin, amentoflavone, luteolin 7-*O*-glucoside, and daidzein exhibit this effect by inhibiting α-amylase and α-glucosidase activity [112]. In human, starch digestion and consequently glucose level can be affected through inhibition of α-amylase activity by flavonoids as quercetin, quercetagetin, myricetin, fisetin, luteolin, eupafolin and scutellarein, docking of a group of flavonoids showed that hydroxyl group at 7 and 4', 3' or 5'- positions are essential for activity [113].

Quercetin is a common flavonoid in apple, onion, citrus and tea, it was found to activate AMPK that increases glucose uptake by muscles and activates hepatic glucokinase resulting in elevation of insulin level [2, 114], also it can reduce aldose reductase activity [98]. Quercetin-3-*O*-glycoside exerts its activity *via* AMPK activation also [98]. Rutin is an effective antidiabetic flavonoid that exerts its action *via* decreasing carbohydrates absorption, increasing glucose uptake and reducing gluconeogenesis, it can also protect β-cells and increase insulin secretion [115]. Combination of luteolin, apigenin and quercetin was found to enhance β-cells viability [2]. The common hepatoprotective flavonoid of milk thistle; silymarin was found to reduce blood glucose level (BGL) in type 2 diabetic patients (T2DP); recommended dose is 200 mg three times per day, silymarin also reduces hemoglobin A1c, LDL and total cholesterol [99, 116].

Genistein (main soybean constituent) treatment for 98 days reduced BGL in diabetic rats at a dose of 20 mg/kg. It can act by enhancing insulin secretion and protecting β-cells [2, 117]. A dose of 40 to 160 mg isoflavones of soybean reduced body weight and glucose level in postmenopausal diabetic women [102]. 3',5'-Diprenylgenistein, 6,8-diprenylgenistein, alpinumisoflavone, derrone and genistein antidiabetic activity may be attributed to activation of AMPK and glucose transporter GLUT-4 [98]. Kaempferitrin (kaempferol-3,7-*O*-(α--dirhamnoside) was found to have hypoglycemic action at doses of 50, 100, and 200 mg/kg in diabetic rats, this compound represents the major constituent in *Bauhinia forficate* (brazilian orchid tree) leaves n-butanol fraction [118], this action may be attributed to its anti-oxidant activity. Sulfated flavonoids can reduce BGL *via* inhibition of aldose reductase in diabetic mice, they represent the major constituent in *Potentilla discolor* decoction [119].

3.2.2. Phenolics

Polyphenolics like anthocyanins and tannins of fruits as strawberry, raspberry, blueberry, and blackcurrant showed α-amylase and α-glucosidase inhibition action. Red grape and green tea can also inhibit α-amylase due to their tannin contents [120, 121]. In addition to their anti-oxidant activity, polyphenols of *Vaccinium myrtillus* (European blueberry) leaf and *Phaseolus vulgaris* (green bean) seed coat were found to reduce BGL and lipids [122]. Anthocyanins from *Pharbitis nil* (Japanese morning glory) and *Ipomoea batatas* (sweet potato) inhibited α-glucosidase and α-amylase but not sucrase activity [108]. Peonidin, a diacylated anthocyanin from *I. batatas* represents an example for α-glucosidase and α-amylase inhibitors [123]. Procyanidins from the bark extract of maritime pine was found to reduce glucose level in diabetic patients through α-glucosidase inhibition; it did not increase insulin secretion [124]. Salicylates constitute a group of phenolic compounds that belong to willow (Salix species) with known anti-inflammatory effect, the bark of willow is rich in salicin and other salicylates, it was found that salicylates activate AMPK with a positive impact on diabetes and cancer [114]. Resveratrol is another phenolic that reduced BGL in T2DP, this action may be attributed to its Nrf2 activation effect [2, 125].

Curcumin, the main curcuminoid of *Curcuma longa* (turmeric) is known for its pharmaceutical importance [126]. *C. longa* increased insulin secretion in diabetic patients [102]. In streptozotocin induced diabetic mice, curcumin decreased BGL and increased insulin secretion, its combination with bone marrow transplantation regenerated β-islets, decreased pancreatic lipid peroxidation, increased anti-oxidant enzymes activity and ceased inflammatory mediators like TNF-α and IL-1β [127]. Another mechanism of action for curcumin and its demethoxylated analogues; demethoxycurcumin and bis-demethoxycurcumin is α-glucosidase inhibition as indicated in *in vitro* study by Du *et al.* [128]. Curcumin can also decrease insulin resistance and increase glycogen synthesis in rats [93], as a polyphenolic, it may exert its antidiabetic action due to its antioxidant activity and Nrf2 activation [2]. Because of its poor solubility, curcumin was loaded on a polymeric formulation of chitosan, alginate, maltodextrin, pluronic F127, pluronic P123, and tween 80, this formulation was found to decrease BGL [126]. Nanoencapsulated curcumin using chitosan decreased BGL at a dose of 50 mg/kg after a week of treatment in diabetic rats [129]. Similarly, pterostilbene showed antidiabetic effect *via* Nrf2 activation [2].

3.2.3. Xanthones

Xanthones like α-mangostin from *Garcinia mangostana* (purple mangosteen) were found to show antidiabetic action as well as hypolipidimic and anti-inflammatory activities [130]. Mangiferin the main constituent of *Mangifera indica* (mango) [131], was reported to have antidiabetic action, a docking study showed that its action can be attributed to activation of glucokinase enzyme which is responsible for conversion of glucose to glucose-6-phosphate. Mangiferin reduced BGL and increased serum insulin at a dose of 200 mg/kg in diabetic mice after 8 weeks of treatment [132].

3.2.4. Alkaloids

Berberine, an alkaloid isolated from barberry extract, was found to decrease BGL in patients by different mechanisms like stimulating insulin secretion and glycolysis and preventing adipogenesis [133]. Its bioavailability was enhanced 2-4 folds in diabetic mice when administered *via* anhydrous reverse micelle delivery system [134]. Another study showed that berberine can do its hypoglycemic action *via* decreasing free fatty acids [135]. Patients treated with berberine for 3 months at a dose of 0.5 g trice daily showed reduction in fasting and postprandial BGL as well as hemoglobin A1c, triglycerides, LDL cholesterol and total cholesterol. The BGL reduction had started after one week from the beginning of the treatment [136]. In diabetic rats, berberine activated AMP-activated protein kinase resulting in a decrease in energy storage and increase in energy production [137].

3.2.5. Triterpenes

A preparation of ursolic and oleanolic acids obtained from apple peel exhibited hypoglycemic action *via* stimulating glucose uptake in a subclinical trial in the jejunum [138]. Ursolic acid was found to reduce BGL in diabetic rats *via* different mechanisms like sorbitol dehydrogenase and aldose reductase inhibition, decreasing glucose-6-phosphatase activity and increasing glucokinase1, ursolic acid can also decrease cholesterol, triglycerides and free fatty acids [139].

Ginsenoside Re from ginseng was found to decrease fasting BGL in diabetic mice after 12 days of treatment at a dose of 20 mg/kg, the hypoglycemic action lasted for 3 days after treatment [140]. Three weeks treatment of diabetic rats with 50 and 100 mg/kg malonylginsenosides reduced BGL *via* improving insulin sensitivity [141]. Furostanolic-saponin isolated from fenugreek seeds reduced BGL in diabetic patients at a dose of 500 or 1000 mg/day [98]. *In silico* analysis revealed that gymnemagenin, a main constituent of *Gymnema sylvestre* (Gymnema) can induce hypoglycemic action *via* affecting important proteins in carbohydrate metabolic pathway [142].

3.2.6. Sterols

Guggulsterone, a sterol from *Commiphora mukul* (Indian bdellium tree) resin was found to reduce BGL in diabetic rats, it increased plasma insulin, hepatic and muscle glycogen and decreased the expression of G6Pase and PEPCK gluconeogenic genes and LDL cholesterol [143].

3.2.7. Sesquiterpenes

Eremanthin from *Costus speciosus* (crepe ginger) was found to reduce plasma glucose and lipid (cholesterol, LDL-cholesterol and triglyceride) levels in diabetic rats at a dose of 5-20 mg/kg after sixty days of treatment; glycosylated hemoglobin was also decreased at a dose of 20 mg/kg. The compound increased insulin level as well as HDL-cholesterol, serum proteins and glycogen [144].

3.2.8. Monoterpenes

Iridoid glucoside from *Vitex negundo* (Chinese chaste tree) showed a decrease in plasma glucose and glycosylated hemoglobin and increase in insulin and hemoglobin levels suggesting its hypoglycemic action in diabetic rats treated with a dose of 50 mg/kg for 30 days [145].

3.2.9. Essential Oils

Single topical dose of *Foeniculum vulgare* (fennel) nanoemulsion sustained release essential oil preparation (120 mg/kg) reduced plasma glucose level in diabetic rats [146], *trans*-anethole represents the major constituent in its oil followed by fenchone, methyl chavicol, *p*-cymene and limonene [147]. Carvone reduced BGL at a dose of 50 mg/kg (30 days treatment), it elevated insulin level in plasma of diabetic rats [148]. Carvone is a common constituent in many oils like *Carum carvi* (carawy), *Mentha spicata* (spearmint) and *Anethum sowa* (sowa) [149, 150].

3.2.10. Glucosinolates

Glucosinolates constitute a group of natural compounds belonging to Brassicaceae, their hydrolytic products have anticancer acticvity [151]. Sulforaphane, an isothiocyanate (glucosinolate hydrolysis product) was found to participate in diabetes treatment *via* Nrf2 activation [2].

3.2.11. Carbohydrates

Gum Arabic is the dried exudate of *Acacia senegal* and *Acacia seyal*, 16 weeks treatment with a dose of 10 g daily decreased BGL and glycosylated hemoglobin in T2DP, this action can be attributed to glucose absorption inhibition [74]. Guar gum is a polysaccharide obtained from seeds of *Cyamopsis tetragonolobus* [152], it retarded carbohydrates absorption however its effect on BGL is not as good as expected, chemically it is a galactomannan derivative [153]. Phytate (myo-inositol hexaphosphate) is a common constituent in cereals and legumes, it was found to reduce diabetic complications *via* reduction of glycated hemoglobin A1c and advanced glycation end products in diabetic patients after 3 months of treatment [154].

3.2.12. Vitamins

Vitamin E can be obtained from several sources like sunflower, olive oil and nuts [155]; Alpha-tocopherol (20 and 500 mg) was found to exhibit a reduction in BGL and glycated hemoglobin A1c with insulin level elevation in glucose tolerance test in diabetic rats, its anti-oxidant action explains its LDL lowering effect [156].

3.2.13. Miscellaneous Compounds

Isohumulone from hops decreased plasma glucose level in diabetic mice at doses of 32 and 48 mg/day after 4 weeks of treatment. It activated peroxisome proliferator-activated receptors α and γ and decreased both insulin resistance and total fats [157]. MCS-18, an anti-inflammatory compound isolated from *Helleborus purpurascens* (hellebores), it was found to increase pancreatic regulatory T-cells and decrease interferon gamma, this findings explain its anti-diabetic action in type-I autoimmune diabetes [158].

Amorfrutins as dietary products from legumes of *Amorpha fruticosa* (desert false Indigo) with a bibenzyl structure are promising constituents for diabetes treatment by targeting peroxisome proliferator-activated receptor γ with a positive impact on insulin resistance and metabolic parameters [159, 160].

3.2.14. Dietary Fibers

Dietary fibers consisting of yellow mustard mucilage, fenugreek gum and flaxseed mucilage can reduce postprandial glucose levels [161]. Beta-glucan as an oat dietary fiber improved insulin resistance in diabetic patients and consequently control hyperglycemia [162]. Clinically, dietary fibers had been proven to be a natural source that can reduce triglyceride levels with a positive impact on cardiovascular profile of diabetic patients [163]. Increasing soluble fibers intake can decrease glucose as well as LDL-cholesterol levels in healthy individuals [164].

3.2.15. Resin

Propolis (resin of bees) reduced blood glucose level in T2DP at a dose of 900 mg per day for 12 weeks treatment [165]. Propolis can also participate in healing diabetic foot ulcer [166]. *Boswellia serrata* (frankincense) gum resin protected β-cells in diabetic mice recommending its protective effect against T1D [167].

3.2.16. Herbal Material

Camellia sinensis (tea) is the most popular drink all over the world. It is a powerful anti-oxidant plant due to its polyphenolics high content [168]. It is characterized by a prophylactic action against diabetes. Consumption of green tea containing 96.3 mg to 582.8 mg catechins for 12 weeks elevates insulin level and reduces hemoglobin A1c in diabetic patients [102].

Cinnamon is a common plant that is used as a drink and in bakery. It has several pharmaceutical applications. Chemically, it contains phenolic compounds and essential oil [169, 170]. *C. cassia, C. aromaticum*, and *C. zeylanicum* can be used as a food supplement for diabetic patients due to their hypoglycemic effect [171]. In a clinical study to test action of cinnamon on BGL, it was found that cinnamon powder can reduce glucose level as well as lipids such as triglycerides, LDL cholesterol and total cholesterol [172]. In another study on rat model, cinnamon exhibited a decrease in BGL *via* stimulating insulin secretion [173]. Six weeks treatment with *C. cassia* bark extract at doses 50-200 mg/kg decreased BGL, α-glycosidase, cholesterol and triglycerides in diabetic mice while it increased insulin and HDL-cholesterol levels [174]. *C. cassia* aqueous extract decreased BGL, LDL cholesterol, total cholesterol and increased insulin sensitivity in diabetic patients after 2 months of treatment at a dose of 250 mg twice daily [175]. Additionally, cinnamon extract (300 mg/kg) and (600 mg/kg) decreased fasting BGL in diabetic mice, they inhibited hepatic glucose production *via* decreasing gene expression of phosphoenolpyruvate carboxykinase and glucose-6-phosphatase [176]. Polyphenolic oligomer of *C. parthenoxylon* bark reduced fasting BGL in diabetic rats at doses of 100-300 mg/kg after 2 weeks of treatment, its action may be attributed to enhanced insulin activity [177].

Gymnema sylvestre extract is supposed to repair or regenerate β-cells in hyperglycemic patients and increases membrane permeability leading to increase in insulin levels and consequently decrease in BGL, 400 mg of the extract were co-administered daily with an oral hypoglycemic (glibenclamide or tolbutamide) for 18-20 months in T2DP and with insulin therapy for 10-12 months in T1DP to exert this action [178 - 181]. Its powder increased glucose utilization by activating phosphorylase, sorbitol dehydrogenase and gluconeogenic enzymes [182]. Chemically, *G. sylvestre* contains saponins and triterpenoid glycosides [102].

Extract contains several classes of natural products including methyl ester of 9-octadecenoic acid and eicosanoic acid as major constituents decreased BGL in T2DP [183]. *Urtica dioica* (nettle) is supposed to enhance insulin secretion and inhibit α-glucosidase. Clinically, it is safe to use the leaves as a hypoglycemic agent in diabetic patients [102]. Its effect was correlated with the phytochemical composition of flavonoids, fatty acids, tannins, sterols, polysaccharides, scopoletin and isolectins [184]. *Allium cepa* (red onion) exhibited reduction in BGL in T2DP; 100 g of *A. cepa* is the recommended dose to reduce fasting blood glucose [99, 185]. *A. cepa* is rich in polyphenolics and flavonoids. *Capparis spinosa* (flinders rose) can reduce BGL in T2DBP also [186], it contains phenyl propanoids, terpenes, isothiocyanates, alkanes, aldehydes and fatty acids [187, 188].

Capsules of *Juglans regia* (walnut) leaf extract showed decrease in BGL in diabetic patients treated for 3 months at a dose of 100 mg twice daily. It also reduced hemoglobin A1c and elevated insulin level due to its phenols content which are responsible for its antioxidant activity [102, 189, 190].

Astragulus helps in decreasing BGL and hemoglobin A1c in T2DP, it is recommended to use it as adjuvant therapy [191]. Chemical constituents of Astragalus include flavonoids, saponins and polysaccharides [192]. Ginseng contains a special type of triterpenoidal saponins named ginsenosides [193]. Hydrolyzed ginseng extract was found to decrease BGL after 8 weeks of treatment [194]. Intraperitoneal aqueous root extract of *Panax quinquefolius* (american ginseng) was found to reduce fasting blood glucose level at a dose of 300 mg/kg after 12 days of treatment in diabetic rats and the same dose reduced the body weight also [195]. Berry extract of *Panax ginseng* reduced fasting serum glucose level in diabetic patients after 12 weeks of treatment [196] while *P. quinquefolius* reduced BGL and hemoglobin A1c after 8 weeks at a dose of 100 to 200 mg daily. The same action is reported for *Salacia reticulate* at a dose of 240 mg daily after 6 weeks of treatment [99, 103], the activity is attributed to the presence of α-glucosidase inhibitor salacinol [197].

Ocimum sanctum (holybasil) was found to reduce fasting blood glucose in pateints more than 40 years old with metabolic disease, treatment of diabetic patients with the plant leaf powder reduced BGL, LDL, triglycerides and total cholesterol after 3 months at a dose of 2 g daily, it contains several phytoconstituents like tannins, flavonoids, triterpenes and saponins, the plant also has anticonvulsant effect [99, 198, 199]. *Raphia hookeri* (Raffia palm) showed inhibitory action on α-amylase and α-glucosidase. HPLC analysis of the plant extract identified eight phenolic and flavonoid compounds including gallic acid, caffeic acid, chlorogenic acid, catechin, rutin, kaempferol, luteolin and apigenin [200]. Phenolics of *Hordeum vulgare* (barely) exhibited the same inhibitory action [201]. Citrus is known for its high content of flavonoids, limonoids, essential oil and sterols [202]. *Citrus junos* (Yuzu) fruit peel extract was found to reduce fasting blood glucose which recommend using it as a supplement for prediabetics [203]. *In vitro* study of *C. hystrix* (papeda) and *C. maxima* (Pomelo) revealed reduction in BGL by inhibiting α-glucosidase and α-amylase enzymes [204]. *Passiflora edulis* (passion fruit) possess antioxidant activity due to its phenolic contents, at doses of 250 and 500 mg/kg decreased BGL and protect end organs *via* activating anti-oxidant enzymes in diabetic rats [205, 206].

Momordica charantia (bitter melon) can decrease blood glucose by increasing insulin sensitivity in diabetic rats [207], as to its clinical trials its antidiabetic activity is affected by dose, part used, extract type and time of administration [102]. It contains polypeptides that have structural similarity to insulin that is responsible for its activity as an insulin substitute [208]. *Citrullus colocynthis* (colocynth) seed extract (300 mg/kg) decreased BGL in diabetic rats *via* β-cells regeneration. It contains curcurbitacins, colocynthosides, glycosides, flavonoids, essential oils, fatty acids and alkaloids, the plant can be used also as anti-inflammatory, anti-oxidant, anti-microbial and anti-cancer [209, 210]. *Curcuma longa* (turmeric) and *Allium sativum* (garlic) extracts (200 mg each) exhibited a decrease in BGL after 14 weeks treatment, their activity was attributed to curcuminoids and alliin content, respectively [211]. *Zingiber officinale* (ginger) improved insulin sensitivity in diabetic patients and decreased their cholesterol and triglyceride levels, beside its anti-diabetic activity; *Z. officinale* possessed anti-inflammatory and immunomodulatory action, it contains essential oil like gingerol, shagaol and zingiberine [104]. 6-Shogaol and its metabolite 6-paradol enhanced glucose utilization by adipocytes and myotubes resulting in a decrease in BGL [212]. Seed extract of *Oroxylum indicum* (Indian trumpet flower) was found to potentiate acarbose anti-diabetic prophylactic action and decrease its side effects, their mechanism of action targets α-glucosidase, it contains multiple phytochemicals including flavonoids, anthraquinones and iridoides [213, 214]. *Morinda citrifolia* (indian mulberry) fruit extract (300 mg/kg), reduced BGL and increased plasma insulin after 30 days treatment in diabetic rats, the extract contains a wide spectrum of metabolites like alkaloids, flavonoids, triterpenes, vitamins and minerals [215]. Pre-diabetics subjected to 3000 mg daily dose of *Artemisia princeps* (Japanese mugwort) for nine weeks showed lowering of BGL and reduced insulin resistance, it is characterized by high flavonoid content [216, 217]. *Uncaria tomentosa* (Cat's claw) extract reduced BGL in diabetic rats at a dose of 50-400 mg/kg after 21 days of treatment; the extract has a protective action for β-islets and immunomodulatory effect. Phytochemically, it contains indolic and oxindolic alkaloids, sterols, triterpenes and proanthocyanidins [218].

Aloe vera (aloes) juice decreased BGL after one week of treatment at a dose of one tablespoonful, two times per day, the juice reduced triglycerides at the same hypoglycemic dose but after two weeks of treatment [219]. High molecular weight fraction of *Aloe vera* leaves' gel exhibited a reduction in BGL in T2DP after six weeks of treatment at a dose of 0.05 g three times daily, it reduced triglycerides in a shorter period (4 weeks), chemically, it consists of neutral polysaccharides, carbohydrates, proteins, glycoproteins and verectin [220]. *Ximenia Americana* (Tallow wood) root methanolic extract is rich in phenolic compounds like catechins, in addition to its anti-oxidant and hepatoprotective effect; Ximenia has antidiabetic action by reducing BGL and increasing insulin secretion in diabetic rats [221]. Methanolic extract of *Albizia harveyi* bark contains flavon-3-ols and condensed tannins as major constituents, it exhibited similar anti-oxidant, hepatoprotective and antidiabetic activities, by molecular modeling of Albizia major contents to human enzymes, it is suggested that they may exert their antidiabetic action by targeting α-amylase, maltase-glucoamylase, and aldol reductase [222]. *Psidium guajava* (guava) aqueous extract was found to reduce BGL in diabetic patients after 3 weeks treatment at a dose of 500 mg. It contains flavonoids, phenolics and terpenes and recommended as supplement [102, 223]. *Aegle marmelos* (japanese bitter orange) contains coumarins, tannins, alkaloids and carotenoids [224], the leaf decoction potentiated hypoglycemic action of oral hypoglycemic, treatment with this decoction at a dose of 5 g for 16 weeks reduced BGL in diabetic patients [99]. *Nigella sativa* (black seed) seeds oil reduced fasting blood glucose and LDL and elevated HDL in diabetic patients after 6 weeks treatment at a dose of 2.5 mL, two times per day.The seeds increased insulin level after 40 days as it contains volatile oil, isoquinoline and pyrazole alkaloids as nigellamine N-oxide and nigelledine, respectively, in addition to imidazile alkaloids, flavonoids, fatty acids, saponins and cardiac glycosides. *N. sativa* can treat arthritis, inflammation and digestive disorders [99, 225].

Cocos nucifera (coconut) methanolic extract was found to reduce fasting BGL in type 2 diabetic rats [226]; chemically, it contains phenolics like tannins and leucoanthocyanidins in addition to flavonoids, sterols, triterpenes, alkaloids and vitamins, it has several pharmacological activities like anti-inflammatory, antioxidant, antitumor and anthelmentic [227]. *Zizyphus spina-christi* (Christ's thorn jujube) leaves extract is rich in polyphenols and saponins, it can reduce BGL, increase insulin secretion and C-peptide levels, restore glycogen to normal values *via* increasing glucose-6-phosphate dehydrogenase and decreasing glucose-6-phosphatase; *in vitro*, the extract reduced α-amylase activity [228]. *Spergularia rubra* (red sand spurrey) extract showed α-glucosidase inhibition *in vitro* recommending its use as hypoglycemic agent, the extract contains flavonoids as main constituents in addition to organic and fatty acids [229]. *Potentilla discolor* contains flavonoids and triterpenes as major components, the plant flavonoids and triterpenoid extract were found to reduce BGL and glycosylated serum protein in diabetic rats *via* protecting β-cells [230]. Many species of Syzygium (Eugenia) like *S. cumini* have been reported to possess antihypergylcemic activity [231]. Aqueous fraction of *Syzygium alternifolium* seeds exhibited glucose level reduction in both diabetic and normal rats, the ethanolic and hexane fractions of the seeds decreased the glucose level but not the same as the aqueous one. Its flavonoids, alkaloids, sterols, triterpenes and other glycosides and phenolics content possess anti-inflammatory action as well [232, 233]. *S. oleana* pericarp methanolic extract protects β-cells and reduces BGL in T2D [234]. *Scoparia dulcis* (liquorice weed) aqueous extract (200mg/kg) reduced BGL and elevated plasma insulin levels in diabetic rats after 5 days of treatment [235], its leaf extract exhibited reduction in fasting blood glucose and hemoglobin A1c in T2DP without affecting cholesterol and triglycerides when used trice weekly for 3 months [236], the plant possessed other biological activities like analgesic and antimicrobial [237, 238], phytochemical screening of *S. dulcis* indicates the presence of alkaloids, glycosides, tannins and carbohydrates, it contains also scoparic and scopadulic acids in addition to scopadulin and scopadulciol [237]. Fifteen days treatment of diabetic patients with 100 mg *Ficus racemosa* (indian fig tree) bark extract twice daily decreased their BGL [239]. Also, it has antinflammatory and hepatoprotective action beside its analgesic effect. Its phytochemical screening showed flavonoids, tannins, alkaloids, sterols and gums [237]. *Salvia officinalis* (Sage) extract (150 mg, trice daily) reduced BGL and cholesterol levels in diabetic patients, increasing the dose to 500mg, trice daily for 3 months decreased hemoglobin A1c together with glucose level in diabetic patients [102]. The plant contains several phytochemical compounds like phenolics, triterpenes, flavonoids and volatile oil [240].

Lagerstroemi aspeciosa (banaba) aqueous leaf extract reduced BGL in diabetic patients at a dose of 100 mg *via* reduction of gluconeogenesis and glucose uptake enhancement [102]. Additionally, it has antibacterial activity and characterized by the presence of polyphenols like tannins and anthraquinones, flavonoids and saponins [241]. *Theobroma cacao* (cocoa tree) improves insulin resistance in diabetic patients after 15 days treatment at a dose of 100 g daily [102], it showed other activities like anticancer, anti-inflammatory and antimicrobial [242]. *T. cacao* is a source of chocolate and contains polyphenols like catechins and proanthocyanidins and alkaloids like theobromine and caffeine [242, 243]. *Ilex paraguariensis* (yerba mate) reduced BGL, hemoglobin A1c, and LDL cholesterol in diabetic patients, in addition to its polyphenolic components like caffeoylquinic and dicaffeoylquinic acids which are responsible for its antioxidant activity, due to its with the plant contains purine alkaloids and chlorogenic acids [102, 244, 245]. *Trigonella foenum-graecum* (fenugreek) seed exhibited hypoglycemic action, the strength of its effect based on dose and duration of administration, its mode of action targets several mechanisms including enhanced insulin secretion, α-amylase and sucrose inhibition and increasing insulin receptors number [102], it was found to decrease BGL in T1DP after 10 days of treatment if administered at a dose of 50 g daily [106]. Chemically, *T. foenum-graecum* contains trigoneosides (furostanol saponins) and trigonelline alkaloid which are responsible for its hypoglycemic activity [98, 246, 247]. *Coccinia indica* (bimba) fruit and leaf were found to decrease BGL, it is supposed to exert insulin like action; the fiber content of the plant may be responsible for its activity [101]. Leaf extract of *C. indica* exerted its action after 6 weeks treatment at a dose of 500mg/kg in diabetic patients; it can retain levels of lipoprotein lipase, HDL and G-6 phosphatase to normal values, the plant contains flavonoids, alkaloids, sterols and saponins [106, 248]. *Phyllanthus niruri* (gale of the wind) plant preparation decreased BGL at a dose of 5 gm/day in diabetic and non-diabetic hypertensive patients [106], it contains a wide spectrum of phytochemicals including flavonoids, tannins, triterpenes, coumarins, alkaloids, lignans, polyphenols and saponins [249]. *Galinsoga parviflora* (guasca) aqueous ethanolic extract decreased BGL in diabetic rats at a dose of 5mg/kg, chemically, the plant is rich in terpenes and phenolics [250].

Myrmecodia platytyrea ethyl acetate and dichloromethane extracts can inhibit α-amylase activity, this action is attributed to stigmasterol content in these extracts [251]. Chloroform extract of *Nymphaea stellate* (water lily) flower decreased BGL in diabetic rats, the activity attributed to nymphayol that stimulates insulin secretion [252].

Vernonia amygdalina (bitter leaf) chloroform extract exhibited reduction in BGL, GC-MS analysis of the extract showed that linoleic acid, α-linolenic acid and phytols are the major constituents [253].

Glucocorticoids are known to play a role in metabolic pathways.They can affect glucose and fat contents. Methanolic and dichloromethane extracts (50μg/ml) of *Cinnamomum zeylanicum*, *Coffea Arabica* (coffee beans), *Cynara scolymus* (globe artichoke), *Eriobotrya japonica* (Japanese medlar), *Magnolia officinalis* (houpu magnolia) and *Morus alba* (white mulberry) were found to inhibit 11β-hydroxysteroid dehydrogenase 1 and 11β-hydroxysteroid dehydrogenase 2 which are glucocorticoid activators, consequently their antidiabetic effect may be attributed to 11β-hydroxysteroid dehydrogenases inhibition.The activity of the dichloromethane extract was higher than the methanolic extract indicating the lipophilicity of the active material. Leaves of *Eriobotrya japonica* and roasted coffee beans extracts inhibited 11β-hydroxysteroid dehydrogenase1 more than 11β-hydroxysteroid dehydrogenase 2 [254].

Plantago psyllium (psyllium husk) as a dietary fiber source was found to affect diabetic patients positively at a dose of 5g; 3 times per day *via* lowering plasma glucose, triglycerides, cholesterol and LDL cholesterol and elevating HDL cholesterol [255]. A Psyllium dose of 5.1g twice daily exhibited the same effect with reduction in glycosylated hemoglobin A1 [256].

Rice bran exhibited antidiabetic action in both type I and type II diabetic patients *via* reduction of fasting blood glucose and glycosylated hemoglobin and elevation of serum insulin levels, rice bran consists of carbohydrates, tocols, γ-oryzanols, and polyphenols [257]. Maple syrup butanol and ethyl acetate extracts inhibited α-glucosidase and α-amylase activities *in vitro*, this action is attributed to their phenolic contents [258].

3.2.17. Herbal Combination

Combination of *Morus alba*, *Artemisia dracunculus* (tarragon), *Urtica dioica*, *Cinnamomum zeylanicum*, and *Taraxacum officinale* (dandelion) decreased BGL after 12 weeks of diabetic patients treatment [95], in addition to its glucocorticoids, *M. alba* contains flavonoids, stilbenoids and alkaloids [254, 259] while *A. dracunculus* contains flavonoids, essential oil, coumarins and phenolcarbonic acids [260] and *T. officinale* contains flavonoids, coumarins and cinnamic acids [261]. Another combination of *Vitis vinifera* (grape) seed, *Phyllanthus emblica* (indian gooseberry), turmeric and fenugreek seeds were administered twice daily for 12 weeks in a capsulated form reduced BGL in T2DP as well [262]. Grape seeds contain procyanidins and tannins while contains glycosides, tannins, vitamins, amino acids and essential and fatty oils [263, 264].

Chinese oil tea (a mixture of green tea and ginger) was found to reduce BGL in mice; it mainly contains polyphenols and gingerol [265]. *Ravuolfia vomitoria* (rauwolfia) and *Citrus aurantium* (bitter orange) boiled foliage reduced plasma glucose level in diabetic patients after 4 months treatment [266]. *R. vomitoria* is known to contain indol alkaloids [267].

3.2.18. Non-herbal Antidiabetic Material

Probiotic supplements consisting of *Lactobacillus*, *Bifidobacterium* and *Streptococcus* (gut microbiota) reduced plasma glucose level in T2DP [268]. Erythropoietin and spirulina (mass of cyanobacteria) reduced BGL in experimental rats *via* activating β-islets of Langerhans [269]. Mushrooms are rich source of polysaccharides, dietary fibers and proteins that were found to exhibit hypoglycemic activity. However, clinical studies of their effect is still poor and need further research [270, 271]. Honey and fructose-glucose mixture can reduce blood glucose in healthy human without affecting triglyceride level in plasma [272]. Honey was found to stimulate β-cells and consequently lower BGL in T1DP [273].

Royal jelly at a dose of 1000 mg, 3 times per day for eight weeks can reduce BGL [274], it mainly contains sterols and hydrocarbons including fatty acids [275]. Macronutrients (proteins, fats and carbohydrates) were found to exhibit prophylactic effect from gestational diabetes, they can reduce BGL [276].

4. DYSLIPDEMIA

Lipids are heterogeneous group of water insoluble organic compounds including triglycerides, phospholipids and cholesterol [277]. Lipids play vital roles in our bodies as sources of energy, essential fatty acids and fat soluble vitamins. Additionally, phospholipids are indispensable structural components of cell membrane, brain and nervous tissue while cholesterol is the precursor of bile acids, steroid hormones and vitamin D [278]. Inside the body, cholesterol and triglycerides are packed into lipoproteins to be transported through blood. Lipoproteins have complex structure with internal core of cholesterol and triglycerides surrounded by free cholesterol, phospholipids and apolipoprotein. According to the type of apolipoprotein, size of lipoprotein and composition of lipids, plasma lipoproteins are divided into seven classes as chylomicrons, chylomicron remnants, very low density lipoprotein (VLDL), intermediate density lipoprotein (IDL), low density lipoprotein (LDL), high density lipoprotein (HDL), and a lipoprotein. All lipoprotein classes are considered atherogenic except HDL which is an anti-atherogenic agent [279].

Dyslipidemia is an endocrine and metabolic disorder characterized by abnormal blood lipid levels mainly due to overproduction or deficiency of certain lipoproteins [277]. It is associated with increased flux of free fatty acids, high level of triglycerides, LDL, and apoprotein B or low HDL levels [280]. Dyslipidemia seems to be one of the basic features of metabolic syndrome [281].

It does not cause any symptoms but it increases the potential risk of atherosclerotic cardiovascular diseases [277, 282], diabetes [283], acute pancreatitis [284] and chronic kidney diseases [285].

4.1. Pathophysiology of Dyslipidemia

According to the main cause, dyslipidemia can be classified into primary and secondary types. Primary dyslipidemia results from genetic defects in a single or multiple genes which cause either overproduction and decrease elimination of triglycerides and LDL or underproduction and excessive elimination of HDL [286]. On the other hand, secondary dyslipidemia caused by any reason other than genetic disorder. This includes bad life style with no physical activities as well as consumption of excessive food with high content of saturated and trans fats [287]. Additionally, diabetes, excessive alcohol consumption, smoking, anabolic hormones, oral estrogen contraceptives, hypothyroidism and many liver diseases can also be important secondary causes of dyslipidemia [288]. Secondary dyslipidemia includes hypercholesterolemia, hypertriglyceridemia and low HDL level [289]. Both primary and secondary dyslipidemia can interfere with each other, so a person with primary causes of dyslipidemia may not express the disorder unless the presence of other secondary causes and *vice versa* [290].

Recent researches revealed the linkage between dyslipidemia and metabolic syndrome confirming that metabolic syndrome is strongly related to high triglycerides, free fatty acids and VLDL levels while high cholesterol and LDL are not a component of it [280, 291, 292]. Dyslipidemia in metabolic syndrome originated mainly from insulin resistance in adipose tissue of the visceral fats. Those abdominal fats are more metabolically active than subcutaneous tissues. The free fatty acids released from insulin resistant fat cells increase in circulation and inhibit protein kinase activation in muscles. This results in reduction of glucose uptake, elevation of protein kinase activation in the liver and induced lipogenesis and gluconeogenesis [292]. Liver converts free fatty acids into triglycerides which stimulate apolipoprotein B and VLDL cholesterol. The cholesterol ester transfer protein (CETP) facilitates the conversion of VLDL into small dense LDL instead of HDL [293, 294]. Additionally, chylomicrons and VLDL production in both intestine and liver are increased in case of hypertriglyceridemia [286].

4.2. Natural Products and Dyslipidemia

Management of dyslipidemia always includes medications in concomitant with a healthy life style, adequate physical activity and suitable body weight.

Medications of dyslipidemia depend mainly on decreasing plasma total cholesterol, LDL, VLDL and triglycerides and increasing HDL levels. These effects can be achieved by decreasing the intestinal absorption of lipids, enhancing lipid excretion and manipulating the activity of some important enzymes involving lipid metabolism as 3-hydroxy-3-methyl-glutaryl-coenzyme A (HMG-CoA) reductase, beta-hydroxysteroid dehydrogenase, cholesterol-7--hydroxylase, acetyl-coenzyme A, acetyl transferases and lecithin–cholesterol acyltransferase. Statins, fibrates, bile-acid sequestrants and nicotinic acid are considered the most widely used antihyperlipidemic medications [294, 295]. A large number of natural products including pure compounds and extracts have been reported for their antihyperlipidemic activities (Table **3**). They include statins, flavonoids, alkaloids, fatty acids, essential oils, saponins, carotenoids, dietary plants fibers and many other natural product classes (Figs. **5** and **6A - D**).

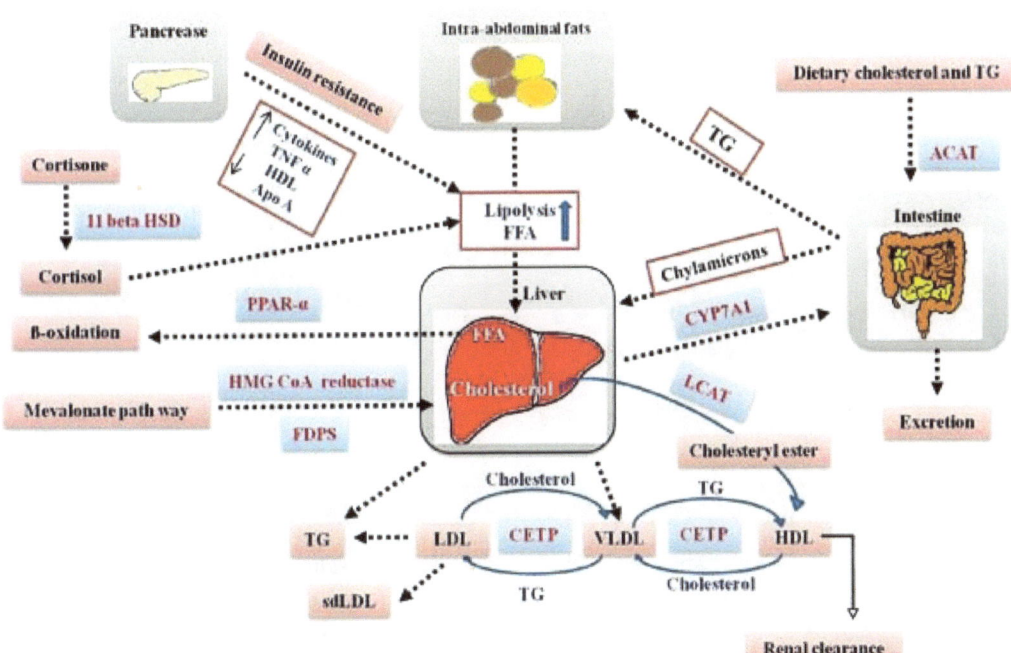

Fig. (5). Targeting dyslipidemia with representative examples of natural products.

Fig. (6A). Chemical structures of some natural compounds with anti-hyperlipidemic activity.

Fig. (6B). Chemical structures of some natural compounds with anti-hyperlipidemic activity.

Fig. (6C). Chemical structures of some natural compounds with anti-hyperlipidemic activity.

Fig. (6D). Chemical structures of some natural compounds with anti-hyperlipidemic activity.

4.2.1. Statins

The majority of cholesterol in our bodies is synthesized by liver so, the inhibition of HMG-CoA reductase (the rate-controlling enzyme in cholesterol synthesis) is considered a very efficient strategy to lower blood cholesterol level and reduce the risk of atherosclerosis and other cardiovascular diseases [296]. Statins are potent HMG-CoA reductase inhibitors by competitive inhibition of the enzyme substrate. Compactin was the first discovered statin which was isolated from the blue-green fungus *Penicillium citrinum* in 1972. After that, a series of statins became available [296, 297]. Another member of naturally occurring statins is lovastatin isolated from *Aspergillus terreus* and *Pleurotus ostreatus*. Lovastatin production was also reported in *Aspergillus niger*, *A. flavus*, *Penicillium* sp., *Trichoderma viride*, *Monascus ruber*, and *Monascus* spp. endophytes [298, 299]. Lovastatin received the approval in the USA in 1987 and is believed to be the first statin approved by the FDA [300]. Moreover, mevastatin is another naturally occurring statin which was isolated from *Penicillium citinium*, *P. cyclopium*, *Pythium ultimum*, and a few strains of *Colletotrichum* spp [301]. It is a specific inhibitor of HMG-CoA reductase and highly effective in lowering plasma cholesterol levels. Simvastatin was produced by an endophytic fungus *Aspergillus terreus*, as a fermentation product [302]. Its intake in concomitant with exercise and low lipid diet is believed to lower elevated blood cholesterol level [303]. Moreover, monacolin K, a natural product with a structure identical to lovastatin, was isolated from red yeast rice (RYR). When *Monascus purpureus* is fermented, it produces red yest rice [304, 305]. RYR is an important food stuff in the daily diet of Chinese people which is used as blood circulation and food digestion stimuli [306]. A large number of clinical trials were carried out on thousands of volunteer patients with hyperlipidemia to investigate the change in lipid profile as well as safety of RYR in a doses ranged from 1.2 to 2.4 g/day. RYR showed significant decrease in total cholesterol especially LDL and triglycerides as well as elevation of HDL [307 - 310]. Moreover it showed 33% decrease in mortality rate with cardiovascular diseases in studies involved 4870 patients who had a history of acute myocardial infarction and increased cholesterol levels and lasted for 4.5 years [311]. On the other hand, studies revealed that long-term therapy with RYR is safe and well-tolerated by patients [312]. In fact, all naturally occurring statins are inactive pro-drugs activated by *in vivo* hydrolysis of the lactone ring [313].

Table 3. Anti-hyperlipidemic activity of some phytoconstituents.

Phytoconstituents	Source	Mechanism
Allyl propyl disulphide and diallyl disulphide	*Allium sativum*	Inhibit 3-hydroxy 3-methylglutaryl coenzyme A (HMG-CoA) reductase activity.

(Table 3) cont.....

Berberine	*Hydrastis canadensis, Coptis chinensis, Berberis* sp.	Activates protein kinase in adipocytes; inhibits Acetyl-coenzyme A acetyl transferases.
Citrus flavonoids (hesperitin, naringenin, tangeretin, nobiletin)	*Citrus* sp.	Inhibit hepatic fatty acid synthesis.
Curcumin	*Curcuma longa*	Increases LDL-receptors in liver; elevate cholesterol 7α-hydroxylase.
Epigallocatechin gallate	*Camelia sinensis*	Inhibits 11 β-hydroxysteroid dehydrogenase.
Fucoxanthin	*Undaria pinnatifida*	Decreases the expression of leptin; promote β-oxidation.
Galactomannan polysaccharide	*Cyamopsis retragonoloba*	Increases cholesterol excretion.
Gingerol	*Zingiber officinale*	Increases leptin, insulin, amylase and lipase.
Glycyrrhizin	*Glycerrhiza glabra*	Inhibits 11 β-hydroxysteroid dehydrogenase.
Isoflavones (melitidin, brutieridin)	*Citrus bergamia*	Inhibit HMG-CoA reductase activity.
Kaempferol	A large number of plants	Inhibits HMG-CoA reductase activity.
Mucilaginous polysaccharides	*Plantago psyllium*	Increase cholesterol excretion.
Omega-3 fatty acids	Fish oil	Peroxisome proliferator activated receptor α.
Phytosterols (sitosterol, campesterol, stigmasterol)	A large number of plants	Reduce the intestinal absorption of cholesterol.
Policosanol	Sugar cane wax	Inhibits hepatic cholesterol synthesis at a step before mevalonate generation.
Quercetin	A large number of plants	Inhibits HMG-CoA reductase; elevate LCAT elevates.
Resveratrol	Grapes and peanuts	Induces apoptosis of fat cells; elevates cholesterol 7α-hydroxylase; inhibits HMG-CoA reductase activity.
Rutin	A large number of plants	Elevates LCAT activities.
Sapogenins	*Trigonella foenum-groecum*	Increase biliary cholesterol excretion.
Silymarin	*Silybum marianum*	Inhibits HMG-CoA reductas activity.
Statins (compactin, lovastatin, simvastatin, mevastatin, monacolin K)	*Aspergillus* sp., *Penicillium* sp., *Monascus purpureus*	Inhibit HMG-CoA reductase by competitive inhibition of the enzyme substrate.

(Table 3) cont.....

Tocotrienols (vitamin E)	palm oil	Increase the conversion of farnesyl to farnesol, which reduces the conversion of farnesyl to squalene and then to cholesterol; inhibit HMGCoA reductase activity.

4.2.2. Flavonoids

Flavonoids are a group of polyphenolic compounds that exert a wide range of biological activities. Citrus flavonoids, including hesperitin, naringenin, tangeretin, and nobiletin have been used as potential therapeutics for the treatment of metabolic disorders as dyslipidemia, insulin resistance, hepatic steatosis, obesity, and atherosclerosis. Many studies revealed a relation between the intake of citrus flavonoid–containing foods and a decreased incidence of cardiovascular diseases. Additionally, many *in vitro* and *in vivo* studies confirmed the lipid-lowering properties of citrus flavonoids. In animal models, addition of citrus flavonoids to rodent diets prevented hepatic steatosis, dyslipidemia, and insulin resistance through the inhibition of hepatic fatty acid synthesis besides their powerful antioxidant and anti-inflammatory effects especially on metabolically important tissues as liver, kidney, adipose and blood vessels [314, 315]. Quercetin and rutin exhibit a hypocholesterolemic effect. Oral administration of rutin to streptozotocin-induced diabetic rats showed a reduction in the levels of lipids in plasma and tissues. Rutin increases HDL and decreases LDL and VLDL. Its effects were attributed to the inhibition of HMG-CoA reductase, and elevation of LCAT activities [316]. The same results were obtained by using quercetin obese zucker rats [317]. On the other hand, isoflavonoids such as formononetin, biochanin A and daidzein have been reported to increase LDL receptor activity in hepatic cells. This biological action is probably due to the effect of flavonoids on sterol regulatory element-binding protein 2 (SREBP-2). Moreover, two isoflavones isolated from *Citrus bergamia* (bergamot orange) juice, melitidin and brutieridin; in addition to kaempferol, naringenin, myricetin had the ability to inhibit HMG-CoA reductase activity [318].

Silymarin is a flavonolignan from *Silybum marianum* (milk thistle) which has been widely used because of its excellent hepatoprotective activities [319]. A significant reduction in blood glucose levels, total cholesterol, LDL cholesterol, and triglyceride was observed in a clinical trial included 25 patients who received 200 mg silymarin three times daily for four months [320].

A significant reduction in triglycerides, total cholesterol and LDL were reported in animals with induced hyperlipidemia after the consumption of flavonoid-rich extracts of *Polygonum perfoliatum* (asiatic tearthumb) tuber [321], *Morus alba* leaves (white mulberry) [322] and *Linaria vulgaris* (common toadflax) herb [323].

4.2.3. Coumarins

Based on animal studies, some pure coumarins such as coumarin, esculetin, umbelliferone and suksdorfin, in addition to extracts rich in coumarins like *Peucedanum japonicum* (coastal hog fennel) and *Mammea Africana* (african mammee apple) may be useful in the treatment of metabolic disorders because of their lipid lowering and antidiabetic effects [324]. Additionally, a study of 17 coumarins of 7-methoxycoumarin and 6,7-dimethoxycoumarin groups showed a potential cholesterol-lowering activities in comparison to the statins [325].

4.2.4. Phenolic Derivatives

Resveratrol is a type of plant phytoalexins. Its highest concentration is found in grapes, peanuts, berries and red wine [326]. It is reported that resveratrol reduces blood lipid levels by multiple mechanisms as HMG-CoA reductase inhibition [327], reversing cholesterol transport by increasing high-density lipoprotein (HDL) levels [328], in addition to adipogenesis prevention by inducing apoptosis of fat cells [329] and activation of cholesterol 7α-hydroxylase that mediates the conversion of cholesterol in 7α-hydroxycholesterol prior to its elimination from plasma through bile [330].

Gingerol is the phenolic pungent constituent of ginger (*Zingiber officinale*). Because of the antihyperlipidemic activity reported for ginger extract, gingerol was assigned for its hypolipidemic activity [331 - 334]. Gingerol oral solution showed a significant decrease in glucose level, body weight, leptin, insulin, amylase, lipase plasma and tissue lipids when compared to normal control in HFD-induced obese rats receiving 75 mg/kg once daily for 30 days [335]. Those results confirmed the result of a previous study which concluded that gingerol (100 mg/kg) significantly decreases plasma triglycerides, free fatty acids and LDL cholesterol [336].

Curcumin is the bioactive compound of turmeric (*Curcuma longa*). A randomized, double-blind, placebo-controlled, crossover trial including 30 obese individuals treated with curcuminoids (1 g/day) for 30 days showed a significant decrease in serum triglycerides. However, curcuminoids showed no significant effect on the total cholesterol, LDL or HDL levels [72]. On the other hand, a previous clinical trial on 10 healthy volunteers receiving 500 mg/day of curcumin for 7 days concluded that curcumin could effectively lower the serum cholesterol [337]. The hypolipidemic effects of curcumin can be attributed to increase in

LDL-receptor mRNA in liver; peroxisome proliferator-activated receptors and enhanced activity of cholesterol-7α-hydroxylase which increases the rate of cholesterol breakdown [338].

4.2.5. Tannins

Epigallocatechin gallate, the most abundant catechin in tea (*Camelia sinensis*) [339], was effective against hypercholesterolemia, obesity and hyperglycemia. Also, it decreased both total cholesterol and LDL-C [340, 341]. This compound is found to be a potent inhibitor of human 11 beta-hydroxysteroid dehydrogenase, a microsomal enzyme that catalyses the conversion of glucocorticoid receptor, and therefore has potential for treatment of various metabolic disorders including dyslipidemia [342].

4.2.6. Alkaloids

Berberine is an isoquinoline alkaloid found in numerous medicinal plants as *Hydrastis canadensis* (orange root), *Coptis chinensis* (Chinese gold thread), *Berberis aquifolium* (oregon grape), *B. vulgaris* (common barberry) and *B. aristata* (indian barberry) [343]. Several animal trials beside a number of clinical trials involving hundreds of patients with dyslipidemia and/or type 2 diabetes mellitus were carried out to investigate the effect of berberine on blood sugar level and lipid profile in doses range from 500 to 1500 mg/day. All studies have confirmed a significant reduction in fasting blood glucose level, HbA1c, total cholesterol and LDL-cholesterol except for HDL which was significantly increased. At the same time, berberine did not show any toxicity at used doses and the major side effects can result from overdose, including mild gastrointestinal discomfort [344 - 347]. The activity of berberine in the treatment of dyslipidemia associated with diabetes may be attributed to the activation of protein kinase in adipocytes and L6 myotubes and facilitated GLUT4 translocation in L6 myotubes *via* phosphatidylinositol 3-kinase so decrease insulin resistant besides, inhibition of ACAT which accelerate the intestinal absorption [348]. Moreover, Berberine probably inhibits the transcription of the mRNA encoding the proprotein convertase subtilisin/kexina type 9 (PCSK9). It is the protein that facilitates the separation of hepatic LDL-R from the cell surface toward the lysosomes where it is usually deteriorated [349]. *Rhizoma coptidis* alkaloids including berberine, palmatine, coptisine, jatrorrhizine and epiberberine exerted hypolipidemic effects in hamsters [350] *via* the inhibition of HMGCoA reductase [351].

The alkaloid-rich extract *Litsea glutinosa* (Indian laurel) bark possessed a significant reduction of triglycerides, total cholesterol and LDL in obese mice with hyperlipidemia. A number of aporphine alkaloids were isolated from this plant as boldine, laurelliptine, laurolitsine and litseglutine. The lipid lowering activity of the extract is related to its stimulating effect of liver and serum lipase which increases the hydrolysis of triglycerides [352]. Additionally, the pyrrolizidine alkaloid-rich extract of *Parinari curatellifolia* (mupundu or mobola plum) seeds also possessed antihyperlipidemic activities [353] in triton-induced hyperlipidemic rats.

4.2.7. Fixed Oils

Fish oil is very rich in long chain omega-3 fatty acids including eicosapentaenoic acid and docosahexaenoic acid. Fish oil can be safely used in the treatment of dyslipidemia *via* reduction of triglycerides levels [354]. The mechanism of action for the hypotriglyceridemic effect has been identified as upregulation of peroxisome proliferator activated receptor α (PPAR-α) in dyslipidemic patients and those with non alcoholic fatty liver disease [355, 356].

Olive oil composed mainly of a monounsaturated fatty acid (oleic acid), possessed antihyperlipidemic activity. The consumption of olive oil by 60 male patients suffering from hyperlipidemia has shown an improvement in their lipid profile [357]. The incorporation of oleic acid in lipoprotein particles generated LDL particles which appear to be more resistant for oxidation [358, 359].

Flaxseed oil comes from the flax plant (*Linum usitatissimum*) contains high levels of alpha-linolenic acid, an omega-3 fatty acid [360]. Oral administration of flaxseed oil in rats and hamsters significantly lowered body weight, liver weight, plasma cholesterol, triglycerides, phospholipids, free fatty acids and lipoproteins [361, 362].

The fixed oil of *Euterpe Oleracea* (açaí palm) was able to reduce the levels of triglycerides, total cholesterol and LDL, as well as to increase HDL in rats with triton-induced dyslipidemia. This effect may be contributed to the high percentage of unsaturated fatty acids (UFA) ranging from 60 to 70% and oleic acid is the majority [363]. Additionally, *Citrullus colocynthis* (colocynth) seed oil was found to decrease body weight significantly. The oral consumption of this oil in rats decreases intestinal absorption of lipids and increases fecal output and fecal lipids. Moreover, a significant decrease in plasma lipids was observed. The oil is composed mainly of hydrocarbons, squalenes, phytosterols and α-tocopherol [364].

Policosanol is a mixture of fatty alcohols derived from sugar cane wax. It has the ability to reduce LDL cholesterol as well as triglycerides. At doses of 20 mg/day, policosanol lowers total cholesterol by 21% and LDL cholesterol by 29% and raises HDL by 15%. The suggested mechanism is that policosanol may inhibit hepatic cholesterol synthesis at a step before mevalonate generation [365].

Tocotrienols (vitamin E) are a naturally occurring derivatives of tocopherols in the vitamin E family. The tocotrienols have more potent antioxidant activity than tocopherols [366]. In a double-blind, 8-week, crossover study involving 25 volunteer, the effects of the tocotrienol-rich fraction of palm oil at 200 mg/day on serum lipids in hypercholesterolemic humans were compared. Total cholesterol fell 15%, LDL 8%, apolipoprotein B 10%, thromboxane 25% and glucose 12% while HDL and TG levels were not significantly changed. These effects could be attributed to increase in the conversion of farnesyl to farnesol, which reduces the conversion of farnesyl to squalene and then to cholesterol. Additionally, the farnesol signals 2 post-transcriptional pathways suppressing HMG-CoA reductase activity. There was a decreased efficiency of translation of the HMGCoA reductase mRNA and a decrease in HMG-CoA reductase protein mass levels. In addition, the LDL receptor protein was augmented, increasing the number of LDL receptors and LDL removal as well as stimulation of apolipoprotein B degradation clearance [367, 368]. Another clinical trial on 36 dyslipidemic patients treated with Palmvitee capsules which contained 112 mg γ-tocotrienol, 60 mg δ-tocotrienol, 48 mg of α-tocotrienol and 40 mg of α-tocopherol was conducted. A significant decrease of total cholesterol, LDL and apolipoprotein B was recorded while there was no significant changes in TG, HDL or apolipoprotein A [369].

4.2.8. Volatile Oils

Anethum graveolans (dill) essential oil, composed mainly of carvone (30%), limonene (33%) and α-phellandrene (20.61%), showed a cholesterol-lowering effect associated with decreasing intestinal absorption of cholesterol, increasing fecal excretion of neutral lipids besides improving the biological antioxidant status by reducing lipid peroxidation in liver and modulating the activities of antioxidant enzymes [370]. Additionally, the essential oil of *Coriandrum sativum* (coriander) fruits possessed a significant hypolipidemic effect due to enhancing bile acid synthesis and increasing the degradation of cholesterol to fecal bile acids. Coriander oil also reduces the activity of the enzyme HMG-CoA, which is the key regulatory enzyme in cholesterol synthesis [371, 372].

Ocimum sanctum (basil) leaves essential oil contains phenylpropanoid compounds in which eugenol and methyl eugenol were the main compounds caused depression in serum lipid profile in hypercholesterolemic rats. Its anti-hyperlipidemic action is primarily due to the suppression of liver lipid synthesis. Phenylpropanoid derivatives especially eugenol, possibly contribute to the lipid-lowering action of the oil [373].

4.2.9. Organosulphur Compounds

Aged black garlic is a product of fermentation of fresh garlic (*Allium sativum*), at high temperature and humidity [374]. In a clinical trial involved 46 patients with hypercholesterolemia, volunteers were treated for 12 weeks with aged black garlic in the form of enteric-coated capsule contains garlic powder equivalent to 9.6 mg allicin. The results showed a significant decrease in total cholesterol and LDL levels, while no change in tiglycerides or HDL levels [375, 376]. On the other hand, another clinical trial was conducted on 30 volunteers with high blood cholesterol levels. The volunteers consumed 5 g raw garlic twice a day for 42 days. Garlic consumption alone can decrease serum lipids in mild hyperlipidemia but it cannot be used as the main therapeutic agent for hyperlipidemia [377]. Additionally, meta-analysis of clinical trials including 1093 hyperlipidemia patients and involved three types garlic including garlic oil, aged black garlic and garlic powder with the doses ranged from 0.3 to 20 g/day. The patients were followed up for 4 weeks to 10 months. As a result, the values of total cholesterol, LDL and HDL have statistical significance compared to control group. However, there was no significant difference of triglycerides [378]. Garlic effect can be attributed to its sulphur compound contents as allyl propyl disulphide and diallyl disulphide. It is suggested that, garlic effect on blood cholesterol level is due to the inhibition of cholesterol synthesis in liver through inhibition of HMG-CoA reductase or other enzymes in addition to increasing the excretion of cholesterol end product [379, 380].

4.2.10. Saponins

Glycyrrhizin is a triterpenoid saponin and is the main and the most important bioactive agent of the subterranean organs of *Glycerriza glabra* (liquorice). It has been reported that glycyrrhizin is a potent inhibitor of 11 β-hydroxysteroid dehydrogenase enzyme; therefore it will has an effect on the treatment of many metabolic disorders including dyslipidemia [381]. A dose of 100 mg/kg given to obese rats showed a significant decrease in free fatty acids, total cholesterol, LDL, and tissue lipid deposition, as well as a significant increase in HDL [382]. Fenugreek (*Trigonella foenum-graecum*) seeds are rich in sapogenins and phytoestrogens. Sapogenins have been shown to increase biliary cholesterol excretion and phytoestrogens indirectly increase thyroid hormones [383]. In a clinical trial involved 30 hypercholesterolemic type II diabetic patients were treated with 25 gm fenugreek seed powder twice daily for 6 weeks, the results showed a significant reduction in serum triglycerides, cholesterol and LDL levels

[384]. The same results were obtained in triton administrated rats treated with 120 mg/kg aqueous fenugreek seed extract. It is suggested that cholesterol excretion increased due to the reaction between the bile acids and fenugreek-derived saponins causing the formation of micelles that are too large for the digestive tract to absorb [385].

4.2.11. Soy Protein (Glycine max)

A clinical trial was performed on 38 individuals (with high blood cholesterol) consuming 47 g soy protein/dya, it showed a decrease in blood cholesterol level and improvement in low-density lipoprotein/high-density lipoprotein ratio [386]. The significant decrease in total cholesterol, low-density lipoprotein and triglycerides associated with soy protein consumption could be attributed to the reduction in the absorption of lipids by fibers [387], in addition to increasing LDL-receptor (LDL-R) expression in human beings [388]. In 1999, health benefits of soy protein in the reduction of coronary heart diseases due to its cholesterol-lowering effect have been approved by FDA [389].

4.2.12. Gums and Dietary Plants Fibers

Myrrh is a natural oleo gum resin extracted from a number of small trees of the genus *Commiphora*. A study on 61 individuals receiving 100 mg of myrrh for 24 weeks, showed a reduction in total cholesterol level by 11.7%, LDL level by 12.7%, triglyceride by 12%, and cholesterol-HDL ratio to 11.1% [390]. Another double-blind study performed on 228 individuals that were treated with 500 mg of myrrh powder three times a day for 12 weeks indicated similarity of this material's effect with that of clofibrate. None of the patients treated with myrrh showed any significant side effects except one patient who showed some gastrointestinal symptoms [391].

The seeds of various species of psyllium (plantago) can be used as antihypercholesterolemic agent due to its contents of mucilaginous polysaccharides [392]. In a study conducted on 75 individuals with hypercholesterolemia, 6 to 8 weeks of the mucilloid of psyllium treatment decreased total cholesterol by 3.5% and low-density lipoprotein cholesterol by 5.1%. Moreover, in an experiment on 125 individuals with type 2 diabetes and hyperlipidemia, 5 g psyllium seeds were taken 3 times per day for 6 weeks tended to decrease the blood glucose level, the total cholesterol, LDL and plasma triglyceride levels, while the HDL level was increased [393].

Guar Gum (*Cyamopsis retragonoloba*) could significantly decrease the blood cholesterol level in laboratory studies on animals as it is rich in galactomannan polysaccharide. This effect was attributed to the effect of this dietary fiber on enterohepatic circulation. It has been stated that guar gum also decreases the fat intake available in foods by affecting the microflora of the gastrointestinal tract [394]. In addition, reports presented in other researches indicated that the lowering of blood cholesterol by guar gum is possibly due to the increase of steroids' excretion in feces and also increase of bile production [395].

Gum acacia is well known as a dietary supplement for its ability to decrease fat deposition in body especially visceral fats. It showed a remarkable reduction in the levels of total cholesterol, LDL, VLDL and triglycerides in human and mice. As other dietary fibers, gum arabic decreases the intestinal absorption besides its beta-hydroxysteroid dehydrogenase inhibitory effect [74].

Oat (*Avena sativa*) as a foodstuff containing high fiber, in addition to different nutritional properties, can decrease the blood cholesterol level. In a study where 152 patients with hyperlipidemia were fed oat diet for 6 weeks, the total cholesterol and low-density lipoprotein levels was decreased [394]. In addition to the antioxidant properties, it inhibits low-density lipoprotein oxidation in a dose dependent manner [395].

4.2.13. Carotenoids

Crocin belongs to a group of natural carotenoid obtained commercially from the dried trifid stigma of the culinary spice *Crocus sativus* (saffron) [396]. Both saffron and crocin decreased the levels of TG, total cholesterol, aspartate transaminase (AST) and alanine transaminase (ALT). In addition, both were able to quench free radicals and protect against oxidation. Saffron, however, was found to be superior to crocin alone. This suggests the presence of other potential active constituents of saffron apart from crocin causing the synergistic effect [397]

Fucoxanthin is a carotenoid from brown algae *Undaria pinnatifida* has beneficial effects on obesity associated with metabolic disorders. Fucoxanthinm according to studies carried on rats fed with a hyperlipidic diet, could protect animals from body weight gain despite of their high fat diet. Additionally, fucoxanthin tends to decrease serum TG, considerably increase HDL in serum, improve insulin resistance, decrease the expression of leptin and promote β oxidation by increasing the expression of UCP-1 which makes the new adipocytes or existing adipocytes more similar to brown fat than to white [398, 399]. Lutein showed significant hypolipidemic, antiatherogenic and antioxidant effects in hyperlipidemic rats in a dose of 50 mg/kg taken for 30 days [400].

4.2.14. Phytosterols

Phytosterols as sitosterol, campesterol and stigmasterol are structurally similar to cholesterol and have been shown to reduce the intestinal absorption of cholesterol by 30-40%. On the other hand, they do not affect plasma concentrations of HDL or triglycerides. Plant sterols are widely found in foods such as nuts, grains, fruits, legumes, and vegetable oils [401, 402]. Previous studies revealed that 0.4 g of vegetable oil sterols eaten twice a day, may reduce the risk of heart disease [403]. Moreover, sterols can reduce serum total cholesterol even in patients treated with statins [404].

4.2.15. Plant Extracts

Cynara cardunculus (artichoke) dry alcoholic extract were given to patients with hypercholesterolemia in a dose of 1.8 mg/day for 6 weeks. A significant decrease in plasma cholesterol and LDL was reported. Compounds present in the leaf of artichoke like cynarin and luteolin may be responsible for this effect [405]. Moreover, 3 g/day of cinnamon powder taken for 8 weeks had significant effects on total cholesterol, LDL and HDL levels compared with controls. The potential mechanism suggested for the hypolipidemic effects of cinnamon was expected to be related to the high content of polyphenols, which inhibit the intestinal absorption of cholesterol. Similarly, *Salvia officinalis* (sage) leaves decoction (sage tea) which is rich in polyphenols especially, rosmarinic acid [406] has achieved improvement in the lipid profile as it decreased the total cholesterol and LDL as well as increased HDL in a study involved 6 healthy females [407]. Additionally, a study conducted on 40 hyperlipidemic associated with type 2 diabetic patients given 500 mg capsule of *S. officinalis* leaf extract 3 times per day for 3 months revealed that the fasting glucose, HbA1c, total cholesterol, triglycerides and LDL were all decreased while, HDL level was increased [408]. In a similar study, 67 hyperlipidemic patients received one 500 mg capsule of sage leaf extract every 8 hours for 2 months exhibited the same results [409]. *Aloe vera* gel, *Houttuynia cordata* (fish mint) alcoholic extract, *Magnifera indica* (mango) leaf extract, *Peperomia pellucida* (pepper elder) extract, *Clerodendrum volubile* (white butterfly) leaf extract and *Moringa oleifera* (drumstick tree) leaf extract were reported to have antihyperlipidemic activities [410 - 415]. Finally, *Nigella sativa* (black seed) extract and its volatile oil were found to be effective in lowering total cholesterol, triglycerides and LDL levels in both animal based trial and a clinical trial involved 30 patients of dyslipidemia [416, 417].

5. OSTEOPOROSIS

The human skeleton represents the internal frame of the body with more than 200 bones which provide the body structure and organs protection. Minerals, such as calcium and phosphorus, are stored in bones as they are essential for their development and stability. Our bones are continuously remodeled throughout the entire life. Bone remodeling (or bone metabolism) is a life-long process in which mature bone tissues are removed (bone resorption) through osteoclasts which break bone tissues down and new bone tissues are formed (bone formation or ossification) through osteoblasts which synthesize bone [418]. The close cooperation between these two processes ensures bone homeostasis. An imbalance in the regulation of bone remodeling processes results in osteoporosis (Fig. 7).

Osteoporosis is a metabolic bone disease that increases the risk of fractures and is characterized by deterioration of bone architecture [419]. It is asymptomatic condition that often remains undiagnosed until it ends with fracture of the spine, pelvis, and/or hip. The prevalence of osteoporosis has increased exponentially in the last decade, especially in postmenopausal women. Osteoporosis-induced low bone density causes more than 10 million fractures annually worldwide [420]. Osteoporosis-related fractures increase health care costs and mortality. The most osteoporosis-associated serious complication is that people become bedridden and this lead to long-term hospitalization [419].

Table 4. Phytoconstituents used in treatment of osteoporosis.

Phytoconstituents	Source	Mechanism
Acerogenin	*Acer nikoense*	Accelerates osteoblast depressionifferentiation by increasing the mRNA expression of BMP-2.
Acetyl-11-keto-beta-boswellic acid	*Boswellia serrata*	Reduces osteoclastogenesis by suppressing the gene expression of NF-kappa B
Albiflorin	Paeoniae Radix	Suppresses oxidative-stress-mediated osteoblast toxicity.
Apocynin	*Apocynum cannabinum*	Decreases RANKL production and increases OPG release.
Baohuoside I	*Epimediium brevicornu*	Increases OPG and decreases RANKL production
Bergapten	*Cnidium monnieri*	Induces the phosphorylation of p38, ERK, the transcription factor SMAD and BMP-2 in osteoblasts
Butein	*Toxicodendron vernicifluum*	Reduces osteoclastogenesis by suppressing the gene expression of NF-kappa B

(Table 4) cont.....

Calebin A	*Curcuma longa*	Decreases NF-κB, RANKL and ROS levels
Cardamonin	*Alpinia katsumadai*	Decreases RANKL production
Coronarin D	*Hedychium coronarium*	Inhibits NF-κB, leading to suppression of osteoclastogenesis
Costunolide	*Saussurea Lappa*	Stimulates the function of osteoblasticcells.
Curcumin	*Curcuma longa*	Decreases NF-κB, RANKL and ROS levels
Echinacoside	Cistanches herba	Increases in ALP activity, COL I and OCN levels and cell proliferation.
Embelin	Marlberry	Suppresses the gene expression of NF-kappa B.
Emodin	Roots and bark of several plants	Accelerates osteoblast differentiation by increasing the mRNA expression.
Gastrodin	*Gastrodia elata*	Protects against oxidative stress-mediated osteoporosis.
Genistein	Soybean	Induces osteogenesis by increasing the nuclear level of ERα protein
Ginsenoside-Rb2	*Panax ginseng*	A potent antioxidant through reduction of oxidative damage and bone-resorbing cytokines.
Guggulsterone	*Commiphora mukul*	Reduces osteoclastogenesis by suppressing the gene expression of NF-kappa B
Honokiol	*Magnolia officinalis*	Elevates cell growth by significantly increasing OPG release and decreasing RANKL production.
Isodeoxyelephantopin	*Elephantopus scaber*	Suppression of NF-kappa B and NF-kappa B - regulated gene expression
Icariin	*Epimedi umbrevicornu*	Increases bone specific matrix proteins such as alkaline phosphatase (ALP) and collagen type I (COL I), reduces osteoporosis and enhances bone healing.
Kirenol	*Siegesbeckia orientalis*	Increases the expression of osteoblast-specific differentiation markers such as osteopontin (OPN), COL I and ALP.
Kobophenol A	*Caragana chamlagu*	Promotes human osteoblast-like cells proliferation.
Lupeol	*Mangifera in dica*	Reduces osteoclastogenesis by suppressing the gene expression of NF-kappa B
Lycopene	Tomato and watermelon	Induces ALP activity and osteoblasts cell proliferation.
Naringin	Citrus species	Improves proliferation and ALP activity.
Oleanolic acid	*Phytolaccaamericana* and *Oleaeuropaea*	Induces key transcription factors associated with osteoblast differentiation

(Table 4) cont.....

Ophiopogonin D	*Ophiopogon japonicas*	Induces ALP activity and calcium mineralization.
Osthole	*Cnidium monnieri*	Reduces osteoporosis by induction of BMP-2.
Psoralen	*Psoralea corylifolia*	Reduces osteoporosis by induction of BMP-2.
Plumbagin	*Nepenthes* and *Drosera*	Reduces osteoclastogenesis by suppressing the gene expression of NF-kappa B.
Quercetin	Fruits and vegetables	Increases ALP activity and up-regulates the osteoblast differentiation.
Resveratrol	Redgrapes and berries	Promotes osteoblastic differentiation.
Rosmarinic acid	*Rosmarinus officinalis*	Inhibits NF-kappa B, leading to revocation of osteoclastogenesis
Rutin	Fruits and vegetables	Increases ALP activity and up-regulates the osteoblast differentiation.
Salidroside	*Rhodiolarosea* (golden root)	Induces mRNA expressions of ALP, OPN and BMPs
Salvianolic acid B	*Salvia miltiorrhiza*	Induces osteogenesis by promoting ERK signaling pathway.
Sweroside	*Cornus officinalis*	Increases ALP activity, osteocalcin (OCN) expression and proliferation
Taxifolin	Conifers	Decreases RANKL gene expression.
Ursolic acid	*Ocimum sanctum*	Reduces osteoclastogenesis by suppressing the gene expression of NF-kappa B.
Vanillic acid	*Sambucus williamsii*	Increases in ALP activity, COL I and OCN levels and cell proliferation.
Vitexdoin F	*Vitex negundo*	Stimulates proliferation and ALP activity in osteoclastic and osteoblast-like cells.

5.1. Pathophysiology of Osteoporosis

Our body is able to maintain bone homeostasis through several factors such as adequate calcium, calcitonin, vitamin D, growth hormone, steroids and parathyroid hormone (PTH) levels. Moreover, several bone marrow-derived membrane and soluble cytokines such as receptor activator of the nuclear factor kappa-B ligand (RANKL) are also involved in regulating bone function.

Osteoporosis can be classified as either primary or secondary [418, 419]. Primary osteoporosis resulted from old age or sex hormones deficiency. Age-related primary osteoporosis can be caused by continuous deterioration of bone trabeculae. Significant reduction in estrogen levels in postmenopausal women or significant accumulation of sex-hormone–binding globulin that inactivates testosterone in men causes primary osteoporosis. Secondary osteoporosis is resulted from excessive alcohol intake, medications or concurrent diseases which can be caused by changes in calcium, vitamin D, steroids or sex hormones levels. For example, excess glucocorticoid production associated with Cushing's syndrome has been found to induce bone loss. Drug-induced secondary osteoporosis has been also reported in several cases such as long-term glucocorticoid therapy required for patients suffering from rheumatoid arthritis, among other inflammatory diseases. In addition, drug-induced secondary osteoporosis has been reported in men receiving androgen-deprivation therapy (ADT) required for patients suffering prostate cancer. Osteoporosis is primarily diagnosed by bone mineral density (BMD) or bone density test. This test is based on using non-invasive dual-energy x-ray for measuring the density of bones.

5.2. Natural Products and Osteoporosis

The ideal strategy for treating osteoporosis, is to increase bone formation by osteoblasts and/or inhibit bone resorption by osteoclasts. Osteoporosis is treated currently by different groups of drugs especially those that inhibit bone resorption, and there are only few drugs available for promoting bone formation. The major conventional drug therapies for treating osteoporosis include bisphosphonates, hormone-replacement therapy, selective estrogen receptor modulators, calcitonin, vitamin D analogs and recombinant human parathyroid hormone [421]. These traditional drugs have some pros as well as cons. For example, while estrogen replacement therapy has been reported to reduce fracture incidence in women suffering from an early menopausal symptoms, its prolonged administration has some complications in increasing the risk of cardiovascular disorders, breast cancer and uterine bleeding [421]. Different natural compound classes that can induce proliferation and differentiation of osteoblasts have been reported for the treatment of osteoporosis (Table **4**). These include flavonoids and their glycosides, phenolic derivatives, phenolic acids and their glycosides, anthraquinones, lignans, terpenoids (monoterpenoids, diterpenoids, sesquiter-penoids and tetraterpenoids), coumarins, diarylheptanoids and steroidal as well as triterpenoidal saponins (Figs. **7** and **8**).

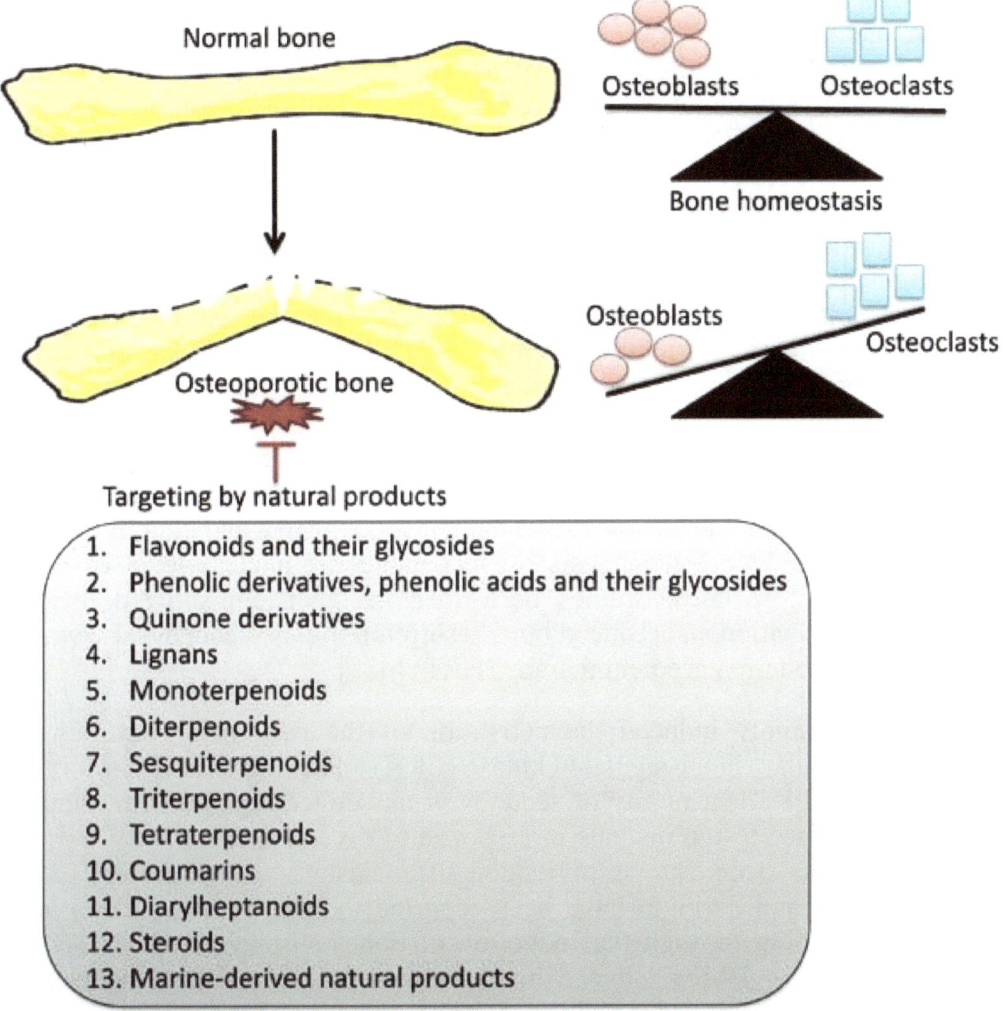

Fig. (7). Targeting osteoporosis with natural products.

5.2.1. Flavonoids and their Glycosides

Several flavones and isoflavones as well as their glycosides have been reported to have anti-osteoporotic activity. Icariin, isolated from *Epimediium brevicornu* (bishop's hat), has been shown to significantly increase bone specific matrix proteins such as alkaline phosphatase (ALP) and collagen type I (COL I) [422]. Additionally, naringin, neoeriocitrin, poncirin and ugonin K significantly improved proliferation and ALP activity in MC3T3-E1 cells (osteoblast precursor cell line derived from *Mus musculus*) [421, 423]. The common flavonoids of most fruits and vegetables, quercetin and rutin, increase ALP activity and up-regulate the osteoblast differentiation of bone marrow-mesenchymal stem cells (BM-MSCs) in a dose dependent manner [424]. Further, quercitrin and taxifolin decreased RANKL gene expression in MC3T3-E1 cells. Sweroside, isolated from *Cornus officinalis*, commonly known as Shan zhu yu, significantly increased ALP activity, osteocalcin (OCN) expression and the proliferation of human osteoblast-like MG-63 cells [421]. Additionally, baohuoside I (icariside-II), icariin, sagittatoside A, epimedin B and puerarin (8-C-glucoside of the isoflavone daidzein) significantly increase OPG and decrease RANKL production [421, 425, 426]. Intriguingly, these flavonoids stimulated estrogen receptors (ER)-dependent osteoblastic functions in osteogenic (UMR-106) cells, but only icariin and sagittatoside A induce estrogen receptors α (ERα) phosphorylation [421]. Estrogen receptors (ERs), members of the ligand regulated nuclear transcription factors superfamily, include estrogen ERα and ERβ, and have been identified in osteoclasts and osteoblasts. Estrogens have indispensable roles in bone homeostasis by coordinating osteoclasts and osteoblasts activities. Therefore, estrogen agonists prevent postmenopausal bone loss. Genistein and ugonin K have been reported to induce osteogenesis by increasing the nuclear level of ERα protein [423, 427]. Clinical studies performed on genistein showed that it increased bone formation and reduced bone resorption in postmenopausal women compared to hormone-replacement therapy (HRT) [428].

Further, icariin rapidly induced the activation of the two major families of MAPKs; extracellular signal-regulated kinase (ERK) and c-Jun N terminal kinase (JNK) [422]. MAPKs is a family of secondary messengers that transfer signals from the cell surface to the nucleus in response to diverse stimuli and MAPKs activation that has been shown to induce osteoblastic differentiation [421]. Moreover, icariin and naringin have been reported to reduce osteoporosis and enhance bone healing through the induction of bone morphogenetic protein-2 (BMP-2) [426, 429]. BMPs induced bone formation *in vivo* by inducing the synthesis of proteoglycan, osteocalcin, collagen type I, fibronectin and ALP activity [421]. Neobava isoflavone promoted osteogenesis by inducing the phosphorylation of p38 kinase of MAPKS family in MC3T3-E1 cells [430]. Additionally, butein, a tetrahydroxychalcone isolated from *Toxicodendron vernicifluum* (Chinese lacquer tree), have been reported to reduce osteoclastogenesis by suppressing the gene expression of NF-kappa B [428].

Fig. (8). Chemical structures of some natural compounds with anti-osteoporotic activity.

5.2.2. Phenolic Derivatives, Phenolic Acids and their Glycosides

Vanillic acid isolated from *Sambucus williamsii* (north china red elder) and echinacoside isolated from *Cistanches herba* (desert ginseng or rou cong rong), have been shown to significantly increase ALP activity, COL I and OCN levels and cell proliferationin osteoblastic MC3T3-E1 cells [431, 432]. Additionally, apocynin, a methoxy-substituted catechol, has been shown to significantly decrease RANKL production and increase OPG release [433]. Salvianolic acid B, a phenolic acid isolated from *Salvia miltiorrhiza* (red sage), induced osteogenesis by promoting ERK signaling pathway in human mesenchymal stem cells (hMSCs) [434].

Resveratrol, a polyphenol stilbenoids (hydroxylated derivatives of 1,2-diphenylethene, stilbene) isolated from red grapes and berries, was shown to promote osteoblastic differentiation in human mesenchymal stem cells *via* ER-dependent extracellular signal-regulated protein kinases 1 and 2 (ERK1/2) activation [435]. Kobophenol A, a stilbenoid tetramer of resveratrol isolated from

Caragana chamlagu (Chinese pea shrub) and *Carex folliculate* (northern long sedge) seeds, promotes human osteoblast-like cells proliferation by inducing ALP and p38 pathway activities as well as potentiating ROS scavenging activity. Salidroside (rhodioloside), phenolic glucoside of tyrosol isolated from *Rhodiola rosea* (golden root) induces the mRNA expressions of ALP, OPN and BMPs [436]. Moreover, 2,3,5,4'-tetrahydroxystilbene-2-O-β-D-glucoside and gastrodin, gastrodigenin glucoside isolated from *Gastrodia elata*(tall gastrodia tuber) and *Galeola faberi* rhizome (Shan shan hu), protect against oxidative stress-mediated osteoporosis by inducing the mRNA expressions of OCN, ALP, and COL I as well as promoting ALP activity, calcium deposition and cell survival [421]. Other phenolic derivatives such as 1'-acetoxychavicol acetate, phenylpropene derivative isolated from *Alpina galangal* commonly called Thaiginger, has been shown to significantly decrease RANKL production [428]. The same mechanism of osteoporosis reduction has been also reported for cardamonin, isolated from *Alpinia katsumadai* known as kat ginger [428]. Obovatol, a biphenolic compound isolated from the bark of *Magnolia obovate* (japanese bigleaf magnolia), gossypin, a pentahydroxy glucosyl flavone isolated from *Hibiscus vitifolius* (rose mallow) and rosmarinic acid, a phenolic acid isolated from *Rosmarinus officinalis* (rosemary), showed a significant inhibitory NF-kappa B, leading to revocation of osteoclastogenesis [428].

5.2.3. Quinone Derivatives

Emodin, an anthraquinone isolated from the roots and bark of several plants, accelerates osteoblast differentiation by increasing the mRNA expression of BMP-2 in MC3T3-E1 cells [437]. Embelin, a hydroxyl benzoquinone with alkyl substitution isolated from *Ardisia japonica* (marlberry), and plumbagin a naphthoquinone derivative isolated from the genera *Nepenthes* and *Drosera* (pitcher plants), have been shown to reduce osteoclastogenesis by suppressing the gene expression of NF-kappa B [428].

5.2.4. Lignans

Honokiol, isolated from the bark of *Magnolia officinalis* (houpu magnolia), has been shown to elevate cell growth by significantly increasing OPG release and decreasing RANKL production in MC3T3-E1 cells [438]. Vitexdoin F, a phenylindene-type lignan isolated from *Vitex negundo* (Chinese chaste tree) seeds, was shown to stimulate proliferation and ALP activity in osteoclastic and osteoblast-like UMR 106 cells.

5.2.5. Monoterpenoids

Albiflorin, a monoterpene isolated from *Paeoniae Radix* (peony root), suppresses oxidative-stress-mediated osteoblast toxicity in MC3T3-E1 cells [439].

5.2.6. Diterpenoids

Kirenol has been reported to increase the expression of osteoblast-specific differentiation markers such as osteopontin (OPN), COL I and ALP as well as significantly reducing osteoporosis by induction of BMP-2 [440]. Curcumin and calebin A, isolated from *Curcuma longa* (turmeric), have been shown to decrease NF-κB, RANKL and ROS levels [428]. Curcumin is considered one of the most widely clinically studied natural products with a high potentiality against a number of bone-related disorders with no side effects. Additionally, coronarin D, a labdane diterpene isolated from *Hedychium* coronarium (butterfly ginger), inhibited NF-κB, leading to suppression of osteoclastogenesis [428].

5.2.7. Sesquiterpenoids

Costunolide, a sesquiterpene lactone isolated from *Saussurea lappa* (costus or kuth root), has been reposted to stimulate the function of osteoblastic MC3T3-E1 cells by increasing cellular mineralization and growth through ERK, PI3K, protein kinase C (PKC) and estrogen receptor (ER) [441]. Isodeoxyelephantopin, a sesquiterpene lactone isolated from *Elephantopus scaber* Linn. (elephant foot) and zerumbone a cyclic sesquiterpene from *Zingiber zerumbethas* (subtropical ginger), have an abolishing activity against osteoclastogenesis *via* suppression of NF-kappa B and NF-kappa B -regulated gene expression [428].

5.2.8. Triterpenoids

Ophiopogonin D, a triterpenoidal saponin isolated from *Ophiopogon japonicas* (mondo grass) roots, induces ALP activity and calcium mineralization in MC3T3-E1 cells. Additionally, acetyl-11-keto-beta-boswellic acid, a pentacyclic triterpene derivative isolated from *Boswellia serrata* (Indian olibanum), ursolic acid, a pentacyclic triterpenoid isolated from *Ocimum sanctum* (holy basil) and lupeol, a triterpenoid isolated from variety of plants, including *Mangifera indica* (mango), *Acacia visco* (viscote blanco and viscote negro) and *Abronia villosa* (desert sand-verbena), have been reported to reduce osteoclastogenesis by suppressing the gene expression of NF-kappa B [428]. Oleanolic acid (oleanic acid), a pentacyclic triterpenoid found in *Phytolacca Americana* (american pokeweed) and *Olea europaea* (olive) showed significant induction of osteocalcin and runt-related transcription factor 2 (RUNX2), a key transcription factor associated with osteoblast differentiation [428].

5.2.9. Tetraterpenoids

Lycopene, a lipid-soluble antioxidant carotenoid found in tomato and watermelon, has been reported to induce ALP activity and osteoblasts cell proliferation [2].

5.2.10. Coumarins

Bergapten and imperatorin, furanocoumarins isolated from *Cnidium monnieri* (osthole, jashoshi, cnidii fructus), induce the phosphorylation of p38, ERK, the transcription factor SMAD and BMP-2 in osteoblasts [442]. Osthole and psoralen, coumarin-like derivatives isolated from *Cnidium monnieri* and *Psoralea corylifolia* (babchi), respectively, significantly reduce osteoporosis by induction of BMP-2 [443, 444].

5.2.11. Diary L Heptanoids

Diary l heptanoids (diphenylheptanoids) consist of two aromatic rings joined by a seven carbons chain (heptane). Acerogenin aaccelerates osteoblast differentiation by increasing the mRNA expression of BMP-2 in MC3T3-E1 cells [445].

5.2.12. Steroids

Ginsenoside-Rb2 (Rb2), 20(S)-protopanaxadiol steroidal glycoside isolated from *Panax ginseng* (Korean ginseng), has potential anti-osteoporosis effects. Rb2 acts as a potent antioxidant through reduction of oxidative damage and bone-resorbing cytokines [446]. Additionally, guggulsterone, a phytosteroid found in the resin of *Commiphora mukul* (guggul tree) and withanolide (withaferin A) a naturally-occurring steroid built on an ergostane skeleton isolated from *Acnistus arborescens* (hollow heart), have been reported to reduce osteoclastogenesis by suppressing the gene expression of NF-kappa B [428].

5.2.13. Marine-derived Natural Products for Osteoporosis

Several marine-derived compounds have been isolated and tested for the iranti-osteoporotic activity. Phorbaketal A, isolated from marine sponge *Phorbas* sp (cushion sponge) and symbioimine, isolated from the marine dinoflagellate *Symbiodinium* sp (zooxanthellae). Symbioimine stimulates osteoblast differentiation and therefore, they are considered good candidates for prevention and treatment of osteoporosis in postmenopausal women. Norzoanthamine, zoanthamine class of marine alkaloids isolated from *Zoanthus* sp (green button polyps), has been reported to induce the formation of the collagen–hydroxyapatite composite that is structure of bone tissue [447]. Mycoepoxydiene, a lactone derivative that is isolated from the marine fungal *Diaporthe* sp., inhibits RANKL-induced osteoclast differentiation and bone loss in mice [447]. Additionally, biselyngbyaside, an 18-membered macrolide glycoside isolated from marine cyanobacteria and fucoxanthin, an oxygenated carotenoid isolated from brown sea algae (*Eisenia bicyclis*, *Laminaria japonica* and *Undaria pinnatifida*) have been reported to promote apoptosis in mature osteoclasts [447]. Largazole, a cyclic depsipeptide isolated from marine cyanobacterium of the genus *Symploca*, exhibits *in vitro* and *in vivo* osteogenic activity through inducing RUNX2 and BMPs expression.

CONCLUDING REMARKS

The incidence of metabolic disorders such as obesity, diabetes mellitus and hyperlipidemia has increased tremendously over the last 10 years. Natural products have raised more attention against many metabolic disorders, owing to their safety, lower cost and toxicity. The use of plant-based formulas is recommended not only for the treatment but also for prophylaxis against metabolism-associated disorders. More clinical studies are essential in the future for in-depth studies of the safety profile as well as the onset and duration of natural products.

CONSENT FOR PUBLICATION

Not applicable.

CONFLICT OF INTEREST

The author confirms that this chapter contents have no conflict of interest.

ACKNOWLEDGEMENTS

The authors would like to thank Prof. Dr. Hesham El-Seedi, Uppsala University, Sweden, for his help and support.

REFERENCES

[1]   Poggiogalle E, Jamshed H, Peterson CM. Circadian regulation of glucose, lipid, and energy metabolism in humans. Metabolism 2018; 84: 11-27.
[http://dx.doi.org/10.1016/j.metabol.2017.11.017] [PMID: 29195759]

[2]   Tabatabaei-Malazy O, Larijani B, Abdollahi M. Targeting metabolic disorders by natural products. J Diabetes Metab Disord 2015; 14(1): 57.
[http://dx.doi.org/10.1186/s40200-015-0184-8] [PMID: 26157708]

[3]   Hotamisligil GS. Inflammation and metabolic disorders. Nature 2006; 444(7121): 860-7.
[http://dx.doi.org/10.1038/nature05485] [PMID: 17167474]

[4]   World Health Organization. World health statistics 2018: monitoring health for the SDGs, sustainable development goals. Geneva: World Health Organization 2018.

[5]   Bays HE, Chapman RH, Grandy S, Group SI. The relationship of body mass index to diabetes mellitus, hypertension and dyslipidaemia: comparison of data from two national surveys. Int J Clin Pract 2007; 61(5): 737-47.
[http://dx.doi.org/10.1111/j.1742-1241.2007.01336.x] [PMID: 17493087]

[6]   Lean ME. Pathophysiology of obesity. Proc Nutr Soc 2000; 59(3): 331-6.
[http://dx.doi.org/10.1017/S0029665100000379] [PMID: 10997648]

[7]   Schwartz MW, Seeley RJ, Zeltser LM, *et al.* Obesity pathogenesis: An endocrine society scientific statement. Endocr Rev 2017; 38(4): 267-96.
[http://dx.doi.org/10.1210/er.2017-00111] [PMID: 28898979]

[8]   Garaulet M, Ordovás JM, Madrid JA. The chronobiology, etiology and pathophysiology of obesity. Int J Obes 2010; 34(12): 1667-83.
[http://dx.doi.org/10.1038/ijo.2010.118] [PMID: 20567242]

[9]   Hedley AA, Ogden CL, Johnson CL, Carroll MD, Curtin LR, Flegal KM. Prevalence of overweight and obesity among US children, adolescents, and adults, 1999-2002. JAMA 2004; 291(23): 2847-50.
[http://dx.doi.org/10.1001/jama.291.23.2847] [PMID: 15199035]

[10]   Rivera CA. Pathophysiology of obesity. Pathophysiology 2008; 15(2): 69-70.
[http://dx.doi.org/10.1016/j.pathophys.2008.04.006] [PMID: 18583111]

[11]   Redinger RN. The pathophysiology of obesity and its clinical manifestations. Gastroenterol Hepatol (N Y) 2007; 3(11): 856-63.
[PMID: 21960798]

[12]   Mingrone G, Castagneto M. The Pathophysiology of obesity.Minimally invasive bariatric and metabolic surgery: principles and technical aspects. Switzerland: Springer 2015; pp. 17-24.
[http://dx.doi.org/10.1007/978-3-319-15356-8_3]

[13]   Waseem T, Mogensen KM, Lautz DB, Robinson MK, Malcolm K, Robinson MD. Pathophysiology of obesity: why surgery remains the most effective treatment. Obes Surg 2007; 17(10): 1389-98.
[http://dx.doi.org/10.1007/s11695-007-9220-1] [PMID: 18000735]

[14]   Erren TC, Reiter RJ. Defining chronodisruption. J Pineal Res 2009; 46(3): 245-7.
[http://dx.doi.org/10.1111/j.1600-079X.2009.00665.x] [PMID: 19215573]

[15]   Hsu Y-W, Chu D-C, Ku P-W, Liou T-H, Chou P. Pharmacotherapy for obesity: past, present and future. J Exp Clin Med 2010; 2(3): 118-23.
[http://dx.doi.org/10.1016/S1878-3317(10)60019-8]

[16]   Gadde KM, Allison DB. Cannabinoid-1 receptor antagonist, rimonabant, for management of obesity and related risks. Circulation 2006; 114(9): 974-84.
[http://dx.doi.org/10.1161/CIRCULATIONAHA.105.596130] [PMID: 16940206]

[17]   Kaur AAD, Goyal A, Kamboj A, Jain U. Treatment of Obesity: An hebal approach. WJPR 2016; 5: 1633-50.

[18]   Atkinson TJ. Central and peripheral neuroendocrine peptides and signalling in appetite regulation: considerations for obesity pharmacotherapy. Obes Rev 2008; 9(2): 108-20.
[http://dx.doi.org/10.1111/j.1467-789X.2007.00412.x] [PMID: 18257752]

[19]   Coll AP, Farooqi IS, O'Rahilly S. The hormonal control of food intake. Cell 2007; 129(2): 251-62.
[http://dx.doi.org/10.1016/j.cell.2007.04.001] [PMID: 17448988]

[20]   Kao YH, Hiipakka RA, Liao S. Modulation of endocrine systems and food intake by green tea *epigallocatechin gallate*. Endocrinology 2000; 141(3): 980-7.
[http://dx.doi.org/10.1210/endo.141.3.7368] [PMID: 10698173]

[21]   Klaus S, Pültz S, Thöne-Reineke C, Wolfram S. *Epigallocatechin gallate* attenuates diet-induced obesity in mice by decreasing energy absorption and increasing fat oxidation. Int J Obes 2005; 29(6): 615-23.
[http://dx.doi.org/10.1038/sj.ijo.0802926] [PMID: 15738931]

[22]   Dulloo AG, Duret C, Rohrer D, *et al.* Efficacy of a green tea extract rich in catechin polyphenols and caffeine in increasing 24-h energy expenditure and fat oxidation in humans. Am J Clin Nutr 1999; 70(6): 1040-5.
[http://dx.doi.org/10.1093/ajcn/70.6.1040] [PMID: 10584049]

[23]   Vermaak I, Hamman JH, Viljoen AM. *Hoodia gordonii*: an up-to-date review of a commercially important anti-obesity plant. Planta Med 2011; 77(11): 1149-60.
[http://dx.doi.org/10.1055/s-0030-1250643] [PMID: 21259185]

[24]   Shukla YJ, Pawar RS, Ding Y, Li X-C, Ferreira D, Khan IA. Pregnane glycosides from *Hoodia gordonii*. Phytochemistry 2009; 70(5): 675-83.
[http://dx.doi.org/10.1016/j.phytochem.2009.02.006] [PMID: 19303614]

[25]   van Heerden FR, Marthinus Horak R, Maharaj VJ, Vleggaar R, Senabe JV, Gunning PJ. An appetite suppressant from Hoodia species. Phytochemistry 2007; 68(20): 2545-53.
[http://dx.doi.org/10.1016/j.phytochem.2007.05.022] [PMID: 17603088]

[26]   Tulp OL, Harbi N, Mihalov J, DerMarderosian A. Effect of Hoodia plant on food intake and body weight in lean and obese LA/Ntul//-cp rats. FASEB J 2001; 15(4): A404.

[27]   Tulp OL, Harbi NA, DerMarderosian A. Effect of Hoodia plant on weight loss in congenic obese LA/Ntul//-cp rats. FASEB J 2002; 16(4): A648.

[28]   Holt S, Taylor TV. *Hoodia gordonii*: An overview of biological and botanical characteristics part I. Townsend Lett 2006; 280: 104-13.

[29]   MacLean DB, Luo L-G. Increased ATP content/production in the hypothalamus may be a signal for energy-sensing of satiety: studies of the anorectic mechanism of a plant steroidal glycoside. Brain Res 2004; 1020(1-2): 1-11.
[http://dx.doi.org/10.1016/j.brainres.2004.04.041] [PMID: 15312781]

[30]   Turner EH, Loftis JM, Blackwell AD. Serotonin a la carte: supplementation with the serotonin precursor 5-hydroxytryptophan. Pharmacol Ther 2006; 109(3): 325-38.
[http://dx.doi.org/10.1016/j.pharmthera.2005.06.004] [PMID: 16023217]

[31]   Amer A, Breu J, McDermott J, Wurtman RJ, Maher TJ. 5-Hydroxy-L-tryptophan suppresses food intake in food-deprived and stressed rats. Pharmacol Biochem Behav 2004; 77(1): 137-43.
[http://dx.doi.org/10.1016/j.pbb.2003.10.011] [PMID: 14724051]

[32]   Yamada J, Ujikawa M, Sugimoto Y. Serum leptin levels after central and systemic injection of a serotonin precursor, 5-hydroxytryptophan, in mice. Eur J Pharmacol 2000; 406(1): 159-62.
[http://dx.doi.org/10.1016/S0014-2999(00)00624-5] [PMID: 11011048]

[33]   Kim JH, Hahm DH, Yang DC, Kim JH, Lee HJ, Shim I. Effect of crude saponin of Korean red ginseng on high-fat diet-induced obesity in the rat. J Pharmacol Sci 2005; 97(1): 124-31.
[http://dx.doi.org/10.1254/jphs.FP0040184] [PMID: 15655288]

[34] Kim JH, Kang SA, Han SM, Shim I. Comparison of the antiobesity effects of the protopanaxadiol- and protopanaxatriol-type saponins of red ginseng. Phytother Res 2009; 23(1): 78-85.
[http://dx.doi.org/10.1002/ptr.2561] [PMID: 18709638]

[35] Zhang WL, Zhu L, Jiang JG. Active ingredients from natural botanicals in the treatment of obesity. Obes Rev 2014; 15(12): 957-67.
[http://dx.doi.org/10.1111/obr.12228] [PMID: 25417736]

[36] Ballinger A, Peikin SR. Orlistat: its current status as an anti-obesity drug. Eur J Pharmacol 2002; 440(2-3): 109-17.
[http://dx.doi.org/10.1016/S0014-2999(02)01422-X] [PMID: 12007529]

[37] Seyedan A, Alshawsh MA, Alshagga MA, Koosha S, Mohamed Z. Medicinal plants and their inhibitory activities against pancreatic lipase: a review. Evid Based Complement Alternat Med 2015; 2015
[http://dx.doi.org/10.1155/2015/973143]

[38] Li F, Li W, Fu H, Zhang Q, Koike K. Pancreatic lipase-inhibiting triterpenoid saponins from fruits of *Acanthopanax senticosus*. Chem Pharm Bull (Tokyo) 2007; 55(7): 1087-9.
[http://dx.doi.org/10.1248/cpb.55.1087] [PMID: 17603209]

[39] Yoshizumi K, Hirano K, Ando H, *et al.* Lupane-type saponins from leaves of *Acanthopanax sessiliflorus* and their inhibitory activity on pancreatic lipase. J Agric Food Chem 2006; 54(2): 335-41.
[http://dx.doi.org/10.1021/jf052047f] [PMID: 16417288]

[40] Karu N, Reifen R, Kerem Z. Weight gain reduction in mice fed *Panax ginseng* saponin, a pancreatic lipase inhibitor. J Agric Food Chem 2007; 55(8): 2824-8.
[http://dx.doi.org/10.1021/jf0628025] [PMID: 17367157]

[41] Han L-K, Zheng Y-N, Yoshikawa M, Okuda H, Kimura Y. Anti-obesity effects of chikusetsusaponins isolated from *Panax japonicus* rhizomes. BMC Complement Altern Med 2005; 5(1): 9.
[http://dx.doi.org/10.1186/1472-6882-5-9] [PMID: 15811191]

[42] Liu W, Zheng Y, Han L, *et al.* Saponins (Ginsenosides) from stems and leaves of *Panax quinquefolium* prevented high-fat diet-induced obesity in mice. Phytomedicine 2008; 15(12): 1140-5.
[http://dx.doi.org/10.1016/j.phymed.2008.07.002] [PMID: 18768305]

[43] Liu R, Zhang J, Liu W, Kimura Y, Zheng Y. Anti-Obesity effects of protopanaxdiol types of Ginsenosides isolated from the leaves of American ginseng (*Panax quinquefolius* L.) in mice fed with a high-fat diet. Fitoterapia 2010; 81(8): 1079-87.
[http://dx.doi.org/10.1016/j.fitote.2010.07.002] [PMID: 20627120]

[44] Kimura H, Ogawa S, Jisaka M, Kimura Y, Katsube T, Yokota K. Identification of novel saponins from edible seeds of Japanese horse chestnut (*Aesculus turbinata* Blume) after treatment with wooden ashes and their nutraceutical activity. J Pharm Biomed Anal 2006; 41(5): 1657-65.
[http://dx.doi.org/10.1016/j.jpba.2006.02.031] [PMID: 16621416]

[45] Hu J-N, Zhu X-M, Han L-K, *et al.* Anti-obesity effects of escins extracted from the seeds of *Aesculus turbinata* BLUME (Hippocastanaceae). Chem Pharm Bull (Tokyo) 2008; 56(1): 12-6.
[http://dx.doi.org/10.1248/cpb.56.12] [PMID: 18175967]

[46] Kimura H, Ogawa S, Katsube T, Jisaka M, Yokota K. Antiobese effects of novel saponins from edible seeds of Japanese horse chestnut (*Aesculus turbinata* BLUME) after treatment with wood ashes. J Agric Food Chem 2008; 56(12): 4783-8.
[http://dx.doi.org/10.1021/jf800340s] [PMID: 18512932]

[47] Moreno DA, Ilic N, Poulev A, Brasaemle DL, Fried SK, Raskin I. Inhibitory effects of grape seed extract on lipases. Nutrition 2003; 19(10): 876-9.
[http://dx.doi.org/10.1016/S0899-9007(03)00167-9] [PMID: 14559324]

[48] Chantre P, Lairon D. Recent findings of green tea extract AR25 (Exolise) and its activity for the treatment of obesity. Phytomedicine 2002; 9(1): 3-8.

[http://dx.doi.org/10.1078/0944-7113-00078] [PMID: 11924761]

[49]   Kovacs EM, Lejeune MP, Nijs I, Westerterp-Plantenga MS. Effects of green tea on weight maintenance after body-weight loss. Br J Nutr 2004; 91(3): 431-7.
[http://dx.doi.org/10.1079/BJN20041061] [PMID: 15005829]

[50]   Yoshikawa M, Shimoda H, Nishida N, Takada M, Matsuda H. *Salacia reticulata* and its polyphenolic constituents with lipase inhibitory and lipolytic activities have mild antiobesity effects in rats. J Nutr 2002; 132(7): 1819-24.
[http://dx.doi.org/10.1093/jn/132.7.1819] [PMID: 12097653]

[51]   Rosen ED, Spiegelman BM. What we talk about when we talk about fat. Cell 2014; 156(1-2): 20-44.
[http://dx.doi.org/10.1016/j.cell.2013.12.012] [PMID: 24439368]

[52]   Wang QA, Tao C, Gupta RK, Scherer PE. Tracking adipogenesis during white adipose tissue development, expansion and regeneration. Nat Med 2013; 19(10): 1338-44.
[http://dx.doi.org/10.1038/nm.3324] [PMID: 23995282]

[53]   Peirce V, Carobbio S, Vidal-Puig A. The different shades of fat. Nature 2014; 510(7503): 76-83.
[http://dx.doi.org/10.1038/nature13477] [PMID: 24899307]

[54]   Ahn J, Lee H, Kim S, Ha T. Curcumin-induced suppression of adipogenic differentiation is accompanied by activation of Wnt/β-catenin signaling. Am J Physiol Cell Physiol 2010; 298(6): C1510-6.
[http://dx.doi.org/10.1152/ajpcell.00369.2009] [PMID: 20357182]

[55]   Ejaz A, Wu D, Kwan P, Meydani M. Curcumin inhibits adipogenesis in 3T3-L1 adipocytes and angiogenesis and obesity in C57/BL mice. J Nutr 2009; 139(5): 919-25.
[http://dx.doi.org/10.3945/jn.108.100966] [PMID: 19297423]

[56]   Martins T, Colaço B, Venâncio C, *et al.* Potential effects of sulforaphane to fight obesity. J Sci Food Agric 2018; 98(8): 2837-44.
[http://dx.doi.org/10.1002/jsfa.8898] [PMID: 29363750]

[57]   Thounaojam MC, Nammi S, Jadeja R. Natural products for the treatment of obesity, metabolic syndrome, and type 2 diabetes. Evid Based Complement Alternat Med 2013; 2013871018
[http://dx.doi.org/10.1155/2013/871018] [PMID: 24368927]

[58]   Baboota RK, Murtaza N, Jagtap S, *et al.* Capsaicin-induced transcriptional changes in hypothalamus and alterations in gut microbial count in high fat diet fed mice. J Nutr Biochem 2014; 25(9): 893-902.
[http://dx.doi.org/10.1016/j.jnutbio.2014.04.004] [PMID: 24917046]

[59]   Baboota RK, Singh DP, Sarma SM, *et al.* Capsaicin induces "brite" phenotype in differentiating 3T3-L1 preadipocytes. PLoS One 2014; 9(7)e103093
[http://dx.doi.org/10.1371/journal.pone.0103093] [PMID: 25072597]

[60]   Ono Y, Hattori E, Fukaya Y, Imai S, Ohizumi Y. Anti-obesity effect of *Nelumbo nucifera* leaves extract in mice and rats. J Ethnopharmacol 2006; 106(2): 238-44.
[http://dx.doi.org/10.1016/j.jep.2005.12.036] [PMID: 16495025]

[61]   Wu C-H, Yang M-Y, Chan K-C, Chung P-J, Ou T-T, Wang C-J. Improvement in high-fat diet-induced obesity and body fat accumulation by a *Nelumbo nucifera* leaf flavonoid-rich extract in mice. J Agric Food Chem 2010; 58(11): 7075-81.
[http://dx.doi.org/10.1021/jf101415v] [PMID: 20481471]

[62]   Gauhar R, Hwang SL, Jeong SS, *et al.* Heat-processed *Gynostemma pentaphyllum* extract improves obesity in ob/ob mice by activating AMP-activated protein kinase. Biotechnol Lett 2012; 34(9): 1607-16.
[http://dx.doi.org/10.1007/s10529-012-0944-1] [PMID: 22576281]

[63]   Nguyen PH, Gauhar R, Hwang SL, *et al.* New dammarane-type glucosides as potential activators of AMP-activated protein kinase (AMPK) from *Gynostemma pentaphyllum.* Bioorg Med Chem 2011; 19(21): 6254-60.

[http://dx.doi.org/10.1016/j.bmc.2011.09.013] [PMID: 21978948]

[64]   Seo JB, Park SW, Choe SS, *et al.* Foenumoside B from *Lysimachia foenum-graecum* inhibits adipocyte differentiation and obesity induced by high-fat diet. Biochem Biophys Res Commun 2012; 417(2): 800-6.
[http://dx.doi.org/10.1016/j.bbrc.2011.12.039] [PMID: 22197824]

[65]   Chen Q, Li ET. Reduced adiposity in bitter melon (*Momordica charantia*) fed rats is associated with lower tissue triglyceride and higher plasma catecholamines. Br J Nutr 2005; 93(5): 747-54.
[http://dx.doi.org/10.1079/BJN20051388] [PMID: 15975176]

[66]   Tan M-J, Ye J-M, Turner N, *et al.* Antidiabetic activities of triterpenoids isolated from bitter melon associated with activation of the AMPK pathway. Chem Biol 2008; 15(3): 263-73.
[http://dx.doi.org/10.1016/j.chembiol.2008.01.013] [PMID: 18355726]

[67]   Kawada T, Suzuki T, Takahashi M, Iwai K. Gastrointestinal absorption and metabolism of capsaicin and dihydrocapsaicin in rats. Toxicol Appl Pharmacol 1984; 72(3): 449-56.
[http://dx.doi.org/10.1016/0041-008X(84)90121-2] [PMID: 6710495]

[68]   Park U-H, Jeong H-S, Jo E-Y, *et al.* Piperine, a component of black pepper, inhibits adipogenesis by antagonizing PPARγ activity in 3T3-L1 cells. J Agric Food Chem 2012; 60(15): 3853-60.
[http://dx.doi.org/10.1021/jf204514a] [PMID: 22463744]

[69]   Watanabe T, Kawada T, Yamamoto M, Iwai K. Capsaicin, a pungent principle of hot red pepper, evokes catecholamine secretion from the adrenal medulla of anesthetized rats. Biochem Biophys Res Commun 1987; 142(1): 259-64.
[http://dx.doi.org/10.1016/0006-291X(87)90479-7] [PMID: 3814133]

[70]   Pérez-Torres I, Ruiz-Ramírez A, Baños G, El-Hafidi M. *Hibiscus sabdariffa* Linnaeus (Malvaceae), curcumin and resveratrol as alternative medicinal agents against metabolic syndrome. Cardiovasc Hematol Agents Med Chem 2013; 11(1): 25-37.
[http://dx.doi.org/10.2174/1871525711311010006] [PMID: 22721439]

[71]   Sahebkar A. Why it is necessary to translate curcumin into clinical practice for the prevention and treatment of metabolic syndrome? Biofactors 2013; 39(2): 197-208.
[http://dx.doi.org/10.1002/biof.1062] [PMID: 23239418]

[72]   Mohammadi A, Sahebkar A, Iranshahi M, *et al.* Effects of supplementation with curcuminoids on dyslipidemia in obese patients: a randomized crossover trial. Phytother Res 2013; 27(3): 374-9.
[http://dx.doi.org/10.1002/ptr.4715] [PMID: 22610853]

[73]   Ahmed AA, Musa HH, Fedail JS, Sifaldin AZ, Musa TH. Gum arabic suppressed diet-induced obesity by alteration the expression of mRNA levels of genes involved in lipid metabolism in mouse liver. Bioact Carbohydr Dietary Fibre 2016; 7: 15-20.
[http://dx.doi.org/10.1016/j.bcdf.2016.01.002]

[74]   Musa HH, Ahmed AA, Musa TH. Chemistry, Biological, and Pharmacological Properties of Gum Arabic.Bioactive Molecules in Food. Springer 2017; pp. 1-18.

[75]   Abourashed EA, El-Alfy AT, Khan IA, Walker L. Ephedra in perspective--a current review. Phytother Res 2003; 17(7): 703-12.
[http://dx.doi.org/10.1002/ptr.1337] [PMID: 12916063]

[76]   Gul R, Jan SU, Faridullah S, Sherani S, Jahan N. Preliminary phytochemical screening, quantitative analysis of alkaloids, and antioxidant activity of crude plant extracts from *Ephedra intermedia* indigenous to Balochistan. ScientificWorldJournal 2017; 20175873648
[http://dx.doi.org/10.1155/2017/5873648] [PMID: 28386582]

[77]   Song M-K, Um J-Y, Jang H-J, Lee B-C. Beneficial effect of dietary *Ephedra sinica* on obesity and glucose intolerance in high-fat diet-fed mice. Exp Ther Med 2012; 3(4): 707-12.
[http://dx.doi.org/10.3892/etm.2012.462] [PMID: 22969956]

[78]   Wang JH, Kim BS, Han K, Kim H. Ephedra-treated donor-derived gut microbiota transplantation

ameliorates high fat diet-induced obesity in rats. Int J Environ Res Public Health 2017; 14(6)E555
[http://dx.doi.org/10.3390/ijerph14060555] [PMID: 28545248]

[79] Kim B-S, Song MY, Kim H. The anti-obesity effect of *Ephedra sinica* through modulation of gut microbiota in obese Korean women. J Ethnopharmacol 2014; 152(3): 532-9.
[http://dx.doi.org/10.1016/j.jep.2014.01.038] [PMID: 24556223]

[80] Bent S, Padula A, Neuhaus J. Safety and efficacy of *citrus aurantium* for weight loss. Am J Cardiol 2004; 94(10): 1359-61.
[http://dx.doi.org/10.1016/j.amjcard.2004.07.137] [PMID: 15541270]

[81] Haaz S, Fontaine KR, Cutter G, Limdi N, Perumean-Chaney S, Allison DB. *Citrus aurantium* and synephrine alkaloids in the treatment of overweight and obesity: an update. Obes Rev 2006; 7(1): 79-88.
[http://dx.doi.org/10.1111/j.1467-789X.2006.00195.x] [PMID: 16436104]

[82] Fugh-Berman A, Myers A. *Citrus aurantium*, an ingredient of dietary supplements marketed for weight loss: current status of clinical and basic research. Exp Biol Med (Maywood) 2004; 229(8): 698-704.
[http://dx.doi.org/10.1177/153537020422900802] [PMID: 15337824]

[83] Calapai G, Firenzuoli F, Saitta A, *et al.* Antiobesity and cardiovascular toxic effects of *Citrus aurantium* extracts in the rat: a preliminary report. Fitoterapia 1999; 70(6): 586-92.
[http://dx.doi.org/10.1016/S0367-326X(99)00093-3]

[84] Jung HA, Jung HJ, Jeong HY, Kwon HJ, Ali MY, Choi JS. Phlorotannins isolated from the edible brown alga *Ecklonia stolonifera* exert anti-adipogenic activity on 3T3-L1 adipocytes by downregulating C/EBPα and PPARγ. Fitoterapia 2014; 92: 260-9.
[http://dx.doi.org/10.1016/j.fitote.2013.12.003] [PMID: 24334103]

[85] Jung HA, Jung HJ, Jeong HY, Kwon HJ, Kim M-S, Choi JS. Anti-adipogenic activity of the edible brown alga *Ecklonia stolonifera* and its constituent fucosterol in 3T3-L1 adipocytes. Arch Pharm Res 2014; 37(6): 713-20.
[http://dx.doi.org/10.1007/s12272-013-0237-9] [PMID: 24014306]

[86] Lee J-H, Jung HA, Kang MJ, Choi JS, Kim G-D. Fucosterol, isolated from *Ecklonia stolonifera*, inhibits adipogenesis through modulation of FoxO1 pathway in 3T3-L1 adipocytes. J Pharm Pharmacol 2017; 69(3): 325-33.
[http://dx.doi.org/10.1111/jphp.12684] [PMID: 28134973]

[87] Kang MC, Ding Y, Kim EA, *et al.* Indole derivatives isolated from brown alga *Sargassum thunbergii* inhibit adipogenesis through AMPK activation in 3T3-L1 preadipocytes. Mar Drugs 2017; 15(4)E119
[http://dx.doi.org/10.3390/md15040119] [PMID: 28417922]

[88] Park YK, Lee TY, Choi JS, *et al.* Inhibition of adipogenesis and leptin production in 3T3-L1 adipocytes by a derivative of meridianin C. Biochem Biophys Res Commun 2014; 452(4): 1078-83.
[http://dx.doi.org/10.1016/j.bbrc.2014.09.050] [PMID: 25245291]

[89] Liang LF, Wang T, Cai YS, *et al.* Brominated polyunsaturated lipids from the Chinese sponge *Xestospongia testudinaria* as a new class of pancreatic lipase inhibitors. Eur J Med Chem 2014; 79: 290-7.
[http://dx.doi.org/10.1016/j.ejmech.2014.04.003] [PMID: 24747066]

[90] Dutta PK, Dutta J, Tripathi VS. Chitin and chitosan: Chemistry, properties and applications. J Sci Ind Res (India) 2004; 63: 20-31.

[91] Peters HPF, Koppert RJ, Boers HM, *et al.* Dose-dependent suppression of hunger by a specific alginate in a low-viscosity drink formulation. Obesity (Silver Spring) 2011; 19(6): 1171-6.
[http://dx.doi.org/10.1038/oby.2011.63] [PMID: 21512509]

[92] Diagnosis and classification of diabetes mellitus. Diabetes Care 2014; 37 (Suppl. 1): S81-90.
[http://dx.doi.org/10.2337/dc14-S081] [PMID: 24357215]

[93]   Rivera-Mancía S, Trujillo J, Chaverri JP. Utility of curcumin for the treatment of diabetes mellitus: Evidence from preclinical and clinical studies. JNIM 2018; 14: 29-41.
[http://dx.doi.org/10.1016/j.jnim.2018.05.001]

[94]   Standards of medical care in diabetes--2014. Diabetes Care 2014; 37 (Suppl. 1): S14-80.
[http://dx.doi.org/10.2337/dc14-S014] [PMID: 24357209]

[95]   Chatterji S, Fogel D. Study of the effect of the herbal composition SR2004 on hemoglobin A1c, fasting blood glucose, and lipids in patients with type 2 diabetes mellitus. Integr Med Res 2018; 7(3): 248-56.
[http://dx.doi.org/10.1016/j.imr.2018.04.002] [PMID: 30271713]

[96]   Tao X, Wang X, Jia W. Using Chinese natural products for diabetes mellitus drug discovery and development. Expert Opin Drug Discov 2007; 2(7): 977-86.
[http://dx.doi.org/10.1517/17460441.2.7.977] [PMID: 23484817]

[97]   Prabhakar PK, Doble M. Mechanism of action of natural products used in the treatment of diabetes mellitus. Chin J Integr Med 2011; 17(8): 563-74.
[http://dx.doi.org/10.1007/s11655-011-0810-3] [PMID: 21826590]

[98]   Hung HY, Qian K, Morris-Natschke SL, Hsu CS, Lee KH. Recent discovery of plant-derived anti-diabetic natural products. Nat Prod Rep 2012; 29(5): 580-606.
[http://dx.doi.org/10.1039/c2np00074a] [PMID: 22491825]

[99]   Ghorbani A. Best herbs for managing diabetes: A review of clinical studies. Braz J Pharm Sci 2013; 49(3): 413-22.
[http://dx.doi.org/10.1590/S1984-82502013000300003]

[100]   Park C, Lee J-S. Mini Review: Natural ingredients for diabetes which are approved by korean FDA. J Biomed Res 2013; 24(1)

[101]   Smith JD, Clinard VB. Natural products for the management of type 2 diabetes mellitus and comorbid conditions. J Am Pharm Assoc (2003) 2014; 54(5): e304-18.
[http://dx.doi.org/10.1331/JAPhA.2014.14537] [PMID: 25107389]

[102]   Ríos JL, Francini F, Schinella GR. Natural products for the treatment of type 2 diabetes mellitus. Planta Med 2015; 81(12-13): 975-94.
[http://dx.doi.org/10.1055/s-0035-1546131] [PMID: 26132858]

[103]   Waltenberger B, Mocan A, Šmejkal K, Heiss EH, Atanasov AG. Natural products to counteract the epidemic of cardiovascular and metabolic disorders. Molecules 2016; 21(6): 807.
[http://dx.doi.org/10.3390/molecules21060807] [PMID: 27338339]

[104]   Ota A, Ulrih NP. An overview of herbal products and secondary metabolites used for management of type two diabetes. Front Pharmacol 2017; 8: 436.
[http://dx.doi.org/10.3389/fphar.2017.00436] [PMID: 28729836]

[105]   Choudhury H, Pandey M, Hua CK, *et al.* An update on natural compounds in the remedy of diabetes mellitus: A systematic review. J Tradit Complement Med 2017; 8(3): 361-76.
[http://dx.doi.org/10.1016/j.jtcme.2017.08.012] [PMID: 29992107]

[106]   Grover JK, Yadav S, Vats V. Medicinal plants of India with anti-diabetic potential. J Ethnopharmacol 2002; 81(1): 81-100.
[http://dx.doi.org/10.1016/S0378-8741(02)00059-4] [PMID: 12020931]

[107]   Chan SM, Ye JM. Strategies for the discovery and development of anti-diabetic drugs from the natural products of traditional medicines. J Pharm Pharm Sci 2013; 16(2): 207-16.
[http://dx.doi.org/10.18433/J3T60G] [PMID: 23958190]

[108]   Matsui T, Ueda T, Oki T, Sugita K, Terahara N, Matsumoto K. alpha-Glucosidase inhibitory action of natural acylated anthocyanins. 1. Survey of natural pigments with potent inhibitory activity. J Agric Food Chem 2001; 49(4): 1948-51.

[http://dx.doi.org/10.1021/jf001251u] [PMID: 11308351]

[109] Matsui T, Ueda T, Oki T, Sugita K, Terahara N, Matsumoto K. alpha-Glucosidase inhibitory action of natural acylated anthocyanins. 2. alpha-Glucosidase inhibition by isolated acylated anthocyanins. J Agric Food Chem 2001; 49(4): 1952-6.
[http://dx.doi.org/10.1021/jf0012502] [PMID: 11308352]

[110] Yadav M. Herbal drugs and phytoconstituents useful for the management of diabetes. Int J Green Pharm 2017; 11(1): S21.

[111] Baldi A, Choudhary N, Kumar S. Nutraceuticals as therapeutic agents for holistic treatment of diabetes. Int J Green Pharm 2013; 7(4): 278.
[http://dx.doi.org/10.4103/0973-8258.122050]

[112] Kim JS, Kwon CS, Son KH. Inhibition of alpha-glucosidase and amylase by luteolin, a flavonoid. Biosci Biotechnol Biochem 2000; 64(11): 2458-61.
[http://dx.doi.org/10.1271/bbb.64.2458] [PMID: 11193416]

[113] Lo Piparo E, Scheib H, Frei N, Williamson G, Grigorov M, Chou CJ. Flavonoids for controlling starch digestion: structural requirements for inhibiting human alpha-amylase. J Med Chem 2008; 51(12): 3555-61.
[http://dx.doi.org/10.1021/jm800115x] [PMID: 18507367]

[114] Hardie DG. AMPK: a target for drugs and natural products with effects on both diabetes and cancer. Diabetes 2013; 62(7): 2164-72.
[http://dx.doi.org/10.2337/db13-0368] [PMID: 23801715]

[115] Ghorbani A. Mechanisms of antidiabetic effects of flavonoid rutin. Biomed Pharmacother 2017; 96: 305-12.
[http://dx.doi.org/10.1016/j.biopha.2017.10.001] [PMID: 29017142]

[116] Ebrahimpour-Koujan S, Gargari BP, Mobasseri M, Valizadeh H, Asghari-Jafarabadi M. Lower glycemic indices and lipid profile among type 2 diabetes mellitus patients who received novel dose of *Silybum marianum* (L.) Gaertn. (silymarin) extract supplement: A Triple-blinded randomized controlled clinical trial. Phytomedicine 2018; 44: 39-44.
[http://dx.doi.org/10.1016/j.phymed.2018.03.050] [PMID: 29895491]

[117] Huang G, Xu J, Lefever DE, Glenn TC, Nagy T, Guo TL. Genistein prevention of hyperglycemia and improvement of glucose tolerance in adult non-obese diabetic mice are associated with alterations of gut microbiome and immune homeostasis. Toxicol Appl Pharmacol 2017; 332: 138-48.
[http://dx.doi.org/10.1016/j.taap.2017.04.009] [PMID: 28412308]

[118] de Sousa E, Zanatta L, Seifriz I, *et al.* Hypoglycemic effect and antioxidant potential of kaempferol-3,7-O-(alpha)-dirhamnoside from *Bauhinia forficata* leaves. J Nat Prod 2004; 67(5): 829-32.
[http://dx.doi.org/10.1021/np030513u] [PMID: 15165145]

[119] Song C, Huang L, Rong L, *et al.* Anti-hyperglycemic effect of *Potentilla discolor* decoction on obese-diabetic (Ob-db) mice and its chemical composition. Fitoterapia 2012; 83(8): 1474-83.
[http://dx.doi.org/10.1016/j.fitote.2012.08.013] [PMID: 22960384]

[120] McDougall GJ, Shpiro F, Dobson P, Smith P, Blake A, Stewart D. Different polyphenolic components of soft fruits inhibit alpha-amylase and alpha-glucosidase. J Agric Food Chem 2005; 53(7): 2760-6.
[http://dx.doi.org/10.1021/jf0489926] [PMID: 15796622]

[121] McDougall GJ, Stewart D. The inhibitory effects of berry polyphenols on digestive enzymes. Biofactors 2005; 23(4): 189-95.
[http://dx.doi.org/10.1002/biof.5520230403] [PMID: 16498205]

[122] Sidorova Y, Shipelin V, Mazo V, Zorin S, Petrov N, Kochetkova A. Hypoglycemic and hypolipidemic effect of *Vaccinium myrtillus* L. leaf and *Phaseolus vulgaris* L. seed coat extracts in diabetic rats. Nutrition 2017; 41: 107-12.
[http://dx.doi.org/10.1016/j.nut.2017.04.010] [PMID: 28760419]

[123]   Matsui T, Ebuchi S, Kobayashi M, *et al.* Anti-hyperglycemic effect of diacylated anthocyanin derived from *Ipomoea batatas* cultivar Ayamurasaki can be achieved through the α-glucosidase inhibitory action. J Agric Food Chem 2002; 50(25): 7244-8.
[http://dx.doi.org/10.1021/jf025913m] [PMID: 12452639]

[124]   Schäfer A, Högger P. Oligomeric procyanidins of French maritime pine bark extract (Pycnogenol) effectively inhibit α-glucosidase. Diabetes Res Clin Pract 2007; 77(1): 41-6.
[http://dx.doi.org/10.1016/j.diabres.2006.10.011] [PMID: 17098323]

[125]   Khodabandehloo H, Seyyedebrahimi S, Esfahani EN, Razi F, Meshkani R. Resveratrol supplementation decreases blood glucose without changing the circulating CD14$^+$CD16$^+$ monocytes and inflammatory cytokines in patients with type 2 diabetes: a randomized, double-blind, placebo-controlled study. Nutr Res 2018; 54: 40-51.
[http://dx.doi.org/10.1016/j.nutres.2018.03.015] [PMID: 29914666]

[126]   Akbar MU, Zia KM, Akash MSH, Nazir A, Zuber M, Ibrahim M. *In-vivo* anti-diabetic and wound healing potential of chitosan/alginate/maltodextrin/pluronic-based mixed polymeric micelles: Curcumin therapeutic potential. Int J Biol Macromol 2018; 120(Pt B): 2418-30.

[127]   El-Azab MF, Attia FM, El-Mowafy AM. Novel role of curcumin combined with bone marrow transplantation in reversing experimental diabetes: Effects on pancreatic islet regeneration, oxidative stress, and inflammatory cytokines. Eur J Pharmacol 2011; 658(1): 41-8.
[http://dx.doi.org/10.1016/j.ejphar.2011.02.010] [PMID: 21349269]

[128]   Du ZY, Liu RR, Shao WY, *et al.* Alpha-glucosidase inhibition of natural curcuminoids and curcumin analogs. Eur J Med Chem 2006; 41(2): 213-8.
[http://dx.doi.org/10.1016/j.ejmech.2005.10.012] [PMID: 16387392]

[129]   Akolade JO, Oloyede HOB, Onyenekwe PC. Encapsulation in chitosan-based polyelectrolyte complexes enhances antidiabetic activity of curcumin. J Funct Foods 2017; 35: 584-94.
[http://dx.doi.org/10.1016/j.jff.2017.06.023]

[130]   Tousian Shandiz H, Razavi BM, Hosseinzadeh H. Review of *Garcinia mangostana* and its xanthones in metabolic syndrome and related complications. Phytother Res 2017; 31(8): 1173-82.
[http://dx.doi.org/10.1002/ptr.5862] [PMID: 28656594]

[131]   Estuningtyas A, Zwicker K, Wahyuni T, Fajri P, Wahidiyat PA, Freisleben SK. Are mangiferin and mangiferin-containing plant extracts helpful for iron-loaded transfusion-dependent and non-transfusion-dependent thalassaemia patients? Biomed Pharmacol J 2018; 11(1): 29-43.
[http://dx.doi.org/10.13005/bpj/1345]

[132]   Min Q, Cai X, Sun W, *et al.* Identification of mangiferin as a potential Glucokinase activator by structure-based virtual ligand screening. Sci Rep 2017; 7: 44681.
[http://dx.doi.org/10.1038/srep44681] [PMID: 28317897]

[133]   Lazavi F, Mirmiran P, Sohrab G, Nikpayam O, Angoorani P, Hedayati M. The barberry juice effects on metabolic factors and oxidative stress in patients with type 2 diabetes: A randomized clinical trial. Complement Ther Clin Pract 2018; 31: 170-4.
[http://dx.doi.org/10.1016/j.ctcp.2018.01.009] [PMID: 29705451]

[134]   Wang T, Wang N, Song H, *et al.* Preparation of an anhydrous reverse micelle delivery system to enhance oral bioavailability and anti-diabetic efficacy of berberine. Eur J Pharm Sci 2011; 44(1-2): 127-35.
[http://dx.doi.org/10.1016/j.ejps.2011.06.015] [PMID: 21742030]

[135]   Gu Y, Zhang Y, Shi X, *et al.* Effect of traditional Chinese medicine berberine on type 2 diabetes based on comprehensive metabonomics. Talanta 2010; 81(3): 766-72.
[http://dx.doi.org/10.1016/j.talanta.2010.01.015] [PMID: 20298851]

[136]   Yin J, Xing H, Ye J. Efficacy of berberine in patients with type 2 diabetes mellitus. Metabolism 2008; 57(5): 712-7.

[http://dx.doi.org/10.1016/j.metabol.2008.01.013] [PMID: 18442638]

[137]   Lee YS, Kim WS, Kim KH, *et al.* Berberine, a natural plant product, activates AMP-activated protein kinase with beneficial metabolic effects in diabetic and insulin-resistant states. Diabetes 2006; 55(8): 2256-64.
        [http://dx.doi.org/10.2337/db06-0006] [PMID: 16873688]

[138]   Gajęcka M, Przybylska-Gornowicz B, Zakłos-Szyda M, *et al.* The influence of a natural triterpene preparation on the gastrointestinal tract of gilts with streptozocin-induced diabetes and on cell metabolic activity. J Funct Foods 2017; 33: 11-20.
        [http://dx.doi.org/10.1016/j.jff.2017.03.019]

[139]   Jang SM, Kim MJ, Choi MS, Kwon EY, Lee MK. Inhibitory effects of ursolic acid on hepatic polyol pathway and glucose production in streptozotocin-induced diabetic mice. Metabolism 2010; 59(4): 512-9.
        [http://dx.doi.org/10.1016/j.metabol.2009.07.040] [PMID: 19846180]

[140]   Xie JT, Mehendale SR, Li X, *et al.* Anti-diabetic effect of ginsenoside Re in ob/ob mice. Biochim Biophys Acta 2005; 1740(3): 319-25.
        [http://dx.doi.org/10.1016/j.bbadis.2004.10.010] [PMID: 15949698]

[141]   Liu Z, Li W, Li X, *et al.* Antidiabetic effects of malonyl ginsenosides from *Panax ginseng* on type 2 diabetic rats induced by high-fat diet and streptozotocin. J Ethnopharmacol 2013; 145(1): 233-40.
        [http://dx.doi.org/10.1016/j.jep.2012.10.058] [PMID: 23147499]

[142]   Rathore PK, Arathy V, Attimarad VS, Kumar P, Roy S. *In-silico* analysis of gymnemagenin from *Gymnema sylvestre* (Retz.) R.Br. with targets related to diabetes. J Theor Biol 2016; 391: 95-101.
        [http://dx.doi.org/10.1016/j.jtbi.2015.12.004] [PMID: 26711684]

[143]   Sharma B, Salunke R, Srivastava S, Majumder C, Roy P. Effects of guggulsterone isolated from *Commiphora mukul* in high fat diet induced diabetic rats. Food Chem Toxicol 2009; 47(10): 2631-9.
        [http://dx.doi.org/10.1016/j.fct.2009.07.021] [PMID: 19635521]

[144]   Eliza J, Daisy P, Ignacimuthu S, Duraipandiyan V. Antidiabetic and antilipidemic effect of eremanthin from *Costus speciosus* (Koen.)Sm., in STZ-induced diabetic rats. Chem Biol Interact 2009; 182(1): 67-72.
        [http://dx.doi.org/10.1016/j.cbi.2009.08.012] [PMID: 19695236]

[145]   Sundaram R, Naresh R, Ranadevan R, Shanthi P, Sachdanandam P. Effect of iridoid glucoside on streptozotocin induced diabetic rats and its role in regulating carbohydrate metabolic enzymes. Eur J Pharmacol 2012; 674(2-3): 460-7.
        [http://dx.doi.org/10.1016/j.ejphar.2011.10.039] [PMID: 22094064]

[146]   Mostafa DM, Abd El-Alim SH, Asfour MH, Al-Okbi SY, Mohamed DA, Awad G. Transdermal nanoemulsions of *Foeniculum vulgare* Mill. essential oil: Preparation, characterization and evaluation of antidiabetic potential. J Drug Deliv Sci Technol 2015; 29: 99-106.
        [http://dx.doi.org/10.1016/j.jddst.2015.06.021]

[147]   Singh G, Maurya S, de Lampasona MP, Catalan C. Chemical constituents, antifungal and antioxidative potential of *Foeniculum vulgare* volatile oil and its acetone extract. Food Control 2006; 17(9): 745-52.
        [http://dx.doi.org/10.1016/j.foodcont.2005.03.010]

[148]   Muruganathan U, Srinivasan S, Indumathi D. Antihyperglycemic effect of carvone: Effect on the levels of glycoprotein components in streptozotocin-induced diabetic rats. J Acute Dis 2013; 2(4): 310-5.
        [http://dx.doi.org/10.1016/S2221-6189(13)60150-X]

[149]   Aggarwal KK, Khanuja SPS, Ahmad A, Santha Kumar TR, Gupta VK, Kumar S. Antimicrobial activity profiles of the two enantiomers of limonene and carvone isolated from the oils of *Mentha spicata* and *Anethum sowa.* Flavour Fragrance J 2002; 17(1): 59-63.
        [http://dx.doi.org/10.1002/ffj.1040]

[150]   Chemat S, Lagha A. AitAmar H, Bartels PV, Chemat F. Comparison of conventional and ultrasound-assisted extraction of carvone and limonene from caraway seeds. Flavour Fragrance J 2004; 19(3): 188-95.
[http://dx.doi.org/10.1002/ffj.1339]

[151]   Mostafa I, Zhu N, Yoo MJ, *et al*. New nodes and edges in the glucosinolate molecular network revealed by proteomics and metabolomics of Arabidopsis *myb28/29* and *cyp79B2/B3* glucosinolate mutants. J Proteomics 2016; 138: 1-19.
[http://dx.doi.org/10.1016/j.jprot.2016.02.012] [PMID: 26915584]

[152]   Thombare N, Jha U, Mishra S, Siddiqui MZ. Guar gum as a promising starting material for diverse applications: A review. Int J Biol Macromol 2016; 88: 361-72.
[http://dx.doi.org/10.1016/j.ijbiomac.2016.04.001] [PMID: 27044346]

[153]   Mansukhani RP, Volino LR, Varghese R. Natural products for the treatment of type 2 diabetes mellitus. Pharmacol Pharm 2014; 5: 487-503.
[http://dx.doi.org/10.4236/pp.2014.55059]

[154]   Sanchis P, Rivera R, Berga F, *et al*. Phytate decreases formation of advanced glycation end-products in patients with type II diabetes: Randomized crossover trial. Sci Rep 2018; 8(1): 9619.
[http://dx.doi.org/10.1038/s41598-018-27853-9] [PMID: 29941991]

[155]   García-Closas R, Berenguer A, José Tormo M, *et al*. Dietary sources of vitamin C, vitamin E and specific carotenoids in Spain. Br J Nutr 2004; 91(6): 1005-11.
[http://dx.doi.org/10.1079/BJN20041130] [PMID: 15182404]

[156]   Paolisso G, Barbieri M, Rosaria Rizzo M, Manzella D. Should we recommend the therapeutical use of vitamin E in diabetic patients? Environ Toxicol Pharmacol 2001; 10(4): 159-65.
[http://dx.doi.org/10.1016/S1382-6689(01)00079-5] [PMID: 21782572]

[157]   Obara K, Mizutani M, Hitomi Y, Yajima H, Kondo K. Isohumulones, the bitter component of beer, improve hyperglycemia and decrease body fat in Japanese subjects with prediabetes. Clin Nutr 2009; 28(3): 278-84.
[http://dx.doi.org/10.1016/j.clnu.2009.03.012] [PMID: 19395131]

[158]   Seifarth C, Littmann L, Resheq Y, *et al*. MCS-18, a novel natural plant product prevents autoimmune diabetes. Immunol Lett 2011; 139(1-2): 58-67.
[http://dx.doi.org/10.1016/j.imlet.2011.04.016] [PMID: 21600928]

[159]   Weidner C, de Groot JC, Prasad A, *et al*. Amorfrutins are potent antidiabetic dietary natural products. Proc Natl Acad Sci USA 2012; 109(19): 7257-62.
[http://dx.doi.org/10.1073/pnas.1116971109] [PMID: 22509006]

[160]   Mitscher LA, Park YH, Alshamma A, Hudson PB, Haas T. Amorfrutin A and B, bibenzyl antimicrobial agents from *Amorpha fruticosa*. Phytochemistry 1981; 20(4): 781-5.
[http://dx.doi.org/10.1016/0031-9422(81)85174-6]

[161]   Kay BA, Trigatti K, MacNeil MB, *et al*. Pudding products enriched with yellow mustard mucilage, fenugreek gum or flaxseed mucilage and matched for simulated intestinal viscosity significantly reduce postprandial peak glucose and insulin in adults at risk for type 2 diabetes. J Funct Foods 2017; 37: 603-11.
[http://dx.doi.org/10.1016/j.jff.2017.08.017]

[162]   Liatis S, Tsapogas P, Chala E, *et al*. The consumption of bread enriched with betaglucan reduces LDL-cholesterol and improves insulin resistance in patients with type 2 diabetes. Diabetes Metab 2009; 35(2): 115-20.
[http://dx.doi.org/10.1016/j.diabet.2008.09.004] [PMID: 19230737]

[163]   Giacco R, Clemente G, Riccardi G. Dietary fibre in treatment of diabetes: myth or reality? Dig Liver Dis 2002; 34 (Suppl. 2): S140-4.
[http://dx.doi.org/10.1016/S1590-8658(02)80182-7] [PMID: 12408458]

[164]   Aller R, de Luis DA, Izaola O, *et al.* Effect of soluble fiber intake in lipid and glucose levels in healthy subjects: a randomized clinical trial. Diabetes Res Clin Pract 2004; 65(1): 7-11.
[http://dx.doi.org/10.1016/j.diabres.2003.11.005] [PMID: 15163472]

[165]   Samadi N, Mozaffari-Khosravi H, Rahmanian M, Askarishahi M. Effects of bee propolis supplementation on glycemic control, lipid profile and insulin resistance indices in patients with type 2 diabetes: a randomized, double-blind clinical trial. J Integr Med 2017; 15(2): 124-34.
[http://dx.doi.org/10.1016/S2095-4964(17)60315-7] [PMID: 28285617]

[166]   Henshaw FR, Bolton T, Nube V, *et al.* Topical application of the bee hive protectant propolis is well tolerated and improves human diabetic foot ulcer healing in a prospective feasibility study. J Diabetes Complications 2014; 28(6): 850-7.
[http://dx.doi.org/10.1016/j.jdiacomp.2014.07.012] [PMID: 25239451]

[167]   Shehata AM, Quintanilla-Fend L, Bettio S, Singh CB, Ammon HP. Prevention of multiple low-dose streptozotocin (MLD-STZ) diabetes in mice by an extract from gum resin of *Boswellia serrata* (BE). Phytomedicine 2011; 18(12): 1037-44.
[http://dx.doi.org/10.1016/j.phymed.2011.06.035] [PMID: 21831620]

[168]   Anesini C, Ferraro GE, Filip R. Total polyphenol content and antioxidant capacity of commercially available tea (*Camellia sinensis*) in Argentina. J Agric Food Chem 2008; 56(19): 9225-9.
[http://dx.doi.org/10.1021/jf8022782] [PMID: 18778031]

[169]   Singh G, Maurya S, DeLampasona MP, Catalan CAN. A comparison of chemical, antioxidant and antimicrobial studies of cinnamon leaf and bark volatile oils, oleoresins and their constituents. Food Chem Toxicol 2007; 45(9): 1650-61.
[http://dx.doi.org/10.1016/j.fct.2007.02.031] [PMID: 17408833]

[170]   Peng X, Cheng K-W, Ma J, *et al.* Cinnamon bark proanthocyanidins as reactive carbonyl scavengers to prevent the formation of advanced glycation endproducts. J Agric Food Chem 2008; 56(6): 1907-11.
[http://dx.doi.org/10.1021/jf073065v] [PMID: 18284204]

[171]   Costello RB, Dwyer JT, Saldanha L, Bailey RL, Merkel J, Wambogo E. Do cinnamon supplements have a role in glycemic control in type 2 diabetes? A narrative review. J Acad Nutr Diet 2016; 116(11): 1794-802.
[http://dx.doi.org/10.1016/j.jand.2016.07.015] [PMID: 27618575]

[172]   Khan A, Safdar M, Ali Khan MM, Khattak KN, Anderson RA. Cinnamon improves glucose and lipids of people with type 2 diabetes. Diabetes Care 2003; 26(12): 3215-8.
[http://dx.doi.org/10.2337/diacare.26.12.3215] [PMID: 14633804]

[173]   Verspohl EJ, Bauer K, Neddermann E. Antidiabetic effect of *Cinnamomum cassia* and *Cinnamomum zeylanicumin vivo* and *in vitro*. Phytother Res 2005; 19(3): 203-6.
[http://dx.doi.org/10.1002/ptr.1643] [PMID: 15934022]

[174]   Kim SH, Hyun SH, Choung SY. Anti-diabetic effect of cinnamon extract on blood glucose in db/db mice. J Ethnopharmacol 2006; 104(1-2): 119-23.
[http://dx.doi.org/10.1016/j.jep.2005.08.059] [PMID: 16213119]

[175]   Anderson RA, Zhan Z, Luo R, *et al.* Cinnamon extract lowers glucose, insulin and cholesterol in people with elevated serum glucose. J Tradit Complement Med 2015; 6(4): 332-6.
[http://dx.doi.org/10.1016/j.jtcme.2015.03.005] [PMID: 27774415]

[176]   Cheng DM, Kuhn P, Poulev A, Rojo LE, Lila MA, Raskin I. *In vivo* and *in vitro* antidiabetic effects of aqueous cinnamon extract and cinnamon polyphenol-enhanced food matrix. Food Chem 2012; 135(4): 2994-3002.
[http://dx.doi.org/10.1016/j.foodchem.2012.06.117] [PMID: 22980902]

[177]   Jia Q, Liu X, Wu X, *et al.* Hypoglycemic activity of a polyphenolic oligomer-rich extract of *Cinnamomum parthenoxylon* bark in normal and streptozotocin-induced diabetic rats. Phytomedicine

2009; 16(8): 744-50.
[http://dx.doi.org/10.1016/j.phymed.2008.12.012] [PMID: 19464860]

[178] Baskaran K, Kizar Ahamath B, Radha Shanmugasundaram K, Shanmugasundaram ER. Antidiabetic effect of a leaf extract from *Gymnema sylvestre* in non-insulin-dependent diabetes mellitus patients. J Ethnopharmacol 1990; 30(3): 295-300.
[http://dx.doi.org/10.1016/0378-8741(90)90108-6] [PMID: 2259217]

[179] Shanmugasundaram ERB, Rajeswari G, Baskaran K, Rajesh Kumar BR, Radha Shanmugasundaram K, Kizar Ahmath B *et al.* Use of *Gymnema sylvestre* leaf extract in the control of blood glucose in insulin-dependent diabetes mellitus. J Ethnopharmacol 1990; 30(3): 281-94.
[http://dx.doi.org/10.1016/0378-8741(90)90107-5] [PMID: 2259216]

[180] Shanmugasundaram ER, Gopinath KL, Radha Shanmugasundaram K, Rajendran VM. Possible regeneration of the islets of Langerhans in streptozotocin-diabetic rats given *Gymnema sylvestre* leaf extracts. J Ethnopharmacol 1990; 30(3): 265-79.
[http://dx.doi.org/10.1016/0378-8741(90)90106-4] [PMID: 2259215]

[181] Persaud SJ, Al-Majed H, Raman A, Jones PM. *Gymnema sylvestre* stimulates insulin release *in vitro* by increased membrane permeability. J Endocrinol 1999; 163(2): 207-12.
[http://dx.doi.org/10.1677/joe.0.1630207] [PMID: 10556769]

[182] Shanmugasundaram KR, Panneerselvam C, Samudram P, Shanmugasundaram ER. Enzyme changes and glucose utilisation in diabetic rabbits: the effect of *Gymnema sylvestre*, R.Br. J Ethnopharmacol 1983; 7(2): 205-34.
[http://dx.doi.org/10.1016/0378-8741(83)90021-1] [PMID: 6865451]

[183] Widjajakusuma EC, Jonosewojo A, Hendriati L, *et al.* Phytochemical screening and preliminary clinical trials of the aqueous extract mixture of *Andrographis paniculata* (Burm. f.) Wall. ex Nees and *Syzygium polyanthum* (Wight.) Walp leaves in metformin treated patients with type 2 diabetes. Phytomedicine 2019; 55: 137-47.
[http://dx.doi.org/10.1016/j.phymed.2018.07.002] [PMID: 30668423]

[184] Asgarpanah J, Mohajerani R. Phytochemistry and pharmacologic properties of *Urtica dioica* L. J Med Plants Res 2012; 6(46): 5714-9.

[185] Akash MS, Rehman K, Chen S. Spice plant *Allium cepa*: dietary supplement for treatment of type 2 diabetes mellitus. Nutrition 2014; 30(10): 1128-37.
[http://dx.doi.org/10.1016/j.nut.2014.02.011] [PMID: 25194613]

[186] Huseini HF, Hasani-Rnjbar S, Nayebi N, *et al.* *Capparis spinosa* L. (Caper) fruit extract in treatment of type 2 diabetic patients: a randomized double-blind placebo-controlled clinical trial. Complement Ther Med 2013; 21(5): 447-52.
[http://dx.doi.org/10.1016/j.ctim.2013.07.003] [PMID: 24050578]

[187] Lachman J, Pronek D, Hejtmankova A, Dudjak J, Pivec V, Faitová K. Total polyphenol and main flavonoid antioxidants in different onion (*Allium cepa* L.) varieties. Hortic Sci (Prague) 2003; 30(4): 142-7.
[http://dx.doi.org/10.17221/3876-HORTSCI]

[188] Afsharypuor S, Jeiran K, Jazy AA. First investigation of the flavour profiles of the leaf, ripe fruit and root of *Capparis spinosa* var. mucronifolia from Iran. Pharm Acta Helv 1998; 72(5): 307-9.
[http://dx.doi.org/10.1016/S0031-6865(97)00023-X]

[189] Abdoli M, Dabaghian FH, Goushegir A, *et al.* Anti-hyperglycemic effect of aqueous extract of *Juglans regia* L. leaf (walnut leaf) on type 2 diabetic patients: A randomized controlled trial. Adv Integr Med 2017; 4(3): 98-102.
[http://dx.doi.org/10.1016/j.aimed.2017.10.001]

[190] Zhang Z, Liao L, Moore J, Wu T, Wang Z. Antioxidant phenolic compounds from walnut kernels (*Juglans regia* L.). Food Chem 2009; 113(1): 160-5.
[http://dx.doi.org/10.1016/j.foodchem.2008.07.061]

[191] Tian H, Lu J, He H, *et al.* The effect of Astragalus as an adjuvant treatment in type 2 diabetes mellitus: A (preliminary) meta-analysis. J Ethnopharmacol 2016; 191: 206-15.
[http://dx.doi.org/10.1016/j.jep.2016.05.062] [PMID: 27269392]

[192] Fu J, Wang Z, Huang L, *et al.* Review of the botanical characteristics, phytochemistry, and pharmacology of *Astragalus membranaceus* (Huangqi). Phytother Res 2014; 28(9): 1275-83.
[http://dx.doi.org/10.1002/ptr.5188] [PMID: 25087616]

[193] Christensen LP. Ginsenosides: Chemistry, Biosynthesis, Analysis, and Potential Health Effects Advances in Food and Nutrition Research. Academic Press 2008; pp. 1-99.

[194] Park SH, Oh MR, Choi EK, *et al.* An 8-wk, randomized, double-blind, placebo-controlled clinical trial for the antidiabetic effects of hydrolyzed ginseng extract. J Ginseng Res 2014; 38(4): 239-43.
[http://dx.doi.org/10.1016/j.jgr.2014.05.006] [PMID: 25379002]

[195] Xie J-T, Wang C-Z, Li X-L, Ni M, Fishbein A, Yuan C-S. Anti-diabetic effect of American ginseng may not be linked to antioxidant activity: comparison between American ginseng and *Scutellaria baicalensis* using an ob/ob mice model. Fitoterapia 2009; 80(5): 306-11.
[http://dx.doi.org/10.1016/j.fitote.2009.04.001] [PMID: 19358881]

[196] Choi HS, Kim S, Kim MJ, *et al.* Efficacy and safety of *Panax ginseng* berry extract on glycemic control: A 12-wk randomized, double-blind, and placebo-controlled clinical trial. J Ginseng Res 2018; 42(1): 90-7.
[http://dx.doi.org/10.1016/j.jgr.2017.01.003] [PMID: 29348727]

[197] Yoshikawa M, Murakami T, Shimada H, *et al.* Salacinol, potent antidiabetic principle with unique thiosugar sulfonium sulfate structure from the Ayurvedic traditional medicine *Salacia reticulata* in Sri Lanka and India. Tetrahedron Lett 1997; 38(48): 8367-70.
[http://dx.doi.org/10.1016/S0040-4039(97)10270-2]

[198] Jamshidi N, Da Costa C, Cohen M. Holybasil (tulsi) lowers fasting glucose and improves lipid profile in adults with metabolic disease: A meta-analysis of randomized clinical trials. J Funct Foods 2018; 45: 47-57.
[http://dx.doi.org/10.1016/j.jff.2018.03.030]

[199] Jaggi RK, Madaan R, Singh B. Anticonvulsant potential of holy basil, *Ocimum sanctum* Linn., and its cultures. Indian J Exp Biol 2003; 41(11): 1329-33.
[PMID: 15332507]

[200] Dada FA, Oyeleye SI, Ogunsuyi OB, *et al.* Phenolic constituents and modulatory effects of Raffia palm leaf (*Raphia hookeri*) extract on carbohydrate hydrolyzing enzymes linked to type-2 diabetes. J Tradit Complement Med 2017; 7(4): 494-500.
[http://dx.doi.org/10.1016/j.jtcme.2017.01.003] [PMID: 29034198]

[201] Ramakrishna R, Sarkar D, Schwarz P, Shetty K. Phenolic linked anti-hyperglycemic bioactives of barley (*Hordeum vulgare* L.) cultivars as nutraceuticals targeting type 2 diabetes. Ind Crops Prod 2017; 107: 509-17.
[http://dx.doi.org/10.1016/j.indcrop.2017.03.033]

[202] Hamdan D, El-Readi MZ, Tahrani A, *et al.* Chemical composition and biological activity of *Citrus jambhiri* Lush. Food Chem 2011; 127(2): 394-403.
[http://dx.doi.org/10.1016/j.foodchem.2010.12.129] [PMID: 23140678]

[203] Hwang J-T, Yang HJ, Ha K-C, So B-O, Choi E-K, Chae S-W. A randomized, double-blind, placebo-controlled clinical trial to investigate the anti-diabetic effect of *Citrus junos* Tanaka peel. J Funct Foods 2015; 18: 532-7.
[http://dx.doi.org/10.1016/j.jff.2015.08.019]

[204] Abirami A, Nagarani G, Siddhuraju P. *In vitro* antioxidant, anti-diabetic, cholinesterase and tyrosinase inhibitory potential of fresh juice from *Citrus hystrix* and *C. maxima* fruits. FSHW 2014; 3(1): 16-25.
[http://dx.doi.org/10.1016/j.fshw.2014.02.001]

[205] Talcott ST, Percival SS, Pittet-Moore J, Celoria C. Phytochemical composition and antioxidant stability of fortified yellow passion fruit (*Passiflora edulis*). J Agric Food Chem 2003; 51(4): 935-41.
[http://dx.doi.org/10.1021/jf020769q] [PMID: 12568552]

[206] Kandandapani S, Balaraman AK, Ahamed HN. Extracts of passion fruit peel and seed of *Passiflora edulis* (Passifloraceae) attenuate oxidative stress in diabetic rats. Chin J Nat Med 2015; 13(9): 680-6.
[http://dx.doi.org/10.1016/S1875-5364(15)30066-2] [PMID: 26412428]

[207] Wang H-Y, Kan W-C, Cheng T-J, Yu S-H, Chang L-H, Chuu J-J. Differential anti-diabetic effects and mechanism of action of charantin-rich extract of Taiwanese *Momordica charantia* between type 1 and type 2 diabetic mice. Food Chem Toxicol 2014; 69: 347-56.
[http://dx.doi.org/10.1016/j.fct.2014.04.008] [PMID: 24751968]

[208] Raman A, Lau C. Anti-diabetic properties and phytochemistry of *Momordica charantia* L. (Cucurbitaceae). Phytomedicine 1996; 2(4): 349-62.
[http://dx.doi.org/10.1016/S0944-7113(96)80080-8] [PMID: 23194773]

[209] Hussain AI, Rathore HA, Sattar MZ, Chatha SA, Sarker SD, Gilani AH. *Citrullus colocynthis* (L.) Schrad (bitter apple fruit): a review of its phytochemistry, pharmacology, traditional uses and nutritional potential. J Ethnopharmacol 2014; 155(1): 54-66.
[http://dx.doi.org/10.1016/j.jep.2014.06.011] [PMID: 24936768]

[210] Oryan A, Hashemnia M, Hamidi A-R, Mohammadalipour A. Effects of hydro-ethanol extract of *Citrullus colocynthis* on blood glucose levels and pathology of organs in alloxan-induced diabetic rats. Asian Pac J Trop Dis 2014; 4(2): 125-30.
[http://dx.doi.org/10.1016/S2222-1808(14)60328-5]

[211] Sukandar EY, Sudjana P, Adnyana IK, Setiawan AS, Yuniarni U. Recent study of turmeric in combination with garlic as antidiabetic agent. Procedia Chem 2014; 13: 44-56.
[http://dx.doi.org/10.1016/j.proche.2014.12.005]

[212] Wei C-K, Tsai Y-H, Korinek M, *et al.* 6-Paradol and 6-shogaol, the pungent compounds of ginger, promote glucose utilization in adipocytes and myotubes, and 6-paradol reduces blood glucose in high-fat diet-fed mice. Int J Mol Sci 2017; 18(1): 168.
[http://dx.doi.org/10.3390/ijms18010168] [PMID: 28106738]

[213] Sun W, Sang Y, Zhang B, *et al.* Synergistic effects of acarbose and an *Oroxylum indicum* seed extract in streptozotocin and high-fat-diet induced prediabetic mice. Biomed Pharmacother 2017; 87: 160-70.
[http://dx.doi.org/10.1016/j.biopha.2016.12.096] [PMID: 28056420]

[214] Harminder SV, Singh V, Chaudhary AK. A Review on the Taxonomy, Ethnobotany, Chemistry and Pharmacology of *Oroxylum indicum* Vent. Indian J Pharm Sci 2011; 73(5): 483-90.
[http://dx.doi.org/10.4103/0250-474X.98981] [PMID: 22923859]

[215] Haque M, Rao USM. Modulatory effect of Mengkudu fruit on the activities of key enzymes of glucose synthesis and utilization pathways of diabetic induced rats. J Pharm Res 2013; 7(1): 53-61.
[http://dx.doi.org/10.1016/j.jopr.2013.01.003]

[216] Jung UJ, Baek NI, Chung HG, *et al.* The anti-diabetic effects of ethanol extract from two variants of *Artemisia princeps* Pampanini in C57BL/KsJ-db/db mice. Food Chem Toxicol 2007; 45(10): 2022-9.
[http://dx.doi.org/10.1016/j.fct.2007.04.021] [PMID: 17574717]

[217] Cho Y-Y, Baek N-I, Chung H-G, *et al.* Randomized controlled trial of Sajabalssuk (*Artemisia princeps* Pampanini) to treat pre-diabetes. Eur J Integr Med 2012; 4(3): e299-308.
[http://dx.doi.org/10.1016/j.eujim.2012.01.009]

[218] Domingues A, Sartori A, Golim MA, *et al.* Prevention of experimental diabetes by *Uncaria tomentosa* extract: Th2 polarization, regulatory T cell preservation or both? J Ethnopharmacol 2011; 137(1): 635-42.
[http://dx.doi.org/10.1016/j.jep.2011.06.021] [PMID: 21718770]

[219] Yongchaiyudha S, Rungpitarangsi V, Bunyapraphatsara N, Chokechaijaroenporn O. Antidiabetic

activity of *Aloe vera* L. juice. I. Clinical trial in new cases of diabetes mellitus. Phytomedicine 1996; 3(3): 241-3.
[http://dx.doi.org/10.1016/S0944-7113(96)80060-2] [PMID: 23195077]

[220] Yagi A, Hegazy S, Kabbash A, Wahab EA. Possible hypoglycemic effect of *Aloe vera* L. high molecular weight fractions on type 2 diabetic patients. Saudi Pharm J 2009; 17(3): 209-15.
[http://dx.doi.org/10.1016/j.jsps.2009.08.007] [PMID: 23964163]

[221] Sobeh M, Mahmoud MF, Abdelfattah MAO, El-Beshbishy HA, El-Shazly AM, Wink M. Hepatoprotective and hypoglycemic effects of a tannin rich extract from *Ximenia americana* var. caffra root. Phytomedicine 2017; 33: 36-42.
[http://dx.doi.org/10.1016/j.phymed.2017.07.003] [PMID: 28887918]

[222] Sobeh M, Mahmoud MF, Abdelfattah MAO, El-Beshbishy HA, El-Shazly AM, Wink M. *Albizia harveyi*: phytochemical profiling, antioxidant, antidiabetic and hepatoprotective activities of the bark extract. Med Chem Res 2017; 26(12): 3091-105.
[http://dx.doi.org/10.1007/s00044-017-2005-8]

[223] Gutiérrez RMP, Mitchell S, Solis RV. *Psidium guajava*: a review of its traditional uses, phytochemistry and pharmacology. J Ethnopharmacol 2008; 117(1): 1-27.
[http://dx.doi.org/10.1016/j.jep.2008.01.025] [PMID: 18353572]

[224] Ruhil S, Balhara M, Dhankhar S, Chhillar A. *Aegle marmelos* (Linn.) Correa: A potential source of Phytomedicine. J Med Plants Res 2011; 5(9): 1497-507.

[225] Kooti W, Hasanzadeh-Noohi Z, Sharafi-Ahvazi N, Asadi-Samani M, Ashtary-Larky D. Phytochemistry, pharmacology, and therapeutic uses of black seed (*Nigella sativa*). Chin J Nat Med 2016; 14(10): 732-45.
[http://dx.doi.org/10.1016/S1875-5364(16)30088-7] [PMID: 28236403]

[226] Naskar S, Mazumder UK, Pramanik G, *et al.* Evaluation of antihyperglycemic activity of *Cocos nucifera* Linn. on streptozotocin induced type 2 diabetic rats. J Ethnopharmacol 2011; 138(3): 769-73.
[http://dx.doi.org/10.1016/j.jep.2011.10.021] [PMID: 22041106]

[227] Lima EB, Sousa CN, Meneses LN, *et al. Cocos nucifera* (L.) (Arecaceae): A phytochemical and pharmacological review. Braz J Med Biol Res 2015; 48(11): 953-64.
[http://dx.doi.org/10.1590/1414-431x20154773] [PMID: 26292222]

[228] Michel CG, Nesseem DI, Ismail MF. Anti-diabetic activity and stability study of the formulated leaf extract of *Ziziphus spina-christi* (L.) Willd with the influence of seasonal variation. J Ethnopharmacol 2011; 133(1): 53-62.
[http://dx.doi.org/10.1016/j.jep.2010.09.001] [PMID: 20833236]

[229] Vinholes J, Grosso C, Andrade PB, *et al. In vitro* studies to assess the antidiabetic, anti-cholinesterase and antioxidant potential of *Spergularia rubra*. Food Chem 2011; 129(2): 454-62.
[http://dx.doi.org/10.1016/j.foodchem.2011.04.098] [PMID: 30634251]

[230] Zhang L, Yang J, Chen XQ, *et al.* Antidiabetic and antioxidant effects of extracts from *Potentilla discolor* Bunge on diabetic rats induced by high fat diet and streptozotocin. J Ethnopharmacol 2010; 132(2): 518-24.
[http://dx.doi.org/10.1016/j.jep.2010.08.053] [PMID: 20816941]

[231] Pushpangadan P, George V. Biological activities of syzygium cumini and allied species the genus syzygium. CRC Press 2017; pp. 133-62.

[232] Rao BK, Rao CH. Hypoglycemic and antihyperglycemic activity of *Syzygium alternifolium* (Wt.) Walp. seed extracts in normal and diabetic rats. Phytomedicine 2001; 8(2): 88-93.
[http://dx.doi.org/10.1078/0944-7113-00015] [PMID: 11315761]

[233] Vasu K, Govardhan P, Reddy CS, Nath AR, Reddy R. *In-vitro* and *in-vivo* anti-inflammatory activity of *Syzygium alternifolium* (wt) Walp. J Med Plants Res 2012; 6(36): 4995-5001.

[234] Musman M, Safrida S, Kurnianda V, Erlidawati E. Evaluation of Antihyperglycemic Property from

Syzygium oleana (Magnoliopsida: Myrtaceae) Pericarp. Res J Med Plant 2017; 11(100): 106.
[http://dx.doi.org/10.3923/rjmp.2017.100.106]

[235] Latha M, Pari L, Sitasawad S, Bhonde R. Insulin-secretagogue activity and cytoprotective role of the traditional antidiabetic plant *Scoparia dulcis* (Sweet Broomweed). Life Sci 2004; 75(16): 2003-14.
[http://dx.doi.org/10.1016/j.lfs.2004.05.012] [PMID: 15306167]

[236] Senadheera SPAS, Ekanayake S, Wanigatunge C. Anti-hyperglycaemic effects of herbal porridge made of *Scoparia dulcis* leaf extract in diabetics - a randomized crossover clinical trial. BMC Complement Altern Med 2015; 15(1): 410.
[http://dx.doi.org/10.1186/s12906-015-0935-6] [PMID: 26582144]

[237] Zulfiker A, Rahman MM, Hossain MK, Hamid K, Mazumder M, Rana MS. *In vivo* analgesic activity of ethanolic extracts of two medicinal plants-*Scoparia dulcis* L. and *Ficus racemosa* Linn. J Biol Med 2010; 2(2): 42-8.

[238] Latha M, Ramkumar KM, Pari L, Damodaran PN, Rajeshkannan V, Suresh T. Phytochemical and antimicrobial study of an antidiabetic plant: *Scoparia dulcis* L. J Med Food 2006; 9(3): 391-4.
[http://dx.doi.org/10.1089/jmf.2006.9.391] [PMID: 17004904]

[239] Gul-e-Rana , Karim S, Khurhsid R, *et al.* Hypoglycemic activity of *Ficus racemosa* bark in combination with oral hypoglycemic drug in diabetic human. Acta Pol Pharm 2013; 70(6): 1045-9.
[PMID: 24383328]

[240] Behradmanesh S, Derees F, Rafieian-Kopaei M. Effect of *Salvia officinalis* on diabetic patients. J Renal Inj Prev 2013; 2(2): 51-4.
[PMID: 25340127]

[241] Laruan LMV, Balangcod T, Balangcod K, *et al.* Phytochemical and antibacterial study of *Lagerstroemia speciosa* (L.) Pers. and its ethnomedicinal importance to indigenous communities of Benguet Province, Philippines. Indian J Tradit Knowl 2013; 12(3): 379-83.

[242] Wollgast J, Anklam E. Review on polyphenols in *Theobroma cacao*: changes in composition during the manufacture of chocolate and methodology for identification and quantification. Food Res Int 2000; 33(6): 423-47.
[http://dx.doi.org/10.1016/S0963-9969(00)00068-5]

[243] Koyama Y, Tomoda Y, Kato M, Ashihara H. Metabolism of purine bases, nucleosides and alkaloids in theobromine-forming *Theobroma cacao* leaves. Plant Physiol Biochem 2003; 41(11): 977-84.
[http://dx.doi.org/10.1016/j.plaphy.2003.07.002]

[244] Bravo L, Goya L, Lecumberri E. LC/MS characterization of phenolic constituents of mate (*Ilex paraguariensis*, St. Hil.) and its antioxidant activity compared to commonly consumed beverages. Food Res Int 2007; 40(3): 393-405.
[http://dx.doi.org/10.1016/j.foodres.2006.10.016]

[245] Clifford MN, Ramirez-Martinez JR. Chlorogenic acids and purine alkaloids contents of Maté (*Ilex paraguariensis*) leaf and beverage. Food Chem 1990; 35(1): 13-21.
[http://dx.doi.org/10.1016/0308-8146(90)90126-O]

[246] Yoshikawa M, Murakami T, Komatsu H, Murakami N, Yamahara J, Matsuda H. Medicinal foodstuffs. IV. Fenugreek seed. (1): structures of trigoneosides Ia, Ib, IIa, IIb, IIIa, and IIIb, new furostanol saponins from the seeds of Indian *Trigonella foenum-graecum* L. Chem Pharm Bull (Tokyo) 1997; 45(1): 81-7.
[http://dx.doi.org/10.1248/cpb.45.81] [PMID: 9023970]

[247] Abdel-Barry JA, Abdel-Hassan IA, Al-Hakiem MH. Hypoglycaemic and antihyperglycaemic effects of *Trigonella foenum-graecum* leaf in normal and alloxan induced diabetic rats. J Ethnopharmacol 1997; 58(3): 149-55.
[http://dx.doi.org/10.1016/S0378-8741(97)00101-3] [PMID: 9421250]

[248] Deokate U, Khadabadi S. Pharmacology and phytochemistry of *Coccinia indica*. J Pharmacognosy

Phytother 2011; 3(11): 155-9.

[249]   Bagalkotkar G, Sagineedu SR, Saad MS, Stanslas J. Phytochemicals from *Phyllanthus niruri* Linn. and their pharmacological properties: a review. J Pharm Pharmacol 2006; 58(12): 1559-70.
[http://dx.doi.org/10.1211/jpp.58.12.0001] [PMID: 17331318]

[250]   Mostafa I, Abd El-Aziz E, Hafez S, El-Shazly A. Chemical constituents and biological activities of *Galinsoga parviflora* cav. (Asteraceae) from Egypt. Z Natforsch C J Biosci 2013; 68(7-8): 285-92.
[http://dx.doi.org/10.1515/znc-2013-7-805] [PMID: 24066513]

[251]   Agatonovic-Kustrin S, Morton DW, Adam A, Mizaton HH, Zakaria H. High-performance thin-layer chromatographic methods in the evaluation of the antioxidant and anti-hyperglycemic activity of *Myrmecodia platytyrea* as a promising opportunity in diabetes treatment. J Chromatogr A 2017; 1530: 192-6.
[http://dx.doi.org/10.1016/j.chroma.2017.11.012] [PMID: 29132827]

[252]   Subash-Babu P, Ignacimuthu S, Alshatwi AA. Nymphayol increases glucose-stimulated insulin secretion by RIN-5F cells and GLUT4-mediated insulin sensitization in type 2 diabetic rat liver. Chem Biol Interact 2015; 226: 72-81.
[http://dx.doi.org/10.1016/j.cbi.2014.12.011] [PMID: 25499137]

[253]   Atangwho IJ, Egbung GE, Ahmad M, Yam MF, Asmawi MZ. Antioxidant *versus* anti-diabetic properties of leaves from *Vernonia amygdalina* Del. growing in Malaysia. Food Chem 2013; 141(4): 3428-34.
[http://dx.doi.org/10.1016/j.foodchem.2013.06.047] [PMID: 23993503]

[254]   Gumy C, Thurnbichler C, Aubry EM, *et al.* Inhibition of 11β-hydroxysteroid dehydrogenase type 1 by plant extracts used as traditional antidiabetic medicines. Fitoterapia 2009; 80(3): 200-5.
[http://dx.doi.org/10.1016/j.fitote.2009.01.009] [PMID: 19535018]

[255]   Rodríguez-Morán M, Guerrero-Romero F, Lazcano-Burciaga G. Lipid- and glucose-lowering efficacy of *Plantago Psyllium* in type II diabetes. J Diabetes Complications 1998; 12(5): 273-8.
[http://dx.doi.org/10.1016/S1056-8727(98)00003-8] [PMID: 9747644]

[256]   Ziai SA, Larijani B, Akhoondzadeh S, *et al.* Psyllium decreased serum glucose and glycosylated hemoglobin significantly in diabetic outpatients. J Ethnopharmacol 2005; 102(2): 202-7.
[http://dx.doi.org/10.1016/j.jep.2005.06.042] [PMID: 16154305]

[257]   Qureshi AA, Sami SA, Khan FA. Effects of stabilized rice bran, its soluble and fiber fractions on blood glucose levels and serum lipid parameters in humans with diabetes mellitus Types I and II. J Nutr Biochem 2002; 13(3): 175-87.
[http://dx.doi.org/10.1016/S0955-2863(01)00211-X] [PMID: 11893482]

[258]   Apostolidis E, Li L, Lee C, Seeram NP. *In vitro* evaluation of phenolic-enriched maple syrup extracts for inhibition of carbohydrate hydrolyzing enzymes relevant to type 2 diabetes management. J Funct Foods 2011; 3(2): 100-6.
[http://dx.doi.org/10.1016/j.jff.2011.03.003]

[259]   Chan EW, Lye PY, Wong SK. Phytochemistry, pharmacology, and clinical trials of *Morus alba*. Chin J Nat Med 2016; 14(1): 17-30.
[PMID: 26850343]

[260]   Obolskiy D, Pischel I, Feistel B, Glotov N, Heinrich M. *Artemisia dracunculus* L. (tarragon): a critical review of its traditional use, chemical composition, pharmacology, and safety. J Agric Food Chem 2011; 59(21): 11367-84.
[http://dx.doi.org/10.1021/jf202277w] [PMID: 21942448]

[261]   Williams CA, Goldstone F, Greenham J. Flavonoids, cinnamic acids and coumarins from the different tissues and medicinal preparations of *Taraxacum officinale*. Phytochemistry 1996; 42(1): 121-7.
[http://dx.doi.org/10.1016/0031-9422(95)00865-9] [PMID: 8728061]

[262]   Banerji S, Banerjee S. A formulation of grape seed, Indian gooseberry, turmeric and fenugreek helps

controlling type 2 diabetes mellitus in advanced-stage patients. Eur J Integr Med 2016; 8(5): 645-53.
[http://dx.doi.org/10.1016/j.eujim.2016.06.012]

[263]   Prieur C, Rigaud J, Cheynier V, Moutounet M. Oligomeric and polymeric procyanidins from grape seeds. Phytochemistry 1994; 36(3): 781-4.
[http://dx.doi.org/10.1016/S0031-9422(00)89817-9] [PMID: 7765690]

[264]   Gaire BP, Subedi L. Phytochemistry, pharmacology and medicinal properties of *Phyllanthus emblica* Linn. Chin J Integr Med 2014; 1-8.
[http://dx.doi.org/10.1007/s11655-014-1984-2] [PMID: 25491539]

[265]   Lin R, He X, Chen H, *et al.* Oil tea improves glucose and lipid levels and alters gut microbiota in type 2 diabetic mice. Nutr Res 2018; 57: 67-77.
[http://dx.doi.org/10.1016/j.nutres.2018.05.004] [PMID: 30122197]

[266]   Campbell-Tofte JIA, Mølgaard P, Josefsen K, *et al.* Randomized and double-blinded pilot clinical study of the safety and anti-diabetic efficacy of the Rauvolfia-Citrus tea, as used in Nigerian traditional medicine. J Ethnopharmacol 2011; 133(2): 402-11.
[http://dx.doi.org/10.1016/j.jep.2010.10.013] [PMID: 20955771]

[267]   Amer MM, Court WE. Leaf alkaloids of *Rauwolfia vomitoria.* Phytochemistry 1980; 19(8): 1833-6.
[http://dx.doi.org/10.1016/S0031-9422(00)83823-6]

[268]   Razmpoosh E, Javadi A, Ejtahed HS, Mirmiran P, Javadi M, Yousefinejad A. The effect of probiotic supplementation on glycemic control and lipid profile in patients with type 2 diabetes: A randomized placebo controlled trial. Diabetes Metab Syndr 2019; 13(1): 175-82.
[http://dx.doi.org/10.1016/j.dsx.2018.08.008] [PMID: 30641692]

[269]   El-Desouki NI, Tabl GA, Abdel-Aziz KK, Salim EI, Nazeeh N. Improvement in beta-islets of Langerhans in alloxan-induced diabetic rats by erythropoietin and spirulina. J Basic Appl Zool 2015; 71: 20-31.
[http://dx.doi.org/10.1016/j.jobaz.2015.04.003]

[270]   De Silva DD, Rapior S, Hyde KD, Bahkali AH. Medicinal mushrooms in prevention and control of diabetes mellitus. Fungal Divers 2012; 56(1): 1-29.
[http://dx.doi.org/10.1007/s13225-012-0187-4] [PMID: 23097638]

[271]   Perera PK, Li Y. Mushrooms as a functional food mediator in preventing and ameliorating diabetes. FFHD 2011; 1(4): 161-71.
[http://dx.doi.org/10.31989/ffhd.v1i4.133]

[272]   Despland C, Walther B, Kast C, *et al.* A randomized-controlled clinical trial of high fructose diets from either Robinia honey or free fructose and glucose in healthy normal weight males. Clin Nutr ESPEN 2017; 19: 16-22.
[http://dx.doi.org/10.1016/j.clnesp.2017.01.009]

[273]   Abdulrhman M, El Hefnawy M, Ali R, Abdel Hamid I, Abou El-Goud A, Refai D. Effects of honey, sucrose and glucose on blood glucose and C-peptide in patients with type 1 diabetes mellitus. Complement Ther Clin Pract 2013; 19(1): 15-9.
[http://dx.doi.org/10.1016/j.ctcp.2012.08.002] [PMID: 23337559]

[274]   Khoshpey B, Djazayeri S, Amiri F, *et al.* Effect of royal jelly intake on serum glucose, Apolipoprotein AI (ApoA-I), Apolipoprotein B (ApoB) and ApoB/ApoA-I ratios in patients with type 2 diabetes: a randomized, double-blind clinical trial study. Can J Diabetes 2016; 40(4): 324-8.
[http://dx.doi.org/10.1016/j.jcjd.2016.01.003] [PMID: 27026221]

[275]   Lercker G, Capella P, Conte LS, Ruini F, Giordani G. Components of Royal Jelly II. The Lipid Fraction, Hydrocarbons and Sterols. J Apic Res 1982; 21(3): 178-84.
[http://dx.doi.org/10.1080/00218839.1982.11100538]

[276]   Li L, Xu J, Zhu W, *et al.* Effect of a macronutrient preload on blood glucose level and pregnancy outcome in gestational diabetes. J Clin Transl Endocrinol 2016; 5: 36-41.

[http://dx.doi.org/10.1016/j.jcte.2016.04.001] [PMID: 29067233]

[277] Devi SA, Jyothi B. Dyslipidemia in Metabolic Syndrome: an Overview of Lipoprotein-Related Disorders. Int J Cardiol 2017; 4(1): 7.

[278] Diet and health: implications for reducing chronic disease risk. National Academies Press 1989.

[279] Feingold KR, Grunfeld C. Introduction to Lipids and Lipoproteins.Endotext South Dartmouth (MA): MDText com, Inc. Feingold, KR 2018.

[280] Kolovou GD, Anagnostopoulou KK, Cokkinos DV. Pathophysiology of dyslipidaemia in the metabolic syndrome. Postgrad Med J 2005; 81(956): 358-66.
[http://dx.doi.org/10.1136/pgmj.2004.025601] [PMID: 15937200]

[281] Blaton V, Korita I, Bulo A. How is metabolic syndrome related to dyslipidemia? EJIFCC 2007; 18(1): 15-22.
[PMID: 29632463]

[282] Halpern A, Mancini MC, Magalhães ME, *et al.* Metabolic syndrome, dyslipidemia, hypertension and type 2 diabetes in youth: from diagnosis to treatment. Diabetol Metab Syndr 2010; 2(1): 55.
[http://dx.doi.org/10.1186/1758-5996-2-55] [PMID: 20718958]

[283] Ginsberg HN, Zhang YL, Hernandez-Ono A. Metabolic syndrome: focus on dyslipidemia. Obesity (Silver Spring) 2006; 14 Suppl 1(S2): 41S-9S.
[http://dx.doi.org/10.1038/oby.2006.281]

[284] Grundy SM, Grundy SM. An International Atherosclerosis Society Position Paper: global recommendations for the management of dyslipidemia. J Clin Lipidol 2013; 7(6): 561-5.
[http://dx.doi.org/10.1016/j.jacl.2013.10.001] [PMID: 24314355]

[285] Vaziri ND. Dyslipidemia of chronic renal failure: the nature, mechanisms, and potential consequences. Am J Physiol Renal Physiol 2006; 290(2): F262-72.
[http://dx.doi.org/10.1152/ajprenal.00099.2005] [PMID: 16403839]

[286] Shah AS, Wilson DP. Primary hypertriglyceridemia in children and adolescents. J Clin Lipidol 2015; 9(5) (Suppl.): S20-8.
[http://dx.doi.org/10.1016/j.jacl.2015.04.004] [PMID: 26343209]

[287] Barnard RJ. Effects of life-style modification on serum lipids. Arch Intern Med 1991; 151(7): 1389-94.
[http://dx.doi.org/10.1001/archinte.1991.00400070141019] [PMID: 2064490]

[288] Vodnala D, Rubenfire M, Brook RD. Secondary causes of dyslipidemia. Am J Cardiol 2012; 110(6): 823-5.
[http://dx.doi.org/10.1016/j.amjcard.2012.04.062] [PMID: 22658245]

[289] Blackett PR, Wilson DP, McNeal C. Secondary Hypertriglyceridemia.Endotext South Dartmouth (MA): MDText com, Inc. Feingold, KR 2018.

[290] Hegele RA, Ginsberg HN, Chapman MJ, *et al.* The polygenic nature of hypertriglyceridaemia: implications for definition, diagnosis, and management. Lancet Diabetes Endocrinol 2014; 2(8): 655-66.
[http://dx.doi.org/10.1016/S2213-8587(13)70191-8] [PMID: 24731657]

[291] Hu FB, Stampfer MJ, Haffner SM, Solomon CG, Willett WC, Manson JE. Elevated risk of cardiovascular disease prior to clinical diagnosis of type 2 diabetes. Diabetes Care 2002; 25(7): 1129-34.
[http://dx.doi.org/10.2337/diacare.25.7.1129] [PMID: 12087009]

[292] Rochlani Y, Pothineni NV, Kovelamudi S, Mehta JL. Metabolic syndrome: pathophysiology, management, and modulation by natural compounds. Ther Adv Cardiovasc Dis 2017; 11(8): 215-25.
[http://dx.doi.org/10.1177/1753944717711379] [PMID: 28639538]

[293] Chehade JM, Gladysz M, Mooradian AD. Dyslipidemia in type 2 diabetes: prevalence,

pathophysiology, and management. Drugs 2013; 73(4): 327-39.
[http://dx.doi.org/10.1007/s40265-013-0023-5] [PMID: 23479408]

[294] Mooradian AD. Dyslipidemia in type 2 diabetes mellitus. Nat Clin Pract Endocrinol Metab 2009; 5(3): 150-9.
[PMID: 19229235]

[295] Rader DJ, Daugherty A. Translating molecular discoveries into new therapies for atherosclerosis. Nature 2008; 451(7181): 904-13.
[http://dx.doi.org/10.1038/nature06796] [PMID: 18288179]

[296] Endo A. A gift from nature: the birth of the statins. Nat Med 2008; 14(10): 1050-2.
[http://dx.doi.org/10.1038/nm1008-1050] [PMID: 18841147]

[297] Tobert JA. Lovastatin and beyond: the history of the HMG-CoA reductase inhibitors. Nat Rev Drug Discov 2003; 2(7): 517-26.
[http://dx.doi.org/10.1038/nrd1112] [PMID: 12815379]

[298] Alberts AW. Discovery, biochemistry and biology of lovastatin. Am J Cardiol 1988; 62(15): 10J-5J.
[http://dx.doi.org/10.1016/0002-9149(88)90002-1] [PMID: 3055919]

[299] Bizukojc M, Ledakowicz S. A macrokinetic modelling of the biosynthesis of lovastatin by *Aspergillus terreus.* J Biotechnol 2007; 130(4): 422-35.
[http://dx.doi.org/10.1016/j.jbiotec.2007.05.007] [PMID: 17602773]

[300] Endo A. The origin of the statins. 2004. Atheroscler Suppl 2004; 5(3): 125-30.
[http://dx.doi.org/10.1016/j.atherosclerosissup.2004.08.033] [PMID: 15531285]

[301] Endo A, Negishi Y, Iwashita T, Mizukawa K, Hirama M. Biosynthesis of ML-236B (compactin) and monacolin K. J Antibiot (Tokyo) 1985; 38(3): 444-8.
[http://dx.doi.org/10.7164/antibiotics.38.444] [PMID: 4008338]

[302] Afuah A. Innovation management: strategies, implementation and profits 2003.

[303] Becker DJ, Gordon RY, Morris PB, *et al.* Simvastatin *vs* therapeutic lifestyle changes and supplements: randomized primary prevention trial. Mayo Clin Proc 2008; 83(7): 758-64.
[http://dx.doi.org/10.4065/83.7.758] [PMID: 18613992]

[304] Ma J, Li Y, Ye Q, *et al.* Constituents of red yeast rice, a traditional Chinese food and medicine. J Agric Food Chem 2000; 48(11): 5220-5.
[http://dx.doi.org/10.1021/jf000338c] [PMID: 11087463]

[305] Li C, Zhu Y, Wang Y, Zhu J-S, Chang J, Kritchevsky D. *Monascus purpureus*-fermented rice (red yeast rice): a natural food product that lowers blood cholesterol in animal models of hypercholesterolemia. Nutr Res 1998; 18(1): 71-81.
[http://dx.doi.org/10.1016/S0271-5317(97)00201-7]

[306] Burnham T, Sjweain S, Short R. Monascus The Review of Natural Products. St Louis, MO: Facts and Comparisons 1997.

[307] Wang J, Lu Z, Chi J, *et al.* Multicenter clinical trial of the serum lipid-lowering effects of a *Monascus purpureus* (red yeast) rice preparation from traditional Chinese medicine. Curr Ther Res Clin Exp 1997; 58(12): 964-78.
[http://dx.doi.org/10.1016/S0011-393X(97)80063-X]

[308] Becker DJ, Gordon RY, Halbert SC, French B, Morris PB, Rader DJ. Red yeast rice for dyslipidemia in statin-intolerant patients: a randomized trial. Ann Intern Med 2009; 150(12): 830-9, W147-9.
[http://dx.doi.org/10.7326/0003-4819-150-12-200906160-00006]

[309] Halbert SC, French B, Gordon RY, *et al.* Tolerability of red yeast rice (2,400 mg twice daily) *versus* pravastatin (20 mg twice daily) in patients with previous statin intolerance. Am J Cardiol 2010; 105(2): 198-204.
[http://dx.doi.org/10.1016/j.amjcard.2009.08.672] [PMID: 20102918]

[310]　Moriarty PM, Roth EM, Karns A, *et al.* Effects of Xuezhikang in patients with dyslipidemia: a multicenter, randomized, placebo-controlled study. J Clin Lipidol 2014; 8(6): 568-75.
[http://dx.doi.org/10.1016/j.jacl.2014.09.002] [PMID: 25499939]

[311]　Lin CC, Li TC, Lai MM. Efficacy and safety of *Monascus purpureus* Went rice in subjects with hyperlipidemia. Eur J Endocrinol 2005; 153(5): 679-86.
[http://dx.doi.org/10.1530/eje.1.02012] [PMID: 16260426]

[312]　Lu Z, Kou W, Du B, *et al.* Effect of Xuezhikang, an extract from red yeast Chinese rice, on coronary events in a Chinese population with previous myocardial infarction. Am J Cardiol 2008; 101(12): 1689-93.
[http://dx.doi.org/10.1016/j.amjcard.2008.02.056] [PMID: 18549841]

[313]　Cenedella RJ, Kuszak JR, Al-Ghoul KJ, Qin S, Sexton PS. Discordant expression of the sterol pathway in lens underlies simvastatin-induced cataracts in Chbb: Thom rats. J Lipid Res 2003; 44(1): 198-211.
[http://dx.doi.org/10.1194/jlr.M200002-JLR200] [PMID: 12518039]

[314]　Mulvihill EE, Burke AC, Huff MW. Citrus flavonoids as regulators of lipoprotein metabolism and atherosclerosis. Annu Rev Nutr 2016; 36: 275-99.
[http://dx.doi.org/10.1146/annurev-nutr-071715-050718] [PMID: 27146015]

[315]　Burke AC, Sutherland BG, Telford DE, *et al.* Intervention with citrus flavonoids reverses obesity and improves metabolic syndrome and atherosclerosis in obese *Ldlr*$^{-/-}$ mice. J Lipid Res 2018; 59(9): 1714-28.
[http://dx.doi.org/10.1194/jlr.M087387] [PMID: 30008441]

[316]　Stanely Mainzen Prince P, Kannan NK. Protective effect of rutin on lipids, lipoproteins, lipid metabolizing enzymes and glycoproteins in streptozotocin-induced diabetic rats. J Pharm Pharmacol 2006; 58(10): 1373-83.
[http://dx.doi.org/10.1211/jpp.58.10.0011] [PMID: 17034661]

[317]　Rivera L, Morón R, Sánchez M, Zarzuelo A, Galisteo M. Quercetin ameliorates metabolic syndrome and improves the inflammatory status in obese Zucker rats. Obesity (Silver Spring) 2008; 16(9): 2081-7.
[http://dx.doi.org/10.1038/oby.2008.315] [PMID: 18551111]

[318]　Zeka K, Ruparelia K, Arroo RR, Budriesi R, Micucci M. Flavonoids and their metabolites: Prevention in cardiovascular diseases and diabetes. Diseases 2017; 5(3): 19.
[http://dx.doi.org/10.3390/diseases5030019]

[319]　Dixit N, Baboota S, Kohli K, Ahmad S, Ali J. Silymarin: A review of pharmacological aspects and bioavailability enhancement approaches. Indian J Pharmacol 2007; 39(4): 172.
[http://dx.doi.org/10.4103/0253-7613.36534]

[320]　Huseini HF, Larijani B, Heshmat R, *et al.* The efficacy of *Silybum marianum* (L.) Gaertn. (silymarin) in the treatment of type II diabetes: a randomized, double-blind, placebo-controlled, clinical trial. Phytother Res 2006; 20(12): 1036-9.
[http://dx.doi.org/10.1002/ptr.1988] [PMID: 17072885]

[321]　Wang J, Wang Y, Xu C, *et al.* Effects of total flavonoids extracted from *Polygonum perfoliatum* L. on hypolipidemic and antioxidant in hyperlipidemia rats induced by high-fat diet. Int J Clin Exp Med 2018; 11(7): 6758-66.

[322]　Chen J, Li X. Hypolipidemic effect of flavonoids from mulberry leaves in triton WR-1339 induced hyperlipidemic mice. Asia Pac J Clin Nutr 2007; 16 Suppl 1(S1): 290-4.

[323]　Kuang W, Zhang X, Lan Z. Flavonoids extracted from *Linaria vulgaris* protect against hyperlipidemia and hepatic steatosis induced by western-type diet in mice. Arch Pharm Res 2018; 41(12): 1190-8.
[http://dx.doi.org/10.1007/s12272-017-0941-y] [PMID: 28770537]

[324]　Macias Alonso M, Marrero JG, Cordova Guerrero I, Perez Sánchez C, Osegueda Robles S. Coumarins

and metabolic syndrome: Brief Report. Med Res Arch 2017; 5(11)

[325] Choi W-S, Chang S-H, Kim J-E, Lee S-E. Hypolipidemic effects of scoparone and its coumarin analogues in hyperlipidemia rats induced by high fat diet. J Korean Soc Appl Biol Chem 2013; 56(6): 647-53.
[http://dx.doi.org/10.1007/s13765-013-3157-y]

[326] Augustin MA, Sanguansri L, Lockett T. Nano- and micro-encapsulated systems for enhancing the delivery of resveratrol. Ann N Y Acad Sci 2013; 1290(1): 107-12.
[http://dx.doi.org/10.1111/nyas.12130] [PMID: 23855472]

[327] Cho IJ, Ahn JY, Kim S, Choi MS, Ha TY. Resveratrol attenuates the expression of HMG-CoA reductase mRNA in hamsters. Biochem Biophys Res Commun 2008; 367(1): 190-4.
[http://dx.doi.org/10.1016/j.bbrc.2007.12.140] [PMID: 18166149]

[328] Berrougui H, Grenier G, Loued S, Drouin G, Khalil A. A new insight into resveratrol as an atheroprotective compound: inhibition of lipid peroxidation and enhancement of cholesterol efflux. Atherosclerosis 2009; 207(2): 420-7.
[http://dx.doi.org/10.1016/j.atherosclerosis.2009.05.017] [PMID: 19552907]

[329] Mader I, Wabitsch M, Debatin KM, Fischer-Posovszky P, Fulda S. Identification of a novel proapoptotic function of resveratrol in fat cells: SIRT1-independent sensitization to TRAIL-induced apoptosis. FASEB J 2010; 24(6): 1997-2009.
[http://dx.doi.org/10.1096/fj.09-142943] [PMID: 20097879]

[330] Chen Q, Wang E, Ma L, Zhai P. Dietary resveratrol increases the expression of hepatic 7α-hydroxylase and ameliorates hypercholesterolemia in high-fat fed C57BL/6J mice. Lipids Health Dis 2012; 11(1): 56.
[http://dx.doi.org/10.1186/1476-511X-11-56] [PMID: 22607622]

[331] Paul P, Islam M, Mustari A, Khan M. Hypolipidemic effect of ginger extract in vanaspati fed rats. Bangl J Vet Med 2012; 10(1&2): 93-6.

[332] Alizadeh-Navaei R, Roozbeh F, Saravi M, Pouramir M, Jalali F, Moghadamnia AA. Investigation of the effect of ginger on the lipid levels. A double blind controlled clinical trial. Saudi Med J 2008; 29(9): 1280-4.
[PMID: 18813412]

[333] Elshater A, Salman MM, Moussa MM. Effect of ginger extract consumption on levels of blood glucose, lipid profile and kidney functions in alloxan induced-diabetic rats. Egypt Acad J Biol Sci 2009; 2(1): 153-62.
[http://dx.doi.org/10.21608/eajbsa.2009.15515]

[334] Stoilova I, Krastanov A, Stoyanova A, Denev P, Gargova S. Antioxidant activity of a ginger extract (*Zingiber officinale*). Food Chem 2007; 102(3): 764-70.
[http://dx.doi.org/10.1016/j.foodchem.2006.06.023]

[335] Saravanan G, Ponmurugan P, Deepa MA, Senthilkumar B. Anti-obesity action of gingerol: effect on lipid profile, insulin, leptin, amylase and lipase in male obese rats induced by a high-fat diet. J Sci Food Agric 2014; 94(14): 2972-7.
[http://dx.doi.org/10.1002/jsfa.6642] [PMID: 24615565]

[336] Singh AB, Singh N, Maurya R, Srivastava AK. Anti-hyperglycaemic, lipid lowering and anti-oxidant properties of [6]-gingerol in db/db mice. Int J Med Med Sci 2009; 1(12): 536-44.

[337] Soni KB, Kuttan R. Effect of oral curcumin administration on serum peroxides and cholesterol levels in human volunteers. Indian J Physiol Pharmacol 1992; 36(4): 273-5.
[PMID: 1291482]

[338] Peschel D, Koerting R, Nass N. Curcumin induces changes in expression of genes involved in cholesterol homeostasis. J Nutr Biochem 2007; 18(2): 113-9.
[http://dx.doi.org/10.1016/j.jnutbio.2006.03.007] [PMID: 16713233]

[339] Legeay S, Rodier M, Fillon L, Faure S, Clere N. *Epigallocatechin gallate*: A review of its beneficial properties to prevent metabolic syndrome. Nutrients 2015; 7(7): 5443-68.
[http://dx.doi.org/10.3390/nu7075230] [PMID: 26198245]

[340] Hintzpeter J, Stapelfeld C, Loerz C, Martin H-J, Maser E. Green tea and one of its constituents, Epigallocatechine-3-gallate, are potent inhibitors of human 11β-hydroxysteroid dehydrogenase type 1. PLoS One 2014; 9(1)e84468
[http://dx.doi.org/10.1371/journal.pone.0084468] [PMID: 24404164]

[341] Bursill CA, Roach PD. Modulation of cholesterol metabolism by the green tea polyphenol (-)-*epigallocatechin gallate* in cultured human liver (HepG2) cells. J Agric Food Chem 2006; 54(5): 1621-6.
[http://dx.doi.org/10.1021/jf051736o] [PMID: 16506810]

[342] Alam MA, Juraimi AS, Rafii MY, *et al*. Evaluation of antioxidant compounds, antioxidant activities, and mineral composition of 13 collected purslane (*Portulaca oleracea* L.) accessions. BioMed Res Int 2014; 2014296063
[http://dx.doi.org/10.1155/2014/296063] [PMID: 24579078]

[343] Amritpal S, Sanjiv D, Navpreet K, Jaswinder S. Berberine: alkaloid with wide spectrum of pharmacological activities. J Nat Prod (India) 2010; 3: 64-75.

[344] Zhang Y, Li X, Zou D, *et al*. Treatment of type 2 diabetes and dyslipidemia with the natural plant alkaloid berberine. J Clin Endocrinol Metab 2008; 93(7): 2559-65.
[http://dx.doi.org/10.1210/jc.2007-2404] [PMID: 18397984]

[345] Dong H, Zhao Y, Zhao L, Lu F. The effects of berberine on blood lipids: a systemic review and meta-analysis of randomized controlled trials. Planta Med 2013; 79(6): 437-46.
[http://dx.doi.org/10.1055/s-0032-1328321] [PMID: 23512497]

[346] Gu S, Cao B, Sun R, *et al*. A metabolomic and pharmacokinetic study on the mechanism underlying the lipid-lowering effect of orally administered berberine. Mol Biosyst 2015; 11(2): 463-74.
[http://dx.doi.org/10.1039/C4MB00500G] [PMID: 25411028]

[347] Wang Y, Yi X, Ghanam K, Zhang S, Zhao T, Zhu X. Berberine decreases cholesterol levels in rats through multiple mechanisms, including inhibition of cholesterol absorption. Metabolism 2014; 63(9): 1167-77.
[http://dx.doi.org/10.1016/j.metabol.2014.05.013] [PMID: 25002181]

[348] Pal P, Gandhi H, Giridhar R, Yadav MR. ACAT inhibitors: the search for novel cholesterol lowering agents. Mini Rev Med Chem 2013; 13(8): 1195-219.
[http://dx.doi.org/10.2174/1389557511313080007] [PMID: 23198718]

[349] Kong W, Wei J, Abidi P, *et al*. Berberine is a novel cholesterol-lowering drug working through a unique mechanism distinct from statins. Nat Med 2004; 10(12): 1344-51.
[http://dx.doi.org/10.1038/nm1135] [PMID: 15531889]

[350] Kou S, Han B, Wang Y, *et al*. Synergetic cholesterol-lowering effects of main alkaloids from *Rhizoma Coptidis* in HepG2 cells and hypercholesterolemia hamsters. Life Sci 2016; 151: 50-60.
[http://dx.doi.org/10.1016/j.lfs.2016.02.046] [PMID: 26876917]

[351] He K, Hu Y, Ma H, *et al*. *Rhizoma Coptidis* alkaloids alleviate hyperlipidemia in B6 mice by modulating gut microbiota and bile acid pathways. Biochim Biophys Acta 2016; 1862(9): 1696-709.
[http://dx.doi.org/10.1016/j.bbadis.2016.06.006] [PMID: 27287254]

[352] Zhang X, Jin Y, Wu Y, *et al*. Anti-hyperglycemic and anti-hyperlipidemia effects of the alkaloid-rich extract from barks of *Litsea glutinosa* in ob/ob mice. Sci Rep 2018; 8(1): 12646.
[http://dx.doi.org/10.1038/s41598-018-30823-w] [PMID: 30140027]

[353] Manuwa TR, Akinmoladun AC, Crown OO, Komolafe K, Olaleye MT. Toxicological assessment and ameliorative effects of *Parinari curatellifolia* alkaloids on triton-induced hyperlipidemia and atherogenicity in rats. P Natl A Sci India B 2017; 87(2): 611-23.

[354] Calder PC. n-3 Fatty acids and cardiovascular disease: evidence explained and mechanisms explored. Clin Sci (Lond) 2004; 107(1): 1-11.
[http://dx.doi.org/10.1042/CS20040119] [PMID: 15132735]

[355] Schmidt S, Willers J, Stahl F, *et al.* Regulation of lipid metabolism-related gene expression in whole blood cells of normo- and dyslipidemic men after fish oil supplementation. Lipids Health Dis 2012; 11(1): 172.
[http://dx.doi.org/10.1186/1476-511X-11-172] [PMID: 23241455]

[356] Qin Y, Zhou Y, Chen SH, *et al.* Fish oil supplements lower serum lipids and glucose in correlation with a reduction in plasma fibroblast growth factor 21 and prostaglandin E2 in nonalcoholic fatty liver disease associated with hyperlipidemia: A randomized clinical trial. PLoS One 2015; 10(7)e0133496
[http://dx.doi.org/10.1371/journal.pone.0133496] [PMID: 26226139]

[357] Hasan SN, Singh D, Siddiqui SS, Kulshreshtha M, Aggarwal T. Effects of olive oil on lipid profile in hyperlipidaemic patients. Natl J Med Res 2013; 3(4): 312-4.

[358] Cullinen K. Olive oil in the treatment of hypercholesterolemia. Med Health R I 2006; 89(3): 113.
[PMID: 16596937]

[359] Martínez-González MÁ, Sánchez-Villegas A. The emerging role of Mediterranean diets in cardiovascular epidemiology: monounsaturated fats, olive oil, red wine or the whole pattern? Eur J Epidemiol 2004; 19(1): 9-13.
[http://dx.doi.org/10.1023/B:EJEP.0000013351.60227.7b] [PMID: 15012018]

[360] Goyal A, Sharma V, Upadhyay N, Gill S, Sihag M. Flax and flaxseed oil: an ancient medicine & modern functional food. J Food Sci Technol 2014; 51(9): 1633-53.
[http://dx.doi.org/10.1007/s13197-013-1247-9] [PMID: 25190822]

[361] Vijaimohan K, Jainu M, Sabitha KE, Subramaniyam S, Anandhan C, Shyamala Devi CS. Beneficial effects of alpha linolenic acid rich flaxseed oil on growth performance and hepatic cholesterol metabolism in high fat diet fed rats. Life Sci 2006; 79(5): 448-54.
[http://dx.doi.org/10.1016/j.lfs.2006.01.025] [PMID: 16490217]

[362] Hussein SA, El-Senosi YA, Ragab MR, Hammad MM. Beneficial effect of flaxseed oil on lipid metabolism in high cholesterol diet fed rats. BVMJ 2014; 27: 290-301.

[363] E Souza BSF, Carvalho HO, Ferreira IM, *et al.* Effect of the treatment with *Euterpe oleracea* Mart. oil in rats with Triton-induced dyslipidemia. Biomed Pharmacother 2017; 90: 542-7.
[http://dx.doi.org/10.1016/j.biopha.2017.04.005] [PMID: 28402923]

[364] Amamou F, Bouafia M, Chabane-Sari D, Meziane R, Nani A. *Citrullus colocynthis*: a desert plant native in Algeria, effects of fixed oil on blood homeostasis in Wistar rat. JNPR 2011; 1: 1-7.

[365] Gouni-Berthold I, Berthold HK. Policosanol: clinical pharmacology and therapeutic significance of a new lipid-lowering agent. Am Heart J 2002; 143(2): 356-65.
[http://dx.doi.org/10.1067/mhj.2002.119997] [PMID: 11835043]

[366] Serbinova E, Kagan V, Han D, Packer L. Free radical recycling and intramembrane mobility in the antioxidant properties of alpha-tocopherol and alpha-tocotrienol. Free Radic Biol Med 1991; 10(5): 263-75.
[http://dx.doi.org/10.1016/0891-5849(91)90033-Y] [PMID: 1649783]

[367] Correll CC, Ng L, Edwards PA. Identification of farnesol as the non-sterol derivative of mevalonic acid required for the accelerated degradation of 3-hydroxy-3-methylglutaryl-coenzyme A reductase. J Biol Chem 1994; 269(26): 17390-3.
[PMID: 8021239]

[368] Qureshi AA, Qureshi N, Wright JJ, *et al.* Lowering of serum cholesterol in hypercholesterolemic humans by tocotrienols (palmvitee). Am J Clin Nutr 1991; 53(4) (Suppl.): 1021S-6S.
[http://dx.doi.org/10.1093/ajcn/53.4.1021S] [PMID: 2012010]

[369] Qureshi AA, Bradlow BA, Brace L, *et al.* Response of hypercholesterolemic subjects to administration of tocotrienols. Lipids 1995; 30(12): 1171-7.
[http://dx.doi.org/10.1007/BF02536620] [PMID: 8614309]

[370] Hajhashemi V, Abbasi N. Hypolipidemic activity of *Anethum graveolens* in rats. Phytother Res 2008; 22(3): 372-5.
[http://dx.doi.org/10.1002/ptr.2329] [PMID: 18058989]

[371] Lal AA, Kumar T, Murthy PB, Pillai KS. Hypolipidemic effect of *Coriandrum sativum* L. in triton-induced hyperlipidemic rats. Indian J Exp Biol 2004; 42(9): 909-12.
[PMID: 15462185]

[372] Rajeshwari U, Shobha I, Andallu B. Comparison of aniseeds and coriander seeds for antidiabetic, hypolipidemic and antioxidant activities. Spatula DD 2011; 1(1): 9-16.
[http://dx.doi.org/10.5455/spatula.20110106123144]

[373] Suanarunsawat T, Ayutthaya WDN, Songsa T, Rattanamahaphoom J. Anti-lipidemic actions of essential oil extracted from *Ocimum sanctum* L. leaves in rats fed with high cholesterol diet. J Appl Biomed 2009; 7(1)
[http://dx.doi.org/10.32725/jab.2009.004]

[374] Kimura S, Tung YC, Pan MH, Su NW, Lai YJ, Cheng KC. Black garlic: A critical review of its production, bioactivity, and application. Yao Wu Shi Pin Fen Xi 2017; 25(1): 62-70.
[http://dx.doi.org/10.1016/j.jfda.2016.11.003] [PMID: 28911544]

[375] Kim I, Kim J-Y, Hwang Y-J, *et al.* The beneficial effects of aged black garlic extract on obesity and hyperlipidemia in rats fed a high-fat diet. J Med Plants Res 2011; 5(14): 3159-68.

[376] Kannar D, Wattanapenpaiboon N, Savige GS, Wahlqvist ML. Hypocholesterolemic effect of an enteric-coated garlic supplement. J Am Coll Nutr 2001; 20(3): 225-31.
[http://dx.doi.org/10.1080/07315724.2001.10719036] [PMID: 11444418]

[377] Mahmoodi M, Islami MR, Asadi Karam GR, *et al.* Study of the effects of raw garlic consumption on the level of lipids and other blood biochemical factors in hyperlipidemic individuals. Pak J Pharm Sci 2006; 19(4): 295-8.
[PMID: 17105707]

[378] Sun YE, Wang W, Qin J. Anti-hyperlipidemia of garlic by reducing the level of total cholesterol and low-density lipoprotein: A meta-analysis. Medicine (Baltimore) 2018; 97(18)e0255
[http://dx.doi.org/10.1097/MD.0000000000010255] [PMID: 29718835]

[379] Choudhary R. Beneficial effect of *Allium sativum* and *Allium tuberosum* on experimental hyperlipidemia and atherosclerosis. Pak J Physiol 2008; 4(2): 7-10.

[380] Yeh YY, Liu L. Cholesterol-lowering effect of garlic extracts and organosulfur compounds: human and animal studies. J Nutr 2001; 131(3s): 989S-93S.
[http://dx.doi.org/10.1093/jn/131.3.989S] [PMID: 11238803]

[381] Isbrucker RA, Burdock GA. Risk and safety assessment on the consumption of Licorice root (*Glycyrrhiza sp.*), its extract and powder as a food ingredient, with emphasis on the pharmacology and toxicology of glycyrrhizin. Regul Toxicol Pharmacol 2006; 46(3): 167-92.
[http://dx.doi.org/10.1016/j.yrtph.2006.06.002] [PMID: 16884839]

[382] Eu CH, Lim WY, Ton SH, bin Abdul Kadir K. Glycyrrhizic acid improved lipoprotein lipase expression, insulin sensitivity, serum lipid and lipid deposition in high-fat diet-induced obese rats. Lipids Health Dis 2010; 9(1): 81.
[http://dx.doi.org/10.1186/1476-511X-9-81] [PMID: 20670429]

[383] Bahmani M, Mirhoseini M, Shirzad H, Sedighi M, Shahinfard N, Rafieian-Kopaei M. A review on promising natural agents effective on hyperlipidemia. J Evid Based Complementary Altern Med 2015; 20(3): 228-38.
[http://dx.doi.org/10.1177/2156587214568457] [PMID: 25633423]

[384]   Moosa ASM, Rashid MU, Asadi A, Ara N, Uddin MM, Ferdaus A. Hypolipidemic effects of fenugreek seed powder. Bangladesh J Pharmacol 2006; 1(2): 64-7.

[385]   Saxena B, Saxena U. Antihyperlipidemic activity of fenugreek (*Trigonella foenum graecum*) seeds extract in triton and high fat diet induced hyperlipidemic model: Apotent anti-atherosclerotic agent. Pharmacologyonline 2009; 2: 616-24.

[386]   Anderson JW, Johnstone BM, Cook-Newell ME. Meta-analysis of the effects of soy protein intake on serum lipids. N Engl J Med 1995; 333(5): 276-82.
        [http://dx.doi.org/10.1056/NEJM199508033330502] [PMID: 7596371]

[387]   Nijjar PS, Burke FM, Bloesch A, Rader DJ. Role of dietary supplements in lowering low-density lipoprotein cholesterol: a review. J Clin Lipidol 2010; 4(4): 248-58.
        [http://dx.doi.org/10.1016/j.jacl.2010.07.001] [PMID: 21122657]

[388]   Baum JA, Teng H, Erdman JW Jr, *et al.* Long-term intake of soy protein improves blood lipid profiles and increases mononuclear cell low-density-lipoprotein receptor messenger RNA in hypercholesterolemic, postmenopausal women. Am J Clin Nutr 1998; 68(3): 545-51.
        [http://dx.doi.org/10.1093/ajcn/68.3.545] [PMID: 9734729]

[389]   Agrawal S, Thomson SR, Shivaprakash G. Nutraceuticals in dyslipidemia: an alternative approach. Asian J Pharm Clin Res 2017; 10(1): 38-42.
        [http://dx.doi.org/10.22159/ajpcr.2017.v10i1.15360]

[390]   Singh RB, Niaz MA, Ghosh S. Hypolipidemic and antioxidant effects of *Commiphora mukul* as an adjunct to dietary therapy in patients with hypercholesterolemia. Cardiovasc Drugs Ther 1994; 8(4): 659-64.
        [http://dx.doi.org/10.1007/BF00877420] [PMID: 7848901]

[391]   Nityanand S, Srivastava JS, Asthana OP. Clinical trials with gugulipid. A new hypolipidaemic agent. J Assoc Physicians India 1989; 37(5): 323-8.
        [PMID: 2693440]

[392]   Madgulkar AR, Rao MR, Warrier D. Characterization of Psyllium (*Plantago ovata*) polysaccharide and its uses. In: Ramawat KG, Merillon JM, Eds. Polysaccharides. 2014; pp. 872-90.
        [http://dx.doi.org/10.1007/978-3-319-03751-6_49-1]

[393]   Bell LP, Hectorne K, Reynolds H, Balm TK, Hunninghake DB. Cholesterol-lowering effects of psyllium hydrophilic mucilloid. Adjunct therapy to a prudent diet for patients with mild to moderate hypercholesterolemia. JAMA 1989; 261(23): 3419-23.
        [http://dx.doi.org/10.1001/jama.1989.03420230073029] [PMID: 2724486]

[394]   Seal CJ, Mathers JC. Comparative gastrointestinal and plasma cholesterol responses of rats fed on cholesterol-free diets supplemented with guar gum and sodium alginate. Br J Nutr 2001; 85(3): 317-24.
        [http://dx.doi.org/10.1079/BJN2000250] [PMID: 11299077]

[395]   Maisonnier S, Gomez J, Brée A, Berri C, Baéza E, Carré B. Effects of microflora status, dietary bile salts and guar gum on lipid digestibility, intestinal bile salts, and histomorphology in broiler chickens. Poult Sci 2003; 82(5): 805-14.
        [http://dx.doi.org/10.1093/ps/82.5.805] [PMID: 12762404]

[396]   Singla RK, Bhat VG. Crocin: an overview. IGJPS 2011; 1(4): 281-6.

[397]   Asdaq SMB, Inamdar MN. Potential of *Crocus sativus* (saffron) and its constituent, crocin, as hypolipidemic and antioxidant in rats. Appl Biochem Biotechnol 2010; 162(2): 358-72.
        [http://dx.doi.org/10.1007/s12010-009-8740-7] [PMID: 19672721]

[398]   Grasa-López A, Miliar-García Á, Quevedo-Corona L, *et al.* *Undaria pinnatifida* and fucoxanthin ameliorate lipogenesis and markers of both inflammation and cardiovascular dysfunction in an animal model of diet-induced obesity. Mar Drugs 2016; 14(8): 148.
        [http://dx.doi.org/10.3390/md14080148] [PMID: 27527189]

[399] Maeda H, Hosokawa M, Sashima T, Funayama K, Miyashita K. Fucoxanthin from edible seaweed, *Undaria pinnatifida*, shows antiobesity effect through UCP1 expression in white adipose tissues. Biochem Biophys Res Commun 2005; 332(2): 392-7.
[http://dx.doi.org/10.1016/j.bbrc.2005.05.002] [PMID: 15896707]

[400] Narayanamurthy U, Anandhi M, Manimekalai K. Effect of lutein on lipid profile in hypercholesterolemic rats. Int J Basic Clin Pharmacol 2018; 7(5): 859-65.
[http://dx.doi.org/10.18203/2319-2003.ijbcp20181625]

[401] Micallef MA, Garg ML. The lipid-lowering effects of phytosterols and (n-3) polyunsaturated fatty acids are synergistic and complementary in hyperlipidemic men and women. J Nutr 2008; 138(6): 1086-90.
[http://dx.doi.org/10.1093/jn/138.6.1086] [PMID: 18492838]

[402] St Jean N. Lowering Cholesterol: through the use of plant sterols and stanols 2008.http://digitalcommons.uri.edu/srhonorsprog/82

[403] Houston M, Sparks W. Effect of combination pantethine, plant sterols, green tea extract, delta-tocotrienol and phytolens on lipid profiles in patients with hyperlipidemia. JANA 2010; 13(1): 15-20.

[404] Simons LA. Additive effect of plant sterol-ester margarine and cerivastatin in lowering low-density lipoprotein cholesterol in primary hypercholesterolemia. Am J Cardiol 2002; 90(7): 737-40.
[http://dx.doi.org/10.1016/S0002-9149(02)02600-0] [PMID: 12356387]

[405] Englisch W, Beckers C, Unkauf M, Ruepp M, Zinserling V. Efficacy of Artichoke dry extract in patients with hyperlipoproteinemia. Arzneimittelforschung 2000; 50(3): 260-5.
[PMID: 10758778]

[406] Daniela T. [*Salvia officinalis* l. I. Botanic characteristics, composition, use and cultivation]. Cesk Farm 1993; 42(3): 111-6.
[PMID: 8402963]

[407] Sá CM, Ramos AA, Azevedo MF, Lima CF, Fernandes-Ferreira M, Pereira-Wilson C. Sage tea drinking improves lipid profile and antioxidant defences in humans. Int J Mol Sci 2009; 10(9): 3937-50.
[http://dx.doi.org/10.3390/ijms10093937] [PMID: 19865527]

[408] Kianbakht S, Dabaghian FH. Improved glycemic control and lipid profile in hyperlipidemic type 2 diabetic patients consuming *Salvia officinalis* L. leaf extract: a randomized placebo. Controlled clinical trial. Complement Ther Med 2013; 21(5): 441-6.
[http://dx.doi.org/10.1016/j.ctim.2013.07.004] [PMID: 24050577]

[409] Kianbakht S, Abasi B, Perham M, Hashem Dabaghian F. Antihyperlipidemic effects of *Salvia officinalis* L. leaf extract in patients with hyperlipidemia: a randomized double-blind placebo-controlled clinical trial. Phytother Res 2011; 25(12): 1849-53.
[http://dx.doi.org/10.1002/ptr.3506] [PMID: 21506190]

[410] Dana N, Javanmard SH, Asgary S, Asnaashari H, Abdian N. The effect of *Aloe vera* leaf gel on fatty streak formation in hypercholesterolemic rabbits. J Res Med Sci 2012; 17(5): 439-42.
[PMID: 23626607]

[411] Poolsil P, Promprom W, Talubmook C. Anti-hyperglycemic and anti-hyperlipidemic effects of extract from *Houttuynia cordata* Thumb. in streptozotocin-induced diabetic rats. Pharmacogn J 2017; 9(3)
[http://dx.doi.org/10.5530/pj.2017.3.65]

[412] Shah K, Patel M, Shah S, Chauhan K, Parmar P, Patel N. Antihyperlipidemic activity of *Mangifera indica* l. leaf extract on rats fed with high cholesterol diet. Pharm Sin 2010; 1(2): 156-61.

[413] Mazroatul C, Deni GD, Habibi NA, Saputri GF. Anti-hypercholesterolemia activity of ethanol extract *Peperomia pellucid.* Alchemy. Jurnal Penelitian Kimia 2016; 12(1): 88-94.
[http://dx.doi.org/10.20961/alchemy.12.1.948.88-94]

[414] Akinpelu B, Apata J, Iwalewa E, Oyedapo O. Evaluation of anti-hyperlipidemic potential of ethanolic leaf extract of *Clerodendrum volubile* P. Beauv. IJS 2016; 18(3): 789-800.

[415] Jain PG, Patil SD, Haswani NG, Girase MV, Surana SJ. Hypolipidemic activity of *Moringa oleifera* Lam., Moringaceae, on high fat diet induced hyperlipidemia in albino rats. Rev Bras Farmacogn 2010; 20(6): 969-73.
[http://dx.doi.org/10.1590/S0102-695X2010005000038]

[416] Ahmad S, Beg ZH. Elucidation of mechanisms of actions of thymoquinone-enriched methanolic and volatile oil extracts from *Nigella sativa* against cardiovascular risk parameters in experimental hyperlipidemia. Lipids Health Dis 2013; 12(1): 86.
[http://dx.doi.org/10.1186/1476-511X-12-86] [PMID: 23758650]

[417] Rasheed A, Siddiqui M, Khan JA. Therapeutic evaluation of Kalonji (*Nigella sativa*) in dyslipidemia-A randomized control trial. Med J Islamic World Acad Sci 2014; 22(3): 111-6.
[http://dx.doi.org/10.12816/0008181]

[418] Raggatt LJ, Partridge NC. Cellular and molecular mechanisms of bone remodeling. J Biol Chem 2010; 285(33): 25103-8.
[http://dx.doi.org/10.1074/jbc.R109.041087] [PMID: 20501658]

[419] Tu KN, Lie JD, Wan CKV, *et al.* Osteoporosis: A review of treatment options. P&T 2018; 43(2): 92-104.
[PMID: 29386866]

[420] Johnell O, Kanis JA. An estimate of the worldwide prevalence and disability associated with osteoporotic fractures. Osteoporos Int 2006; 17(12): 1726-33.
[http://dx.doi.org/10.1007/s00198-006-0172-4] [PMID: 16983459]

[421] An J, Yang H, Zhang Q, *et al.* Natural products for treatment of osteoporosis: The effects and mechanisms on promoting osteoblast-mediated bone formation. Life Sci 2016; 147: 46-58.
[http://dx.doi.org/10.1016/j.lfs.2016.01.024] [PMID: 26796578]

[422] Song L, Zhao J, Zhang X, Li H, Zhou Y. Icariin induces osteoblast proliferation, differentiation and mineralization through estrogen receptor-mediated ERK and JNK signal activation. Eur J Pharmacol 2013; 714(1-3): 15-22.
[http://dx.doi.org/10.1016/j.ejphar.2013.05.039] [PMID: 23764463]

[423] Lee CH, Huang YL, Liao JF, Chiou WF. Ugonin K-stimulated osteogenesis involves estrogen receptor-dependent activation of non-classical Src signaling pathway and classical pathway. Eur J Pharmacol 2012; 676(1-3): 26-33.
[http://dx.doi.org/10.1016/j.ejphar.2011.12.001] [PMID: 22192930]

[424] Srivastava S, Bankar R, Roy P. Assessment of the role of flavonoids for inducing osteoblast differentiation in isolated mouse bone marrow derived mesenchymal stem cells. Phytomedicine 2013; 20(8-9): 683-90.
[http://dx.doi.org/10.1016/j.phymed.2013.03.001] [PMID: 23570998]

[425] Tiyasatkulkovit W, Charoenphandhu N, Wongdee K, Thongbunchoo J, Krishnamra N, Malaivijitnond S. Upregulation of osteoblastic differentiation marker mRNA expression in osteoblast-like UMR106 cells by puerarin and phytoestrogens from *Pueraria mirifica*. Phytomedicine 2012; 19(13): 1147-55.
[http://dx.doi.org/10.1016/j.phymed.2012.07.010] [PMID: 22951392]

[426] Hsieh TP, Sheu SY, Sun JS, Chen MH, Liu MH. Icariin isolated from *Epimedium pubescens* regulates osteoblasts anabolism through BMP-2, SMAD4, and Cbfa1 expression. Phytomedicine 2010; 17(6): 414-23.
[http://dx.doi.org/10.1016/j.phymed.2009.08.007] [PMID: 19747809]

[427] Liao MH, Tai YT, Cherng YG, *et al.* Genistein induces oestrogen receptor-α gene expression in osteoblasts through the activation of mitogen-activated protein kinases/NF-κB/activator protein-1 and promotes cell mineralisation. Br J Nutr 2014; 111(1): 55-63.

[http://dx.doi.org/10.1017/S0007114513002043] [PMID: 23829885]

[428]   Pandey MK, Gupta SC, Karelia D, Gilhooley PJ, Shakibaei M, Aggarwal BB. Dietary nutraceuticals as backbone for bone health. Biotechnol Adv 2018; 36(6): 1633-48.
[http://dx.doi.org/10.1016/j.biotechadv.2018.03.014] [PMID: 29597029]

[429]   Wu JB, Fong YC, Tsai HY, Chen YF, Tsuzuki M, Tang CH. Naringin-induced bone morphogenetic protein-2 expression *via* PI3K, Akt, c-Fos/c-Jun and AP-1 pathway in osteoblasts. Eur J Pharmacol 2008; 588(2-3): 333-41.
[http://dx.doi.org/10.1016/j.ejphar.2008.04.030] [PMID: 18495116]

[430]   Don MJ, Lin LC, Chiou WF. Neobavaisoflavone stimulates osteogenesis *via* p38-mediated up-regulation of transcription factors and osteoid genes expression in MC3T3-E1 cells. Phytomedicine 2012; 19(6): 551-61.
[http://dx.doi.org/10.1016/j.phymed.2012.01.006] [PMID: 22397994]

[431]   Li F, Yang Y, Zhu P, *et al.* Echinacoside promotes bone regeneration by increasing OPG/RANKL ratio in MC3T3-E1 cells. Fitoterapia 2012; 83(8): 1443-50.
[http://dx.doi.org/10.1016/j.fitote.2012.08.008] [PMID: 22951288]

[432]   Xiao HH, Gao QG, Zhang Y, *et al.* Vanillic acid exerts oestrogen-like activities in osteoblast-like UMR 106 cells through MAP kinase (MEK/ERK)-mediated ER signaling pathway. J Steroid Biochem Mol Biol 2014; 144(Pt B): 382-91.

[433]   Lee YS, Choi EM. Apocynin stimulates osteoblast differentiation and inhibits bone-resorbing mediators in MC3T3-E1 cells. Cell Immunol 2011; 270(2): 224-9.
[http://dx.doi.org/10.1016/j.cellimm.2011.05.011] [PMID: 21683946]

[434]   Xu D, Xu L, Zhou C, *et al.* Salvianolic acid B promotes osteogenesis of human mesenchymal stem cells through activating ERK signaling pathway. Int J Biochem Cell Biol 2014; 51: 1-9.
[http://dx.doi.org/10.1016/j.biocel.2014.03.005] [PMID: 24657587]

[435]   Dai Z, Li Y, Quarles LD, *et al.* Resveratrol enhances proliferation and osteoblastic differentiation in human mesenchymal stem cells *via* ER-dependent ERK1/2 activation. Phytomedicine 2007; 14(12): 806-14.
[http://dx.doi.org/10.1016/j.phymed.2007.04.003] [PMID: 17689939]

[436]   Chen JJ, Zhang NF, Mao GX, *et al.* Salidroside stimulates osteoblast differentiation through BMP signaling pathway. Food Chem Toxicol 2013; 62: 499-505.
[http://dx.doi.org/10.1016/j.fct.2013.09.019] [PMID: 24055767]

[437]   Lee SU, Shin HK, Min YK, Kim SH. Emodin accelerates osteoblast differentiation through phosphatidylinositol 3-kinase activation and bone morphogenetic protein-2 gene expression. Int Immunopharmacol 2008; 8(5): 741-7.
[http://dx.doi.org/10.1016/j.intimp.2008.01.027] [PMID: 18387517]

[438]   Choi EM. Honokiol isolated from *Magnolia officinalis* stimulates osteoblast function and inhibits the release of bone-resorbing mediators. Int Immunopharmacol 2011; 11(10): 1541-5.
[http://dx.doi.org/10.1016/j.intimp.2011.05.011] [PMID: 21621646]

[439]   Suh KS, Choi EM, Lee YS, Kim YS. Protective effect of albiflorin against oxidative-stress-mediated toxicity in osteoblast-like MC3T3-E1 cells. Fitoterapia 2013; 89: 33-41.
[http://dx.doi.org/10.1016/j.fitote.2013.05.016] [PMID: 23707745]

[440]   Kim MB, Song Y, Hwang JK. Kirenol stimulates osteoblast differentiation through activation of the BMP and Wnt/β-catenin signaling pathways in MC3T3-E1 cells. Fitoterapia 2014; 98: 59-65.
[http://dx.doi.org/10.1016/j.fitote.2014.07.013] [PMID: 25062891]

[441]   Lee YS, Choi EM. Costunolide stimulates the function of osteoblastic MC3T3-E1 cells. Int Immunopharmacol 2011; 11(6): 712-8.
[http://dx.doi.org/10.1016/j.intimp.2011.01.018] [PMID: 21296696]

[442]   Tang CH, Yang RS, Chien MY, Chen CC, Fu WM. Enhancement of bone morphogenetic protein-2

expression and bone formation by coumarin derivatives *via* p38 and ERK-dependent pathway in osteoblasts. Eur J Pharmacol 2008; 579(1-3): 40-9.
[http://dx.doi.org/10.1016/j.ejphar.2007.10.013] [PMID: 17980360]

[443] Tang DZ, Yang F, Yang Z, *et al.* Psoralen stimulates osteoblast differentiation through activation of BMP signaling. Biochem Biophys Res Commun 2011; 405(2): 256-61.
[http://dx.doi.org/10.1016/j.bbrc.2011.01.021] [PMID: 21219873]

[444] Tang DZ, Hou W, Zhou Q, *et al.* Osthole stimulates osteoblast differentiation and bone formation by activation of beta-catenin-BMP signaling. J Bone Miner Res 2010; 25(6): 1234-45.
[http://dx.doi.org/10.1002/jbmr.21] [PMID: 20200936]

[445] Kihara T, Ichikawa S, Yonezawa T, *et al.* Acerogenin A, a natural compound isolated from *Acer nikoense* Maxim, stimulates osteoblast differentiation through bone morphogenetic protein action. Biochem Biophys Res Commun 2011; 406(2): 211-7.
[http://dx.doi.org/10.1016/j.bbrc.2011.02.017] [PMID: 21303661]

[446] Huang Q, Gao B, Jie Q, *et al.* Ginsenoside-Rb2 displays anti-osteoporosis effects through reducing oxidative damage and bone-resorbing cytokines during osteogenesis. Bone 2014; 66: 306-14.
[http://dx.doi.org/10.1016/j.bone.2014.06.010] [PMID: 24933344]

[447] Senthilkumar K, Venkatesan J, Kim S-K. Marine derived natural products for osteoporosis. Biomedicine & Preventive Nutrition 2014; 4(1): 1-7.
[http://dx.doi.org/10.1016/j.bionut.2013.12.005]

CHAPTER 3

Fluorine-containing Drugs and Drug Candidates Derived from Natural Products

Chunlin Zhuang[1], Yuelin Wu[2], Wannian Zhang[1,3] and Zhenyuan Miao[1,*]

[1] *School of Pharmacy, Second Military Medical University, 325 Guohe Road, Shanghai 200433, China*

[2] *School of Chemical and Environmental Engineering, Shanghai Institute of Technology, 100 Haiquan Road, Shanghai201418, China*

[3] *School of Pharmacy, Ningxia Medical University, Yinchuan750004, China*

Abstract: The incorporation of covalent fluorine has been widely used as an effective strategy in medicinal chemistry for drug discovery. The introduction of fluorine into a molecule can significantly influence conformation, lipophilicity, pKa, metabolism, and pharmacokinetic properties. In 1955, the first fluorinated drug fludrocortisone has been approved in the market for the treatment of the adrenogenital syndrome, postural hypotension, and adrenal insufficiency. Since then, 218 small-molecule drugs with at least one fluorine atom have been launched by U.S. FDA by the end of 2018. Therefore, this chapter is expected to summarize the fluorine-containing natural products in clinical development to the medicinal chemistry community.

Keywords: Antiproliferative, Antiviral, Anti-inflammatory, Clinical Development, Drug Discovery, Fluorinated Drug, Medicinal Chemistry, Natural Product, Nucleosides, Small-molecule, Steroids.

1. INTRODUCTION

As alternatives to chloroform for inhaled general anesthetics in 1950s, the potential of fluorine modulating the properties of bioactive compounds was discovered, which could be a common place use in medicinal chemistry. Obviously, the improved understanding of fluorine in medicinal chemistry, synthetic methods and fluorinated building blocks has promoted the utilization of fluorine in modern drug discovery. Up to now, there are a significant number of clinical candidates and marketed natural products containing multiple fluorine substituents conferring different properties and performing different roles [1, 2].

---

* **Corresponding Author Zhenyuan Miao:** School of Pharmacy, Second Military Medical University, 325 Guohe Road, Shanghai, 200433, China; Tel: 02181871241; E-mail: miaozhenyuan@hotmail.com

Atta-ur-Rahman, Shazia Anjum and Hesham Al-Seedi (Eds.)
All rights reserved-© 2020 Bentham Science Publishers

For instance, the fluorinated nucleoside analogue sofosbuvir, was approved in 2013 for treatment of patients with chronic hepatitis C virus [3], while the trifluorinated fluticasone propionate was marketed as an anti-asthma drug targeting glucocorticoid receptor [4].

In this chapter, we discuss impacts of incorporating covalent fluorine into natural products including lipophilicity, pKa, conformational changes, metabolism, and fluorine interaction with molecular targets. A survey of fluorine-containing natural product in marketed drugs and detailed cases of fluorine-containing natural products for different diseases in clinical trials are also summarized.

2. IMPACT OF FLUORINE

Modulation of pK_a may change the bioavailability by affecting the absorption process. In a drug molecule, the pK_a may change the lipophilicity profile due to the pH dependence of the distribution coefficient, which has a close relationship with solubility, permeability, and protein binding. Therefore, pK_a can change the potency, selectivity, toxicity, and pharmacokinetic (PK) properties of a molecule [5 - 8]. Fluorine, the most electronegative element, is commonly used in medicinal chemistry to modulate the pK_a of proximal functionality and the electron density of aromatic or heteroaromatic rings [9 - 11]. In linear aliphatic systems, the influence of fluorine substitution is additive. A prototypic example is provided by the series of β-fluorinated ethylamines with a systematic basicity reduction of ΔpKa ~ -1.7 per fluorine substituent: $CH_3CH_2NH_3^+$ (pKa = 10.7), $CH_2FCH_2NH_3^+$ (pKa = 9.0), $CHF_2CH_2NH_3^+$ (pKa = 7.3), $CF_3CH_2NH_3^+$ (pKa = 5.7). A similar basicity reduction can also be observed in cyclic amines, such as in piperidine, with ΔpKa ~ -1.8 on average for β-fluoropiperidine and ΔpKa ~ -3.7 (~ 2 x -1.8) for β,β-difluoropiperidine. However, for cyclic amines, stereochemical aspects are also important. Thus, the basicity reduction for β-fluorine in axial position is markedly lower (ΔpKa ~ -1.4) than for an equatorial βfluorine substituent (ΔpKa ~ -2.3) [11, 12]. In aromatic/heteroaromatic systems, the effect of fluorine substitution is quite different. The inductive electron-withdrawing effect of fluorine is counterbalanced by a resonance component, which the electron-withdrawing effect is less than chlorine [13 - 15].

In aliphatic systems, fluorination usually decreases the lipophilicity due to its strong electron-withdrawing capabilities [16]. Fluorination of a terminal methyl group typically leading to a reduction in the lipophilicity follows the series mono-fluorination ≈ di-fluorination > tri-fluorination [17]. In aromatic fluorination, the lipophilicity is increased in most cases except some α-fluorinated carbonyl compounds [16].

The steric effect of fluorine is marginal as the atom with a van der Waals radius of 1.47 Å is very close to the 1.20 Å for hydrogen [18 - 20]. Fluorine is the most electronegative element with a Pauling electronegativity of 3.98, which is higher than hydrogen (2.20), oxygen (3.44) and carbon (2.55). Strong electronic modification leads to a highly polarized C−F bond for hyperconjugation. For instance, 1,2-difluoroethane adopt preferentially a *gauche* rather than *anti* conformation. In the *gauche* conformation, the two electronegative fluorine atoms are antiperiplanar to a C–H bond. Hyperconjugative interactions stabilize this conformation by the low-lying C−F σ* orbitals accepting electron density from adjacent C–H σ bonds [21 - 23]. Therefore, fluorine on the carbon atom positioned to another electronegative group may significantly influence conformation and play an important role in lead optimization.

Fluorine is commonly applied to address issues associated with poor metabolic stability because of the strength of the C−F bond [24 - 26]. As a bioisostere, fluorine is frequently included in carbonyl-containing moieties. Fluorine substitution, in both aromatic and aliphatic system, reduces metabolism by decreasing oxidation [24, 27].

In public X-ray crystal structure database, it is found that a close interaction of fluorine with an amide carbonyl is not uncommon [28, 29]. A smaller angle, associated with a closer contact distance, is observed in the C−F to C=O angle, which typically lies between 100° and 140°. The energy of this interaction has been estimated ranging from 0.2 to 0.38 kcal·mol^{-1} [30], which may lead to a dramatic increase in the potency of a compound [31]. It is an issue of continuing debate that fluorine acts as a hydrogen-bond acceptor (HBA) [32 - 37]. Numbers of C−F···H−X close contacts have been crystallographically observed in the Protein Database Bank and the Cambridge Structural Database [32 - 42]. Predictive models have also been used to support fluorine as a weak hydrogen-bond acceptor [34 - 37, 43 - 45]. It is generally acknowledged that the fluorine's HBA capacity is significantly weaker than oxygen and hard to recognize from other dominant forces. Therefore, in most publications, the C−F···H−X interactions are described as either hydrogen bonding or multipolar interaction [12].

3. FLUORINE-CONTAINING DRUGS APPROVED BY THE FDA THAT ARE DERIVED FROM NATURAL PRODUCTS

The first fluorinated drug fludrocortisone was approved to the market for the treatment of the adrenogenital syndrome, postural hypotension, and adrenal insufficiency in 1955. Since then, 218 small-molecule drugs with at least one fluorine atom have been launched by U.S. FDA by the end of 2018 [http://www.fda.gov].

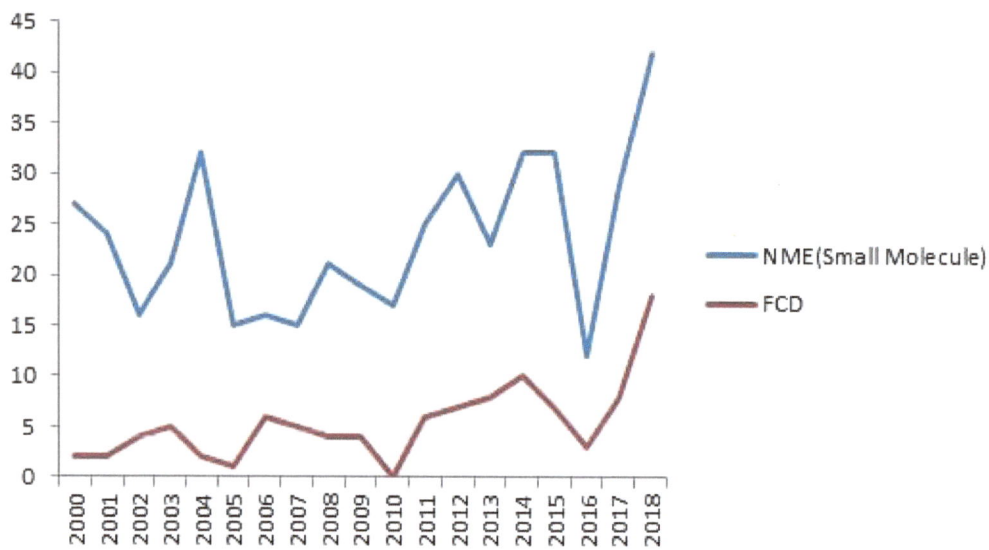

Fig. (1). The annual number of fluorine-containing drugs (FCDs).

The number of new molecule entities (NMEs) has ranged from 10 to 30 per year from 2000 to 2018 (Fig. **1**). During this period, the annual number of fluorine-containing drugs (FCDs) of NMEs followed a similar trend, and in 2018 it reached a maximum level of 18. In total, 102 small-molecule FCDs were approved in the past 19 years with the average percentage of 23.89% among the new molecule entities.

As shown in Fig. (**2**), an increased percentage of FCDs was found from 2006 to 2018 due to increased application of fluorine strategy and the improved synthetic methodologies of organic fluorine compounds. Especially in 2018, 42.86% of the approved NMEs contained fluorine atom in their structures.

Statistically, 51 FDA approved fluorinated drugs are derived from natural products (Figs. **3-7**). Among them, several fluorinated drugs are top-selling products, such as the anti-inflammatory fluorinated steroid luticasone propionate and anti-viral sofosbuvir [https://www.drugs.com/stats/top100]. These fluorinated compounds are derived from steroids (Figs. **3-5**), nucleosides (Fig. **6**), alkaloids, amino acids or prostaglandins (Fig. **7**).

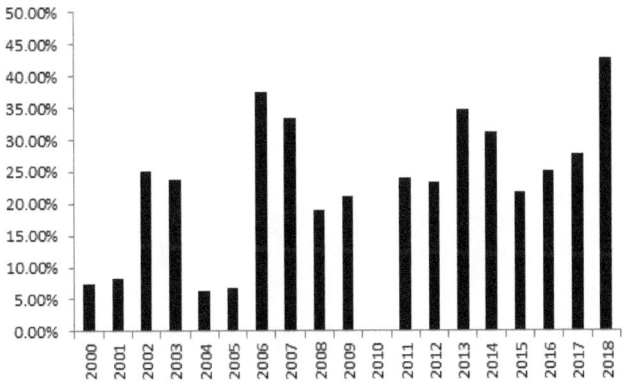

Fig. (2). The percentage fluorine-containing drug in the annual small molecule NMEs.

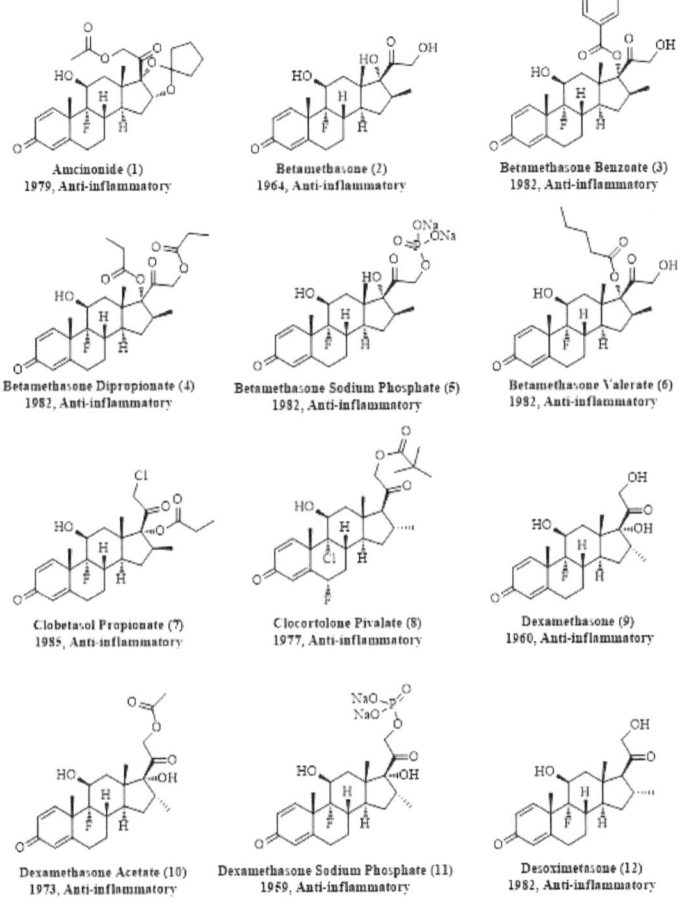

Fig. (3). Fluorinated corticosteroid drugs.

Diflorasone Diacetate (13)
1978, Anti-inflammatory

Difluprednate (14)
2008, Anti-inflammatory

Dutasteride (15)
2001, Anti-prostatic

Fludrocortisone (16)
1955, Mineralocorticoid

Flumethasone Pivalate (17)
1982, Anti-inflammatory

Flunisolide (18)
1984, Anti-inflammatory

Fluocinolone Acetonide (19)
1982, Anti-inflammatory

Fluocinonide (20)
1984, Anti-inflammatory

Fluorometholone Acetate (21)
1986, Anti-inflammatory

Fluorometholone (22)
1982, Antineoplastic

Fluprednisolone (23)
1982, Anti-inflammatory

Flurandrenolide (24)
1963, Anti-inflammatory

Fig. (4). Fluorinated corticosteroid drugs.

Fluticasone Furoate (25)
2007, Glucocorticoid

Fluticasone Propionate (26)
1990, Anti-inflammatory

Fulvestrant (27)
2002, Estrogen antagonist

Halcinonide (28)
1974, Anti-inflammatory

Halobetasol Propionate (29)
1990, Vasoconstrictor agent

Paramethasone Acetate (30)
1982, Anti-inflammatory

Triamcinolone Acetonide (31)
1959, Anti-inflammatory

Triamcinolone Hexacetonide (32)
1969, Anti-inflammatory

Fig. (5). Fluorinated corticosteroid drugs.

3.1. Fluorinated Steroids

It is common for medicinal chemistry community that natural products play valuable role in their direct utilization or the novel lead scaffold [46, 47]. As mentioned in David J. Newman' recent review, 85 small-molecule anticancer drugs (49% of the total approved small molecule in anticancer therapy) were either natural products or derived from natural products from around the 1940s to 2014 [47]. Among the fluorinated pharmaceuticals, a number of the fluorinated steroids shown in (Figs. **3-5**) were launched with anti-cancer and anti-inflammatory properties after the first fluorinated steroid fludrocortisone (**16**) had been discovered with less side-effect [48]. Most of these fluorinated steroids had been approved by FDA before 1990 and these are a few examples of fluorinated steroids currently in service. In this review, we will focus on the drugs launched in the recent years although these fluorinated steroids have played an important role for human health.

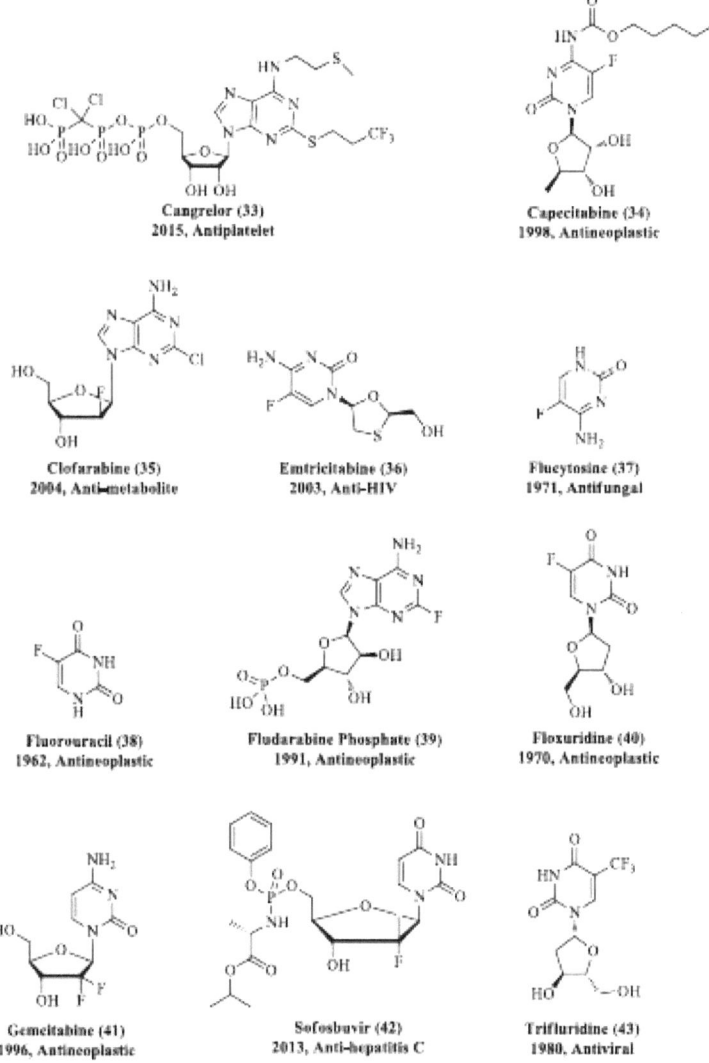

Fig. (6). Fluorinated nucleoside drugs.

Eflornithine (44)
1990, Antineoplastic

Fluciclovine (45)
2016, PET imaging

Fludeoxyglucose F-18 (46)
2004, Diagnostic

Lubiprostone (47)
2006, Opioid-induced constipation

Tafluprost (48)
2012, Ocular hypertension

Travoprost (49)
2001, Antihypertensive

Valrubicin (50)
1998, Antineoplastic

Vorapaxar (51)
2014, Anti-platelet

Fig. (7). Other representative fluorinated nature product derived drugs.

Recently, four steroid drugs, namely, difluprednate (**14**), dutasteride (**15**), fluticasone propionate (**26**) and fulvestrant (**27**), as depicted in (Figs. **4-5**), respectively have entered in market [49 - 52]. Difluprednate (**14**) was approved in 2008 as a fluorinated prednisolone derivative for the treatment of the post-operative ocular inflammation and pain [51, 52]. Dutasteride (**15**) was developed by GlaxoSmithKline as a 5α-reductase inhibitor for the treatment of enlarged prostate. It can decrease the levels of androgen sex hormone dihydrotestosterone

(DHT) in blood [49]. It is structurally different from the other fluorinated steroids with ditrifluoromethylphenyl group in the side chain. Another fluorinated prednisolone derivative, fluticasone propionate (**26**), is used to relieve inflammatory and pruritic symptoms of dermatoses and psoriasis, and is administered orally for the treatment of asthma in combination with salmeterol xinafoate [4]. Fulvestrant (**27**) has been developed as an estrogen receptor antagonist for treating hormone receptor (HR)-positive metastatic breast cancer as a second-line therapy [50]. It has a unique pentafluoro-substituted side chain on the position 7 of the steroid.

These launched fluorinated steroids have a profound impact on the modern pharmaceutical market. Five fluorinated steroids for the treatment of respiratory disorders, urology and oncology have been listed on the top 200 pharmaceutical retail sales in 2016 from the statistics by Njardarson's group from the University of Arizona [http://njardarson.lab.arizona.edu/content/top-pharmaceuticals-poster]. Advair (salmeterol xinafoate and fluticasone propionate), Avodart (dutasteride), Breo Ellipta (fluticasone furonate and vilanterol) and Flovent (fluticasone propionate), were developed by GlaxoSmithKline (GSK) and Faslodex (fulvestrant) was developed AstraZeneca, respectively. Luticasone propionate alone or combined with salmeterol xinafoate made $5.1 billion in sales in 2016 as one of the fluorine-containing blockbuster drugs.

3.2. Fluorinated Nucleosides

Most of nucleoside drugs are developed for the treatment of the diseases closely related with DNA or RNA, such as cancer, fungal and viral infection. Fluorouracil (**38**), the first fluorinated nucleoside drug, was approved in 1962 as the thymidilate synthase inhibitor as depicted in (Fig. **6**). Although fluorouracil has been used for the treatment of numerous cancers, the study of its prodrugs is still a hot field aiming to reduce undesired side effects. For example, capecitabine (**34**) and floxuridine (**40**) were launched in 1998 and 1970 respectively [53, 54]. Capecitabine (**34**), a prodrug of fluorouracil as first-line therapy, is used for the treatment of metastatic colorectal cancer with less side effects. It is an orally administered drug and selectively activated in tumor tissue to obtain the active fluorouracil *via* a three-step enzymatic cascade reaction.

A novel, non-thienopyridine adenosine triphosphate (ATP) fluorinated analogue cangrelor (**33**) has been launched in 2015, which reversibly inhibited the P2Y12 receptor [55]. Cangrelor (**33**) offers potent platelet inhibition and reduces the risk of thrombotic cardiovascular events in patients with coronary artery disease undergoing percutaneous coronary intervention. Furthermore, cangrelor's fast-onset pharmacologic profile is favorable to maintain platelet inhibition in patients requiring premature discontinuation of an oral P2Y12 receptor inhibitor before surgery.

Fluorinated 2',3'-dideoxy-3'-thiacytidine analogue emtricitabine (**36**) was approved by FDA in 2003. Emtricitabine (**36**) competitively inhibits reverse transcriptase and incorporated into nascent viral DNA [56]. It is an orally administered nucleoside drug and uses clinically in combination with other antiretroviral drugs for the treatment of HIV infection. Flucytosine (**37**), a synthetic antimycotic drug, is mechanistically inhibited the synthesis of RNA and DNA. This drug is converted to the metabolite 5-fluorodeoxyuridine *in vivo* [57]. The combinational use of flucytosine (**37**) with the other antifungal drugs is a prevalent therapy for fungal infection owing to its relatively less antifungal efficacy and susceptibility to resistance.

Fludarabine is a 2-fluoro derivative of adenine arabinoside and the added fluorine atom enables it to inhibit adenosine deaminase which is overexpressed in lymphocytes [58, 59]. Fludarabine is used as a single agent or in combination with other drugs for the treatment of chronic lymphocytic leukemia (CCL). The limited solubility and difficulties in its formulation led to the development of fludarabine phosphate as a prodrug. Fludarabine triphosphate (**39**), the active metabolite with cytotoxicity, is formed from fludarabine by deoxycytidine kinase or deoxyguanine kinase *in vivo*.

Except for these fluorine substituents on the uridine, purine and pyrimidine ring, fluorine can be introduced on the ribose of nucleoside. Gemcitabine (2',2'-difluoro-deoxycytidine, **41**) is a fluorinated nucleoside analog approved for the treatment of various solid tumors [60]. It acts as a prodrug being converted to diphosphate and triphosphate by sequential phosphorylation. The gemcitabine diphosphate can inhibit DNA synthesis enzyme ribonucleotide reductase and the triphosphate acted as a deoxycytidine triphosphate-competitive substrate that inhibited DNA chain elongation. Furthermore, gemcitabine is a good radio-sensitizer by a gemcitabine-induced cell-cycle redistribution and depletion of phosphorylated deoxynucleotides [61]. Clofarabine (**35**), a fluorinated nucleoside analogue on the position of ribose, was approved in 2004 as an antimetabolic drug showing good efficacy in the treatment of pediatric, adult lymphoid and myeloid leukemia [62]. Compared with fludarabine, clofarabine exhibits the equivalent pharmacokinetic properties and reduces the potential for dose-limiting toxicity. In December 2013, FDA approved Gilead's new product sofosbuvir (**42**) in combination with other agents for the treatment of chronic hepatitis C virus (HCV). The non-structural protein 5B (NS5B) polymerase inhibitor sofosbuvir (**42**) is orally active fluorinated uridine nucleotide analogue. It metabolizes in the body to the active triphosphate, which is incorporated into the growing HCV ribonucleic acid chain and acts as a chain terminator [63].

Trifluridine (**43**) with a trifluoromethyl group on the uridine is an antiviral drug for the treatment of herpes simplex virus infection in eyes. It is a mechanism-based thymidilate synthase inhibitor, but also a substrate to other enzymes involved in thymidine phosphorylation and DNA incorporation, resulting in cytocidal effects due to DNA strand breaks.

3.3. Other Fluorinated Drugs Derived from Natural Products

Positron emission tomography (PET) is a powerful imaging technique in clinic, providing valuable information for disease diagnosis with radiotracers. The first radiotracer ^{18}F-fluorodeoxyglucose (^{18}F-FDG) [64] was developed for human PET studies in 2004. ^{18}F-FDG (2-deoxy-2-(^{18}F)fluoro-*D*-glucose), with the positron-emitting radionuclide fluorine-18 substituted for the hydroxyl group at C-2 position of the glucose, is widely used to diagnose and monitor the therapeutic effects in patients. However, the false-positives sometimes occur because FDG is a non-specific tumor tracer. The pursuit of the novel small molecule PET drug continued to be booming in drug discovery. Numerous new small molecule PET radiotracers such as ^{11}C-choline [65], ^{13}N-ammonia [66], ^{18}F-florbetapir [67], ^{18}F-florbetaben [68], ^{18}F-flutemetamol [69] and ^{18}F-fluciclovine(**45**) [70] (Fig. **7**) have been approved in the recent decades. Recently, the first example of ^{18}F radiolabeled amino acid derived radiotracers fluciclovine (**45**) was launched by FDA [70]. Fluciclovine (**45**) is useful for detection of recurrent prostate carcinoma due to upregulation of amino acid transport and metabolism in prostate and other cancers. In prostate cancers, fluciclovine PET exhibits more sensitivity, specificity and accuracy than other radiotracers such as ^{111}In-capromab-pendetide, another fluorinated amino acid drug eflornithine (**44**) is specific irreversible ornithine decarboxylase inhibitor and has been used in the chemotherapy and chemoprevention of glioblastoma and colorectal carcinoma [71]. Except for the tumor therapy, it indicates desired result for the treatment of malaria tropica, AIDS, *Pneumocystis jirovecii* infections and *Trypanosoma gambiens*.

Chronic pain affects a number of adults in the world and opioid drugs are commonly used to treat these patients. However, the effectiveness is often limited by side effects, such as constipation. Recently, lubiprostone (**47**) is approved for the treatment of opioid-induced constipation [72]. As a fluorinated prostaglandin E1 derivative, lubiprostone (**47**) activates type 2 chloride channels without any change of the concentration of sodium ion and potassium ion in serum. In the gastrointestinal epithelium cells, Lubiprostone (**47**) selectively activates chloride channels of the apical membrane, leading to an increased fluid secretion. Clinical trials indicates that lubiprostone (**47**) is generally well tolerated and no serious adverse events are observed.

Tafluprost (**48**) is a fluorinated prostaglandin $F_{2\alpha}$ ($PGF_{2\alpha}$) analogue used as an ocular hypotensive drug and exhibits a high and selective binding affinity towards the prostaglandin F receptor [73]. It blocks the metabolic degradation of prostaglandin for the introduction of difluoro substitution. Tafluprost (**48**) is an ester-prodrug facilitating corneal penetration and delivery of the active tafluprost acid to the aqueous humor. Tafluprost (**48**) has a selective affinity for the prostanoid FP receptor, which is 2.8 times higher than latanoprost [74]. Tafluprost (**48**) was approved by FDA in 2012 and used to manipulate the progression of glaucoma for the treatment of ocular hypertension. Travoprost (**49**), another trifluoromethyl substituted prostaglandin analogue, is also an ester-prodrug and can be hydrolysed in the cornea to the biologically metabolic free acid by the esterases [75]. Similar to other $PGF_{2\alpha}$ analogue, such as tafluprost (**48**) and latanoprost, travoprost (**49**) have a greater affinity for the prostaglandin F receptor than latanoprost with increasing outflow of aqueous fluid from the eye and thus cutting down the intraocular pressure.

Valrubicin (**50**) is an N-trifluoroacetyl substituted anthracycline derivative and has been introduced into market in 1998 for bladder cancer therapy [76]. As the second generation anthracycline, valrubicin (**50**) exhibits the highly effective cytostatic effect and results in a reduced proliferation of cancer cells. Vorapaxar (**51**), derived from the natural product himbacine, is a selective and reversible antagonist of the PAR-1 with a long half-life. It inhibits thrombin-induced and thrombin receptor agonist peptide and induces platelet aggregation with a different pathway than other antiplatelet drugs such as aspirin and P2Y12 inhibitors. Vorapaxar (**51**) is used for the patients with a history of myocardial infarction or peripheral arterial disease.

4. FLUORINE-CONTAINING DRUG CANDIDATES DERIVED FROM NATURAL PRODUCTS IN CLINICAL TRIALS

4.1. Overview

From 2008 to 2013, a total of 25 fluorinated drugs derived from natural products have been approved for the treatment of antitumor, antibacterial, antiparasitic and type-2 diabetes [47]. Besides, many fluorinated drugs derived natural products are present in clinic trials and numerous fluorinated candidates are in the drug development [1]. Herein, we summarize these fluorinated molecules which are found with antitumor, antiviral, antimalarial and anti-inflammatory activities [2].

4.2. Antiproliferative Agents

Camptothecin (**52**), a pentacyclic alkaloid isolated from the Chinese tree *Camptotheca acuminate*, shows potent antitumor activities with the mechanism of inhibition of DNA topoisomerase I. Numerous efforts to improve camptothecin pharmacological profile resulted in the discovery of three launched drugs Topotecan, Irinotecan and Belotecan [77 - 80]. Meanwhile, dozens of camptothecin derivatives are in clinical trials under different phases [81 - 86]. Incorporation of fluorine into the camptothecin scaffold has been studied leading to two drug candidates. The water soluble camptothecin derivative exatecan (**53**), fluorinated on the position 11, has been under preclinical evaluation [87] as represented in Table **1** (Clinical trial number: NCT004123). It shows potent antiproliferative activity against a panel of cancer cells including the cancer cells resistant to other camptothecin derivatives. Diflomotecan (**54**), another fluorinated camptothecin derivative with improved stable 7-membered β-hydroxylactone moiety, is currently in phase II (Clinical trial number: NCT008001) [88]. Compared to natural product camptothecin, diflomotecan (**54**) exhibits several advantages, such as increased potency, lower binding to plasma proteins, dual topoisomerase I and II inhibitory activity and reduced toxicity. To investigate the role of fluorine on E-ring, 20-fluorocamptothecin derivatives have been synthesized by the use of Selectfluor or DAST [89]. Unfortunately, these 20-fluorocamptothecin derivatives shows less activity than camptothecin both against cancer cells and the topoisomerase I inhibitory effects. Alternatively, the concept of C=O/C-F bioisosterism has been successfully applied into the E-ring of natural product camptothecin [90, 91]. The novel fluorinated camptothecin derivatives demonstrate potent antitumor activity both *in vitro* and *in vivo* with improved stability in phosphate buffer compared with camptothecin.

Table 1. Representative Fluorine-containing Drug Candidates Derived from Natural Products in Clinical Trials

No.	Natural Product	Fluorinated Derivative	Activity	Clinical Stage
1	Camptothecin (52)	Exatecan (53)	Antiproliferative	Phase III

(Table 1) cont.....

No.	Natural Product	Fluorinated Derivative	Activity	Clinical Stage
2	Camptothecin (52)	Diflomotecan (54)	Antiproliferative	Phase II
3	Vinblastine (55)	Vinflunine (56)	Antiproliferative	Phase III
4	Paclitaxel (57)	4FDT (58)	Antiproliferative	Preclinical
5	Epothilone B (59)	Iso-fludelone (60)	Antiproliferative	Phase I
6	Cytidine (61)	Tezacitabine (62)	Antiproliferative	Phase III
7	Cytidine (61)	Elvucitabine (63)	Antiviral	Phase III

(Table 1) cont.....

No.	Natural Product	Fluorinated Derivative	Activity	Clinical Stage
8	Purine (64)	Alamifovir (65)	Antiviral	Phase II
9	Erythromycin (66)	Solithromycin (67)	Antibiotic	Phase II
10	Vitamin D3 (68)	Elocalcitol (69)	Benign prostatic hyperplasia	Phase II
11	Dehydroepiandrosterone (70)	Fluasterone (71)	Carcinogenesis prevention	Phase II
12	Pregnanolone (72)	CCD-3693 (73)	Sedative-hypnotic	Phase II

Vincristine and vinblastine (**55**) are two dimeric indole-based alkaloids isolated from *Vinca rosea* and indicated noteworthy antitumor activities. These vinca alkaloids interact with tubulin and inhibit polymerization, thus impairing microtubule function as antimitotic agents. Although vinblastine and its analogue vinorelbine have been marketed for cancer therapies, great efforts are still being taken to find new efficacious drugs [92 - 94]. For example, fluorine substitution was introduced and led to difluorodihydrovinorelbine named as vinflunine (**56**) [94]. It shows reduced anticancer activity and microtubule binding than vinblastine *in vitro*. In the *in vivo* assay, increased antitumor activities and depressed cancer cell resistance are observed. Studies have shown that the presence of *gem*-difluoro moiety may be responsible for decreased multidrug resistance because of its hindrance effect of the substrate of P-glycoprotein mediated drug efflux. Encouraged by its broad-spectrum utility and enhanced therapeutic index, vinflunine (**56**) has been advanced into the phase III stage with a single agent or combination with other antineoplastic agents at lower dose (Clinical trial number: NCT0195300).

Paclitaxel (**57**) is another well-known active natural product discovered by Wani and Wall in 1971. Eight years later, Horowitz described its novel mechanism of promoting microtubule polymerization. To date, three NCEs (paclitaxel, docetaxel and cabazitaxel) have been approved for the treatment of various cancers [95 - 97]. These drugs are mainly metabolized in the liver and hydroxylation at the C-3' phenyl and C2 benzoate moiety are the two major metabolic transformations. Thus, fluorine has been introduced to investigate the influences of biological activity for the steric hindrance of oxidative metabolism reaction [98]. Unsurprisingly, the improved activities against a human breast cancer cell are observed compared with paclitaxel and docetaxel. In addition, these fluorinated derivatives exhibit potent activities against multidrug resistant cell lines while both paclitaxel and docetaxel indicated less effect. 4FDT (**58**), one of the fluorinated paclitaxel derivatives with fluorine substitution on meta-position of the C-2 phenyl ring and replacement of one methyl group of the N-ter--butoxycarbonyl unit by a trifluoromethyl group, has shown improved stability. The drug is now under preclinical evaluation for the treatment of hepatocellular carcinoma.

Epothilones (**59**) are a novel class of cytotoxic macrolides isolated from a mycobacterium with similar antitumor activities of clinical taxoids *via* the same mechanism. In contrast to natural taxoids, epothilones indicate remarkable antitumor effects against multidrug resistant cell lines including paclitaxel resistant cell lines [99, 100]. A detailed SAR analysis realizes that the C12/C13 epoxide is a nonessential pharmacophore, leading to the discovery of synthetic derivative desoxyepothilone B with an excellent therapeutic index. The incorporation of both C9/C10 and C12/C13 alkene moieties in epothilone B scaffold results in a significant increase in potency. Iso-fludelone (**60**), its trifluorinated analogue, exhibits an attenuated cytotoxicity and improved stability against metabolic oxidation of the C12/C13 double bond [101]. Compared to former generations of epothilones, the third-generation epothilone B analogue (iso-fludelone, **60**) exhibits increased stability and reduced toxicity and now is under phase I clinical evaluation in patients with advanced solid tumors (Clinical trial number: NCT0137928).

Tezacitabine (**62**) is one of the fluoromethylene deoxycytidine analogues rationally designed as a ribonucleotide reductase inhibitor [102]. It is phosphorylated in cells by the deoxycytidine kinase to generate the diphosphate and triphosphate, then forms the irreversible covalent adduct with the ribonucleotide reductase. A high antiproliferative activity is exhibited and synergistically with the diphosphate and triphosphate products *in vivo*. Tezacitabine (**62**) is now currently in phase III evaluation for the treatment of solid tumors and hematopoietic malignancies.

4.3. Antimicrobial Agents

Nucleoside reverse transcriptase inhibitors are a class of antiretroviral drugs used to treat human immunodeficiency virus (HIV) and in some cases hepatitis B virus (HBV) infection. These drugs are preferred as the first-line drugs because of their long intracellular half-life and high oral bioavailability [103]. However, continuous treatment leads to mutations in reverse transcriptase and causes resistance and cross-resistance to agents. Moreover, these nucleoside reverse transcriptase inhibitors are associated with bone marrow suppression and high mitochondrial toxicity [104]. Elvucitabine (**63**) is a new fluorinated cytidine (**61**) analogue and showed potent antiviral activity [105]. A phase II trial indicates similar efficacy and safety profile in patients compared to an antiretroviral drug lamivudine that is the standard therapy for chronic carriers of the virus. Now elvucitabine is in phase III evaluation for the treatment of HIV and HBV infection.

Alamifovir (**65**) is a bis(trifluoroethoxy) phosphonate purine nucleotide analogue and shows to be active against wild-type as well as lamivudine-resistant HBV [106]. Alamifovir (**65**) is a prodrug and quickly hydrolyzs to its active metabolites monoester, O-desmethyl and free acid with antiviral activity. Compared to reverse transcriptase inhibitors currently in use, compound **65** appears to be a novel mechanism which inhibits the protein priming and the packaging reaction and leads to decrease HBV replication. A phase I trial indicated that alamifovir (**65**) has potent anti-HBV activity with a favorable safety profile and thereby entered into phase II development.

Solithromycin (also named as CEM-101, **67**), a novel fluoroketolide, is under the phase III development for the treatment of community-acquired bacterial pneumonia (CABP) in both intravenous and oral formulations [107]. Solithromycin (**67**) has three ribosomal binding sites instead of two sites on the ribosome of telithromycin. The fluorine at C-2 of solithromycin (**67**) offers the additional binding with increased antimicrobial effectiveness. The structural modifications can improve its ribosomal binding activity and decrease its tendency to known macrolide resistance mechanisms. Solithromycin (**67**) exhibits potent activities against all of the common CABP pathogens *in vitro*, such as macrolide-, penicillin-, and fluoroquinolone-resistant *S. Pneumoniae*, *Haemophilus influenzae* and atypical bacterial pathogens. Compared with levofloxacin and moxifloxacin, solithromycin (**67**) in oral or intravenous demonstrates similar treatment effects in the intention-to-treat patients and may be developed as the fourth-generation macrolides antibiotics.

4.4. Anti-inflammatory Agents

Benign prostatic hyperplasia (BPH) is a disease of urinary system which is a common condition of older people. A gradually increasing prostate gland can cause severe problems of bladder, urinary tract or kidney. The standard medical treatments are selective α1-adrenergic receptor blockers and 5α reductase inhibitors. Recently, it has been shown that vitamin D3 (**68**) receptor agonists indicated the decrease of prostate cell proliferation. A fluorinated vitamin D3 derivative elocalcitol (**69**), also named as BXL-628, reduces prostate volume by the inhibition activity of vitamin D receptor [108]. It inhibits the prostatic growth factors activity, decreases BPH cell proliferation and induces apoptosis without directly acting on the androgen receptor. Thus, elocalcitol (**69**) does not affect sexual function and may represent a novel strategy for the drug development. Now it is in phase II evaluation for the treatment of BPH.

4.5. Miscellaneous

As a natural steroid precursor of androstenedione, dehydroepiandrosterone (**70**) shows antiaging, metabolic and immune-modulating activities. However, its application has been limited because of its side effects of potent hormonal activity. Enormous effort has been made for reducing the undesirable effects. Among them, a synthetic dehydroepiandrosterone analog 16α-fluoro-5-andros-en-17-one is found with decreased adverse hormonal effects of dehydroepiandrosterone (**70**) and indicates the medical treatment in the prevention of mammary and colon carcinogenesis [109]. Except for these cancers, the fluorinated dehydroepiandrosterone analog fluasterone (**71**) exhibits significant protection against human prostate carcinogenesis with less androgenic activity than dehydroepiandrosterone (**70**).

Insomnia is a sleep disorder and resulting in several social problems such as reduced workplace productivity, increased risk of industrial accidents and motor vehicle accidents. The effort to discover desired sedative-hypnotic therapeutics without the side effects of current barbiturates and benzodiazepines is still continued. Recently, the fluorinated neuroactive steroid CCD-3693 (**73**) is found to quickly suppress operant response after oral administration which is similar to the observation of clinically active sedative-hypnotic zolpidem [110]. The preclinical data indicated CCD-3693 (**73**) promotes non-rapid eye movement which is the desired characteristics of novel sedative-hypnotic therapeutic drugs. In addition, CCD-3693 (**73**) exhibits more intrinsically potent in non-rapid eye movement sleep promotion than the endogenous pregnanolone (**72**) without the interference of rapid eye movement sleep and selectively reduces electroencephalogram-defined sleeplessness. Compared with barbiturates and other hypnotics, CCD-3693 (**73**) increases duration of sleep without impacting on the natural status and exhibits clinical advantages for the development of sedative-hypnotic therapeutics.

CONCLUSIONS AND PERSPECTIVES

It is well recognized that nature provides numerous active natural products as efficient lead compounds for further drug development. The introduction of fluorine into lead compound is a successful strategy in drug design and a large number of fluorinated small molecules derived from natural products have advanced to pharmaceutical market for the treatment of cancer, viral and bacterial infection [111, 112]. This important progress promotes the continued use of strategy of fluorine incorporation in drug discovery and development of efficient synthetic methods in fluorine organic chemistry. Fluorine has several impacts on natural products including lipophilicity, pKa, conformational changes, metabolism, and fluorine interaction with molecular targets. However, great endeavor should be stimulated for the understanding of fluorine strategy in medicinal chemistry field. For example, based on the structures of the fluorinated drugs derived from natural products, there are few drugs with five or more fluorine atoms. It is still unclear that how many fluorine atoms are tolerated in the modification of active natural products. Additionally, there is an ongoing debate on the weak hydrogen-bond interactions between the fluorine and targets. More evidence should be explored and provided. In summary, as highlighted in this chapter, the future trend of fluorine in drug discovery derived from natural products will continue to be of great importance.

CONSENT FOR PUBLICATION

Not applicable.

CONFLICT OF INTEREST

The author confirms that this chapter contents have no conflict of interest.

ACKNOWLEDGEMENT

We gratefully acknowledge the support of our program by the National Natural Science Foundation of China (81673352 and 81872791).

REFERENCES

[1] Thomas CJ. Fluorinated natural products with clinical significance. Curr Top Med Chem 2006; 6(14): 1529-43.
[http://dx.doi.org/10.2174/156802606777951109] [PMID: 16918466]

[2] Bégué J-P, Bonnet-Delpon D. Recent advances (1995–2005) in fluorinated pharmaceuticals based on natural products. J Fluor Chem 2006; 127(8): 992-1012.
[http://dx.doi.org/10.1016/j.jfluchem.2006.05.006]

[3] Childs-Kean LM, Hand EO. Simeprevir and sofosbuvir for treatment of chronic hepatitis C infection. Clin Ther 2015; 37(2): 243-67.
[http://dx.doi.org/10.1016/j.clinthera.2014.12.012] [PMID: 25601269]

[4] Papi A, Blasi F, Canonica GW, *et al.* Fluticasone propionate/formoterol: a fixed-combination therapy with flexible dosage. Eur J Intern Med 2014; 25(8): 695-700.
[http://dx.doi.org/10.1016/j.ejim.2014.06.022] [PMID: 25051902]

[5] Meanwell NA. Improving drug candidates by design: a focus on physicochemical properties as a means of improving compound disposition and safety. Chem Res Toxicol 2011; 24(9): 1420-56.
[http://dx.doi.org/10.1021/tx200211v] [PMID: 21790149]

[6] Hopkins AL, Keserü GM, Leeson PD, Rees DC, Reynolds CH. The role of ligand efficiency metrics in drug discovery. Nat Rev Drug Discov 2014; 13(2): 105-21.
[http://dx.doi.org/10.1038/nrd4163] [PMID: 24481311]

[7] Wager TT, Kormos BL, Brady JT, *et al.* Improving the odds of success in drug discovery: choosing the best compounds for *in vivo* toxicology studies. J Med Chem 2013; 56(23): 9771-9.
[http://dx.doi.org/10.1021/jm401485p] [PMID: 24219752]

[8] Tarcsay Á, Keserü GM. Contributions of molecular properties to drug promiscuity. J Med Chem 2013; 56(5): 1789-95.
[http://dx.doi.org/10.1021/jm301514n] [PMID: 23356819]

[9] Shah P, Westwell AD. The role of fluorine in medicinal chemistry. J Enzyme Inhib Med Chem 2007; 22(5): 527-40.
[http://dx.doi.org/10.1080/14756360701425014] [PMID: 18035820]

[10] Alabugin IV, Zeidan TA. Stereoelectronic effects and general trends in hyperconjugative acceptor ability of sigma bonds. J Am Chem Soc 2002; 124(12): 3175-85.
[http://dx.doi.org/10.1021/ja012633z] [PMID: 11902907]

[11] Morgenthaler M, Schweizer E, Hoffmann-Röder A, *et al.* Predicting and tuning physicochemical properties in lead optimization: amine basicities. ChemMedChem 2007; 2(8): 1100-15.
[http://dx.doi.org/10.1002/cmdc.200700059] [PMID: 17530727]

[12] Gillis EP, Eastman KJ, Hill MD, Donnelly DJ, Meanwell NA. Applications of fluorine in medicinal chemistry. J Med Chem 2015; 58(21): 8315-59.
[http://dx.doi.org/10.1021/acs.jmedchem.5b00258] [PMID: 26200936]

[13] Hansch C, Leo A, Unger SH, Kim KH, Nikaitani D, Lien EJ. "Aromatic" substituent constants for structure-activity correlations. J Med Chem 1973; 16(11): 1207-16.
[http://dx.doi.org/10.1021/jm00269a003] [PMID: 4747963]

[14] Corwin. Hansch, A. Leo, Taft RW. A survey of hammett substituent constants and resonance and field parameters. Chem Rev 1991; 91(2): 165-95.

[http://dx.doi.org/10.1021/cr00002a004]

[15] Iwasa J, Fujita T, Hansch C. Substituent constants for aliphatic functions obtained from partition coefficients. J Med Chem 1965; 8: 150-3.
[http://dx.doi.org/10.1021/jm00326a002] [PMID: 14332653]

[16] Smart E. Fluorine Substituent Effects B. (on bioactivity). J Fluor Chem 2001; 109(1): 3-11.
[http://dx.doi.org/10.1016/S0022-1139(01)00375-X]

[17] Huchet QA, Kuhn B, Wagner B, Fischer H, Kansy M, Zimmerli D, *et al.* On the polarity of partially fluorinated methyl groups. J Fluor Chem 2013; 152: 119-28.
[http://dx.doi.org/10.1016/j.jfluchem.2013.02.023]

[18] Böhm HJ, Banner D, Bendels S, *et al.* Fluorine in medicinal chemistry. ChemBioChem 2004; 5(5): 637-43.
[http://dx.doi.org/10.1002/cbic.200301023] [PMID: 15122635]

[19] O'Hagan D. Understanding organofluorine chemistry. An introduction to the C-F bond. Chem Soc Rev 2008; 37(2): 308-19.
[http://dx.doi.org/10.1039/B711844A] [PMID: 18197347]

[20] Raatikainen K, Cametti M, Rissanen K. The subtle balance of weak supramolecular interactions: The hierarchy of halogen and hydrogen bonds in haloanilinium and halopyridinium salts. Beilstein J Org Chem 2010; 6(4): 4.
[http://dx.doi.org/10.3762/bjoc.6.4] [PMID: 20502514]

[21] Purser S, Moore PR, Swallow S, Gouverneur V. Fluorine in medicinal chemistry. Chem Soc Rev 2008; 37(2): 320-30.
[http://dx.doi.org/10.1039/B610213C] [PMID: 18197348]

[22] Buissonneaud DY, Mourik T, O'Hagan D. A DFT Study on the origin of the fluorine gauche effect in substituted fluoroethanes. Tetrahedron 2010; 66(12): 2196-202.
[http://dx.doi.org/10.1016/j.tet.2010.01.049]

[23] O'Hagan D. Organofluorine chemistry: synthesis and conformation of vicinal fluoromethylene motifs. J Org Chem 2012; 77(8): 3689-99.
[http://dx.doi.org/10.1021/jo300044q] [PMID: 22404655]

[24] Park BK, Kitteringham NR, O'Neill PM. Metabolism of fluorine-containing drugs. Annu Rev Pharmacol Toxicol 2001; 41: 443-70.
[http://dx.doi.org/10.1146/annurev.pharmtox.41.1.443] [PMID: 11264465]

[25] Gleeson P, Bravi G, Modi S, Lowe D. ADMET rules of thumb II: A comparison of the effects of common substituents on a range of ADMET parameters. Bioorg Med Chem 2009; 17(16): 5906-19.
[http://dx.doi.org/10.1016/j.bmc.2009.07.002] [PMID: 19632124]

[26] Dossetter AG. A statistical analysis of *in vitro* human microsomal metabolic stability of small phenyl group substituents, leading to improved design sets for parallel SAR exploration of a chemical series. Bioorg Med Chem 2010; 18(12): 4405-14.
[http://dx.doi.org/10.1016/j.bmc.2010.04.077] [PMID: 20510621]

[27] Park BK, Kitteringham NR. Effects of fluorine substitution on drug metabolism: pharmacological and toxicological implications. Drug Metab Rev 1994; 26(3): 605-43.
[http://dx.doi.org/10.3109/03602539408998319] [PMID: 7924905]

[28] Fischer FR, Schweizer WB, Diederich F. Molecular torsion balances: evidence for favorable orthogonal dipolar interactions between organic fluorine and amide groups. Angew Chem Int Ed Engl 2007; 46(43): 8270-3.
[http://dx.doi.org/10.1002/anie.200702497] [PMID: 17899581]

[29] Paulini R, Müller K, Diederich F. Orthogonal multipolar interactions in structural chemistry and biology. Angew Chem Int Ed Engl 2005; 44(12): 1788-805.
[http://dx.doi.org/10.1002/anie.200462213] [PMID: 15706577]

[30]   Hof F, Scofield DM, Schweizer WB, Diederich F. A weak attractive interaction between organic fluorine and an amide group. Angew Chem Int Ed Engl 2004; 43(38): 5056-9.
[http://dx.doi.org/10.1002/anie.200460781] [PMID: 15384111]

[31]   Schweizer E, Hoffmann-Röder A, Olsen JA, *et al.* Multipolar interactions in the D pocket of thrombin: large differences between tricyclic imide and lactam inhibitors. Org Biomol Chem 2006; 4(12): 2364-75.
[http://dx.doi.org/10.1039/B602585D] [PMID: 16763681]

[32]   Dunitz JD, Taylor R. Organic Fluorine Hardly Ever Accepts Hydrogen Bonds. Chemistry 1997; 3(1): 89-98.
[http://dx.doi.org/10.1002/chem.19970030115]

[33]   Dunitz JD. Organic fluorine: odd man out. ChemBioChem 2004; 5(5): 614-21.
[http://dx.doi.org/10.1002/cbic.200300801] [PMID: 15122632]

[34]   Dalvit C, Vulpetti A. Intermolecular and intramolecular hydrogen bonds involving fluorine atoms: implications for recognition, selectivity, and chemical properties. ChemMedChem 2012; 7(2): 262-72.
[http://dx.doi.org/10.1002/cmdc.201100483] [PMID: 22262517]

[35]   Schneider H-J. Hydrogen bonds with fluorine. Studies in solution, in gas phase and by computations, conflicting conclusions from crystallographic analyses. Chem Sci (Camb) 2012; 3(5): 1381-94.
[http://dx.doi.org/10.1039/c2sc00764a]

[36]   Champagne PA, Desroches J, Paquin J-F. Organic Fluorine as a Hydrogen-Bond Acceptor: Recent Examples and Applications. Synthesis 2014; 47(3): 306-22.
[http://dx.doi.org/10.1055/s-0034-1379537]

[37]   Dalvit C, Invernizzi C, Vulpetti A. Fluorine as a hydrogen-bond acceptor: experimental evidence and computational calculations. Chemistry 2014; 20(35): 11058-68.
[http://dx.doi.org/10.1002/chem.201402858] [PMID: 25044441]

[38]   Müller K, Faeh C, Diederich F. Fluorine in pharmaceuticals: looking beyond intuition. Science 2007; 317(5846): 1881-6.
[http://dx.doi.org/10.1126/science.1131943] [PMID: 17901324]

[39]   Seddon KR. Critical Evaluation of C-H···X Hydrogen Bonding in the Crystalline State. Cryst Growth Des 2003; 3(5): 643-61.
[http://dx.doi.org/10.1021/cg034083h]

[40]   Carosati E, Sciabola S, Cruciani G. Hydrogen bonding interactions of covalently bonded fluorine atoms: from crystallographic data to a new angular function in the GRID force field. J Med Chem 2004; 47(21): 5114-25.
[http://dx.doi.org/10.1021/jm0498349] [PMID: 15456255]

[41]   Oria ED, Novoa JJ. On the hydrogen bond nature of the C-H...F interactions in molecular crystals. An exhaustive investigation combining a crystallographic database search and ab initio theoretical calculations. CrystEngComm 2008; 10(4): 423-36.
[http://dx.doi.org/10.1039/b717276c]

[42]   Zhou P, Zou J, Tian F, Shang Z. Fluorine bonding how does it work in protein-ligand interactions? J Chem Inf Model 2009; 49(10): 2344-55.
[http://dx.doi.org/10.1021/ci9002393] [PMID: 19788294]

[43]   Ouvrard C, Berthelot M, Laurence C. The first basicity scale of fluoro-, chloro-, bromo- and iodo-alkanes: Some Cross-comparisons with Simple Alkyl Derivatives of Other Elements. J Chem Soc, Perkin Trans 2 1999; 0(7)
[http://dx.doi.org/10.1039/a901867k]

[44]   Laurence C, Berthelot M. Observations on the strength of hydrogen bonding. Perspect Drug Discov Des 2000; 18(1): 39-60.
[http://dx.doi.org/10.1023/A:1008743229409]

[45] Laurence C, Brameld KA, Graton J, Le Questel JY, Renault E. The pK(BHX) database: toward a better understanding of hydrogen-bond basicity for medicinal chemists. J Med Chem 2009; 52(14): 4073-86.
[http://dx.doi.org/10.1021/jm801331y] [PMID: 19537797]

[46] Butler MS. Natural products to drugs: natural product-derived compounds in clinical trials. Nat Prod Rep 2008; 25(3): 475-516.
[http://dx.doi.org/10.1039/b514294f] [PMID: 18497896]

[47] Newman DJ, Cragg GM. Natural products as sources of new drugs from 1981 to 2014. J Nat Prod 2016; 79(3): 629-61.
[http://dx.doi.org/10.1021/acs.jnatprod.5b01055] [PMID: 26852623]

[48] Fried J, Sabo EF. 9α-Fluoro derivatives of cortisone and hydrocortisone. J Am Chem Soc 1954; 76(5): 1455-6.
[http://dx.doi.org/10.1021/ja01634a101]

[49] van Leeuwen PJ, Kölble K, Huland H, Hambrock T, Barentsz J, Schröder FH. Prostate cancer detection and dutasteride: utility and limitations of prostate-specific antigen in men with previous negative biopsies. Eur Urol 2011; 59(2): 183-90.
[http://dx.doi.org/10.1016/j.eururo.2010.09.035] [PMID: 21130560]

[50] Robertson JF, Lindemann J, Garnett S, *et al*. A good drug made better: the fulvestrant dose-response story. Clin Breast Cancer 2014; 14(6): 381-9.
[http://dx.doi.org/10.1016/j.clbc.2014.06.005] [PMID: 25457991]

[51] Hagan DO. Fluorine in health care: organofluorine containing blockbuster drugs. J Fluor Chem 2010; 131(11): 1071-81.
[http://dx.doi.org/10.1016/j.jfluchem.2010.03.003]

[52] Jasem YA, Thiemann T, Gano L, Oliveira MC. Fluorinated steroids and their derivatives. J Fluor Chem 2016; 185: 48-85.
[http://dx.doi.org/10.1016/j.jfluchem.2016.03.009]

[53] Robak P, Robak T. Older and new purine nucleoside analogs for patients with acute leukemias. Cancer Treat Rev 2013; 39(8): 851-61.
[http://dx.doi.org/10.1016/j.ctrv.2013.03.006] [PMID: 23566572]

[54] Pankiewicz KW. Fluorinated nucleosides. Carbohydr Res 2000; 327(1-2): 87-105.
[http://dx.doi.org/10.1016/S0008-6215(00)00089-6] [PMID: 10968677]

[55] Qamar A, Bhatt DL. Current status of data on cangrelor. Pharmacol Ther 2016; 159: 102-9.
[http://dx.doi.org/10.1016/j.pharmthera.2016.01.004] [PMID: 26802900]

[56] Kabbara WK, Ramadan WH. Emtricitabine/rilpivirine/tenofovir disoproxil fumarate for the treatment of HIV-1 infection in adults. J Infect Public Health 2015; 8(5): 409-17.
[http://dx.doi.org/10.1016/j.jiph.2015.04.020] [PMID: 26001757]

[57] Fang XF, Li D, Tangadanchu VKR, Gopala L, Gao WW, Zhou CH. Novel potentially antifungal hybrids of 5-flucytosine and fluconazole: Design, synthesis and bioactive evaluation. Bioorg Med Chem Lett 2017; 27(22): 4964-9.
[http://dx.doi.org/10.1016/j.bmcl.2017.10.020] [PMID: 29050784]

[58] Astrow AB. Fludarabine in chronic leukaemia. Lancet 1996; 347(9013): 1420-1.
[http://dx.doi.org/10.1016/S0140-6736(96)91675-X] [PMID: 8676619]

[59] Clercq E. Milestones in the discovery of antiviral agents: nucleosides and nucleotides. Acta Pharm Sin B 2012; 2(6): 535-48.
[http://dx.doi.org/10.1016/j.apsb.2012.10.001]

[60] Bastiancich C, Bastiat G, Lagarce F. Gemcitabine and glioblastoma: challenges and current perspectives. Drug Discov Today 2018; 23(2): 416-23.

[http://dx.doi.org/10.1016/j.drudis.2017.10.010] [PMID: 29074439]

[61]   Shewach DS, Lawrence TS. Gemcitabine and radiosensitization in human tumor cells. Invest New Drugs 1996; 14(3): 257-63.
       [http://dx.doi.org/10.1007/BF00194528] [PMID: 8958180]

[62]   Ghanem H, Jabbour E, Faderl S, Ghandhi V, Plunkett W, Kantarjian H. Clofarabine in leukemia. Expert Rev Hematol 2010; 3(1): 15-22.
       [http://dx.doi.org/10.1586/ehm.09.70] [PMID: 21082931]

[63]   Mangia A, Piazzolla V. Overall efficacy and safety results of sofosbuvir-based therapies in phase II and III studies. Dig Liver Dis 2014; 46 (Suppl. 5): S179-85.
       [http://dx.doi.org/10.1016/j.dld.2014.09.026] [PMID: 25458780]

[64]   Schuster DM, Nanni C, Fanti S. PET tracers beyond FDG in prostate cancer. Semin Nucl Med 2016; 46(6): 507-21.
       [http://dx.doi.org/10.1053/j.semnuclmed.2016.07.005] [PMID: 27825431]

[65]   Huang Z, Rui J, Li X, Meng X, Liu Q. Use of ^{11}C-Choline positron emission tomography/computed tomography to investigate the mechanism of choline metabolism in lung cancer. Mol Med Rep 2015; 11(5): 3285-90.
       [http://dx.doi.org/10.3892/mmr.2015.3200] [PMID: 25591716]

[66]   Kawaguchi N, Okayama H, Kawamura G, *et al.* Clinical usefulness of coronary flow reserve ratio for the detection of significant coronary artery disease on ^{13}N-Ammonia positron emission tomography. Circ J 2018; 82(2): 486-93.
       [http://dx.doi.org/10.1253/circj.CJ-17-0745] [PMID: 28954967]

[67]   Renard D, Collombier L, Demattei C, *et al.* Cerebrospinal fluid, MRI, and florbetaben-PET in cerebral amyloid angiopathy-related inflammation. J Alzheimers Dis 2018; 61(3): 1107-17.
       [http://dx.doi.org/10.3233/JAD-170843] [PMID: 29254099]

[68]   Kang K, Yoon U, Hong J, *et al.* Amyloid deposits and idiopathic normal-pressure hydrocephalus: an 18F-Florbetaben study. Eur Neurol 2018; 79(3-4): 192-9.
       [http://dx.doi.org/10.1159/000487133] [PMID: 29566389]

[69]   de Lartigue J. Flutemetamol (18F): a β-amyloid positron emission tomography tracer for Alzheimer's and dementia diagnosis. Drugs Today (Barc) 2014; 50(3): 219-29.
       [http://dx.doi.org/10.1358/dot.2014.050.03.2116672] [PMID: 24696867]

[70]   Yang W, Zhang Y, Fu Z, *et al.* Imaging of proliferation with 18F-FLT PET/CT *versus* 18F-FDG PET/CT in non-small-cell lung cancer. Eur J Nucl Med Mol Imaging 2010; 37(7): 1291-9.
       [http://dx.doi.org/10.1007/s00259-010-1412-6] [PMID: 20309686]

[71]   Burke CA, Dekker E, Samadder NJ, Stoffel E, Cohen A. Efficacy and safety of eflornithine (CPP-1X)/sulindac combination therapy *versus* each as monotherapy in patients with familial adenomatous polyposis (FAP): design and rationale of a randomized, double-blind, Phase III trial. BMC Gastroenterol 2016; 16(1): 87.
       [http://dx.doi.org/10.1186/s12876-016-0494-4] [PMID: 27480131]

[72]   Jamal MM, Adams AB, Jansen JP, Webster LR. A randomized, placebo-controlled trial of lubiprostone for opioid-induced constipation in chronic noncancer pain. Am J Gastroenterol 2015; 110(5): 725-32.
       [http://dx.doi.org/10.1038/ajg.2015.106] [PMID: 25916220]

[73]   Takagi Y, Nakajima T, Shimazaki A, *et al.* Pharmacological characteristics of AFP-168 (tafluprost), a new prostanoid FP receptor agonist, as an ocular hypotensive drug. Exp Eye Res 2004; 78(4): 767-76.
       [http://dx.doi.org/10.1016/j.exer.2003.12.007] [PMID: 15037111]

[74]   Pantcheva MB, Seibold LK, Awadallah NS, Kahook MY. Tafluprost: a novel prostaglandin analog for treatment of glaucoma. Adv Ther 2011; 28(9): 707-15.
       [http://dx.doi.org/10.1007/s12325-011-0055-8] [PMID: 21858491]

[75] Cheng JW, Xi GL, Wei RL, Cai JP, Li Y. Effects of travoprost in the treatment of open-angle glaucoma or ocular hypertension: A systematic review and meta-analysis. Curr Ther Res Clin Exp 2009; 70(4): 335-50.
[http://dx.doi.org/10.1016/j.curtheres.2009.08.006] [PMID: 24683242]

[76] Hajian R, Hossaini P, Mehrayin Z, Woi PM, Shams N. DNA-binding studies of valrubicin as a chemotherapy drug using spectroscopy and electrochemical techniques. J Pharm Anal 2017; 7(3): 176-80.
[http://dx.doi.org/10.1016/j.jpha.2017.01.003] [PMID: 29404035]

[77] Chazin EdeL, Reis RdaR, Junior WT, Moor LF, Vasconcelos TR. An overview on the development of new potentially active camptothecin analogs against cancer. Mini Rev Med Chem 2014; 14(12): 953-62.
[http://dx.doi.org/10.2174/1389557514666141029233037] [PMID: 25355593]

[78] Zhu L, Zhuang C, Lei N, *et al.* Synthesis and preliminary bioevaluation of novel E-ring modified acetal analog of camptothecin as cytotoxic agents. Eur J Med Chem 2012; 56: 1-9.
[http://dx.doi.org/10.1016/j.ejmech.2012.07.050] [PMID: 23084702]

[79] Prijovich ZM, Burnouf PA, Chou HC, *et al.* Synthesis and antitumor properties of BQC-glucuronide, a camptothecin prodrug for selective tumor activation. Mol Pharm 2016; 13(4): 1242-50.
[http://dx.doi.org/10.1021/acs.molpharmaceut.5b00771] [PMID: 26824303]

[80] Wang L, Xie S, Ma L, Chen Y, Lu W. 10-Boronic acid substituted camptothecin as prodrug of SN-38. Eur J Med Chem 2016; 116: 84-9.
[http://dx.doi.org/10.1016/j.ejmech.2016.03.063] [PMID: 27060760]

[81] Wall ME, Wani MC. Camptothecin and taxol: discovery to clinic--thirteenth Bruce F. Cain Memorial Award Lecture. Cancer Res 1995; 55(4): 753-60.
[PMID: 7850785]

[82] Huang M, Gao H, Chen Y, *et al.* Chimmitecan, a novel 9-substituted camptothecin, with improved anticancer pharmacologic profiles *in vitro* and *in vivo.* Clin Cancer Res 2007; 13(4): 1298-307.
[http://dx.doi.org/10.1158/1078-0432.CCR-06-1277] [PMID: 17287296]

[83] Hu J, Wen PY, Abrey LE, *et al.* A phase II trial of oral gimatecan for recurrent glioblastoma. J Neurooncol 2013; 111(3): 347-53.
[http://dx.doi.org/10.1007/s11060-012-1023-0] [PMID: 23232808]

[84] Daud A, Valkov N, Centeno B, *et al.* Phase II trial of karenitecin in patients with malignant melanoma: clinical and translational study. Clin Cancer Res 2005; 11(8): 3009-16.
[http://dx.doi.org/10.1158/1078-0432.CCR-04-1722] [PMID: 15837755]

[85] Tsakalozou E, Adane ED, Liang Y, Arnold SM, Leggas M. Protracted dosing of the lipophilic camptothecin analogue AR-67 in non-small cell lung cancer xenografts and humans. Cancer Chemother Pharmacol 2014; 74(1): 45-54.
[http://dx.doi.org/10.1007/s00280-014-2472-2] [PMID: 24807458]

[86] Hwang JH, Lim MC, Seo SS, Park SY, Kang S. Phase II study of belotecan (CKD 602) as a single agent in patients with recurrent or progressive carcinoma of uterine cervix. Jpn J Clin Oncol 2011; 41(5): 624-9.
[http://dx.doi.org/10.1093/jjco/hyr017] [PMID: 21355002]

[87] Braybrooke JP, Ranson M, Manegold C, *et al.* Phase II study of exatecan mesylate (DX-8951f) as first line therapy for advanced non-small cell lung cancer. Lung Cancer 2003; 41(2): 215-9.
[http://dx.doi.org/10.1016/S0169-5002(03)00190-9] [PMID: 12871785]

[88] Kroep JR, Gelderblom H. Diflomotecan, a promising homocamptothecin for cancer therapy. Expert Opin Investig Drugs 2009; 18(1): 69-75.
[http://dx.doi.org/10.1517/13543780802571674] [PMID: 19053883]

[89] Shibata N, Ishimaru T, Nakamura M, Toru T. 20-Deoxy-20-fluorocamptothecin: Design and Synthesis

of Camptothecin Isostere. Synlett 2004; 14: 2509-12.
[http://dx.doi.org/10.1055/s-2004-834810]

[90]   Miao Z, Zhu L, Dong G, *et al.* A new strategy to improve the metabolic stability of lactone: discovery of (20S,21S)-21-fluorocamptothecins as novel, hydrolytically stable topoisomerase I inhibitors. J Med Chem 2013; 56(20): 7902-10.
[http://dx.doi.org/10.1021/jm400906z] [PMID: 24069881]

[91]   Silvestri R. New prospects for vinblastine analogues as anticancer agents. J Med Chem 2013; 56(3): 625-7.
[http://dx.doi.org/10.1021/jm400002j] [PMID: 23316748]

[92]   Leggans EK, Duncan KK, Barker TJ, Schleicher KD, Boger DL. A remarkable series of vinblastine analogues displaying enhanced activity and an unprecedented tubulin binding steric tolerance: C20′ urea derivatives. J Med Chem 2013; 56(3): 628-39.
[http://dx.doi.org/10.1021/jm3015684] [PMID: 23244701]

[93]   Va P, Campbell EL, Robertson WM, Boger DL. Total synthesis and evaluation of a key series of C5-substituted vinblastine derivatives. J Am Chem Soc 2010; 132(24): 8489-95.
[http://dx.doi.org/10.1021/ja1027748] [PMID: 20518465]

[94]   Genova C, Alama A, Coco S, *et al.* Vinflunine for the treatment of non-small cell lung cancer. Expert Opin Investig Drugs 2016; 25(12): 1447-55.
[http://dx.doi.org/10.1080/13543784.2016.1252331] [PMID: 27771969]

[95]   Kundranda MN, Niu J. Albumin-bound paclitaxel in solid tumors: clinical development and future directions. Drug Des Devel Ther 2015; 9: 3767-77.
[http://dx.doi.org/10.2147/DDDT.S88023] [PMID: 26244011]

[96]   Albany C, Sonpavde G. Docetaxel for the treatment of bladder cancer. Expert Opin Investig Drugs 2015; 24(12): 1657-64.
[http://dx.doi.org/10.1517/13543784.2015.1109626] [PMID: 26535615]

[97]   Vrignaud P, Semiond D, Benning V, Beys E, Bouchard H, Gupta S. Preclinical profile of cabazitaxel. Drug Des Devel Ther 2014; 8: 1851-67.
[http://dx.doi.org/10.2147/DDDT.S64940] [PMID: 25378905]

[98]   Ojima I. Use of fluorine in the medicinal chemistry and chemical biology of bioactive compounds--a case study on fluorinated taxane anticancer agents. ChemBioChem 2004; 5(5): 628-35.
[http://dx.doi.org/10.1002/cbic.200300844] [PMID: 15122634]

[99]   Höfle G, Bedorf N, Steinmetz IH, Schomburg D, Gerth K, Reichenbach H. Epothilone A and B--novel 16-membered macrolides with cytotoxic activity: isolation, crystal structure, and conformation in solution. Angew Chem Int Ed Engl 1996; 35(13-14): 1567-9.
[http://dx.doi.org/10.1002/anie.199615671]

[100]   Rivkin A, Yoshimura F, Gabarda AE, *et al.* Complex target-oriented total synthesis in the drug discovery process: the discovery of a highly promising family of second generation epothilones. J Am Chem Soc 2003; 125(10): 2899-901.
[http://dx.doi.org/10.1021/ja029695p] [PMID: 12617656]

[101]   Christner SM, Parise RA, Levine ED, Rizvi NA, Gounder MM, Beumer JH. Quantitative method for the determination of iso-fludelone (KOS-1803) in human plasma by LC-MS/MS. J Pharm Biomed Anal 2014; 100: 199-204.
[http://dx.doi.org/10.1016/j.jpba.2014.08.007] [PMID: 25168219]

[102]   Taverna P, Rendahl K, Jekic-McMullen D, *et al.* Tezacitabine enhances the DNA-directed effects of fluoropyrimidines in human colon cancer cells and tumor xenografts. Biochem Pharmacol 2007; 73(1): 44-55.
[http://dx.doi.org/10.1016/j.bcp.2006.09.009] [PMID: 17046720]

[103]   Liu P, Sharon A, Chu CK. Fluorinated nucleosides: synthesis and biological implication. J Fluor Chem

2008; 129(9): 743-66.
[http://dx.doi.org/10.1016/j.jfluchem.2008.06.007] [PMID: 19727318]

[104]   Vinogradov SV, Poluektova LY, Makarov E, Gerson T, Senanayake MT. Nano-NRTIs: efficient inhibitors of HIV type-1 in macrophages with a reduced mitochondrial toxicity. Antivir Chem Chemother 2010; 21(1): 1-14.
[http://dx.doi.org/10.3851/IMP1680] [PMID: 21045256]

[105]   Stellbrink HJ. Novel compounds for the treatment of HIV type-1 infection. Antivir Chem Chemother 2009; 19(5): 189-200.
[http://dx.doi.org/10.1177/095632020901900502] [PMID: 19483267]

[106]   Chan C, Abu-Raddad E, Golor G, et al. Clinical pharmacokinetics of alamifovir and its metabolites. Antimicrob Agents Chemother 2005; 49(5): 1813-22.
[http://dx.doi.org/10.1128/AAC.49.5.1813-1822.2005] [PMID: 15855501]

[107]   Furfaro LL, Spiller OB, Keelan JA, Payne MS. *In vitro* activity of solithromycin and its metabolites, CEM-214 and N-acetyl-CEM-101, against 100 clinical Ureaplasma spp. isolates compared with azithromycin. Int J Antimicrob Agents 2015; 46(3): 319-24.
[http://dx.doi.org/10.1016/j.ijantimicag.2015.04.015] [PMID: 26141231]

[108]   Tiwari A. Elocalcitol (BXL-628): a novel, investigational therapy for the therapeutic management of benign prostatic hyperplasia. Expert Opin Investig Drugs 2008; 17(5): 819-24.
[http://dx.doi.org/10.1517/13543784.17.5.819] [PMID: 18447607]

[109]   Burgess JP, Green JS, Hill JM, et al. Identification of [14C]fluasterone metabolites in urine and feces collected from dogs after subcutaneous and oral administration of [14C]fluasterone. Drug Metab Dispos 2009; 37(5): 1089-97.
[http://dx.doi.org/10.1124/dmd.108.023614] [PMID: 19196848]

[110]   Edgar DM, Seidel WF, Gee KW, et al. CCD-3693: an orally bioavailable analog of the endogenous neuroactive steroid, pregnanolone, demonstrates potent sedative hypnotic actions in the rat. J Pharmacol Exp Ther 1997; 282(1): 420-9.
[PMID: 9223583]

[111]   Wang J, Sánchez-Roselló M, Aceña JL, et al. Fluorine in pharmaceutical industry: fluorine-containing drugs introduced to the market in the last decade (2001-2011). Chem Rev 2014; 114(4): 2432-506.
[http://dx.doi.org/10.1021/cr4002879] [PMID: 24299176]

[112]   Wang BC, Wang LJ, Jiang B, et al. Application of fluorine in drug design during 2010-2015 years: a mini-review. Mini Rev Med Chem 2017; 17(8): 683-92.
[http://dx.doi.org/10.2174/1389557515666151016124957] [PMID: 26471967]

CHAPTER 4

Natural Products for the Management of Cardiovascular Diseases

Mohamed A. Salem[1], Mahitab H. El Bishbishy[2], Ahmed Zayed[3], Amr A. Mahrous[4,5], Maha M. Salama[6,7] and Shahira M. Ezzat[2,6,*]

[1] *Department of Pharmacognosy, Faculty of Pharmacy, Menoufia University, Gamal Abd El Nasr st., Shibin Elkom 32511, Menoufia, Egypt*

[2] *Department of Pharmacognosy, Faculty of Pharmacy, October University for Modern Sciences and Arts (MSA), Giza 12451, Egypt*

[3] *Department of Pharmacognosy, College of Pharmacy, Tanta University, El Guish Street, 31527, Tanta, Egypt*

[4] *Department of Pharmacology and Toxicology, Faculty of Pharmacy, Cairo University, Kasr El-Aini Street, Cairo 11562, Egypt*

[5] *Department of Neuroscience, Cell Biology, and Physiology, Wright State University, Dayton, Ohio 45435, USA*

[6] *Department of Pharmacognosy, Faculty of Pharmacy, Cairo University, Kasr El-Aini Street, Cairo 11562, Egypt*

[7] *Department of Pharmacognosy, Faculty of Pharmacy, British University in Egypt, El Sherouk City, Suez Desert Road, Cairo 11837, Egypt*

Abstract: Cardiovascular diseases constitute a serious public health problem. It is estimated that they are responsible for nearly 30% of world mortality. Regardless of the developments in the diagnosis and management of cardiovascular diseases, their incidence rate remains increasing. Therefore, newlines of drugs are needed to manage the expanding population of patients with cardiovascular diseases. Even though the most common existing treatments for cardiovascular diseases are synthetic molecules, natural compounds, of different chemical classes, are also being tested. Medicinal plants have been employed in the treatment of some cardiovascular diseases such as congestive heart failure and hypertension many centuries ago. Recently, the traditional remedies application for the treatment of different disorders is gaining revived popularity. In this chapter, we will investigate the efficacy and safety of natural products under preclinical studies and clinical trials with particular emphasis on their

*Corresponding author Shahira M. Ezzat: Department of Pharmacognosy, Faculty of Pharmacy, Cairo University, Kasr ElAini Street, Cairo 11562, Egypt; Department of Pharmacognosy, Faculty of Pharmacy, October University for Modern Sciences and Arts (MSA), Giza 12451, Egypt; E-mail: shahira.ezzat@pharma.cu.edu.eg

Atta-ur-Rahman, Shazia Anjum and Hesham Al-Seedi (Eds.)

traditional uses and implementations in the primary health care system. The great potential of medicinal plants and herbs will be discussed in light of the rising prevalence of cardiovascular diseases as one of the most devastating global health problems.

Keywords: Angina, Cardiovascular diseases, Clinical trials, Hypertension, Heart failure, Ischemic heart diseases, Natural products.

1. INTRODUCTION

According to the World Health Organization (WHO) definition, cardiovascular diseases (CVD) are the diseases associated with the heart and/or the blood vessels [1]. Most common Cardiovascular disease (CVD) types include Hypertension, Angina Pectoris, Atherosclerosis, Ischemic Heart Disease and Cerebral and Venous Insufficiency.

There are many cardiovascular risk factors for the development and evolution of CVD. According to "European guidelines on cardiovascular disease prevention in clinical practice" which were published by the European Society of Cardiology, there are two main categories of cardiovascular risk factor: modifiable and non-modifiable factors [2, 3]. As for modifiable cardiovascular risk factors; they include smoking, limited physical activity, inappropriate diet, overweight and obesity or disturbed lipid profile. Non-modifiable individual risk factors include genetic factors, sex, age or family history. Tobacco use is a major risk factor for CVD as well as chronic respiratory diseases and cancer. Several reports showed that proper nutrition, active physical lifestyle and avoiding tobacco are able to decrease CVD risk [4, 5].

The incidence rate of cardiovascular diseases worldwide has increased drastically during the last years. Cardiovascular diseases are considered one of the four main non-communicable diseases (NCDs) accounting for serious threats next to diabetes, cancer and chronic respiratory disease [6]. The WHO estimated that more than 40 million deaths occurred in 2016 due to NCDs, of which 17.9 million deaths were caused by cardiovascular diseases, accounting for 44% of all NCD deaths [6]. Therefore, CVD are ranked as the leading cause of death worldwide.

CVD are presently one of the major causes of death worldwide. The current strategic approaches for the treatment of CVD diseases involve many effective drugs. However, the majority of these drugs have low safety profile and lead to serious side effects. Natural products have constantly been considered a treasured source for innovation of novel drug leads. Growing evidence suggests that numerous natural compounds are invaluable sources of CVD remedies. In this review, the prevalence and the pathophysiology of CVD disorders are discussed. Additionally, the great impact of medicinal plants and natural compounds for the prevention and treatment of CVD disorders is addressed. Special emphasis is laid on plant-derived products which are in pre-clinical or clinical trials.

2. ISCHEMIC HEART DISEASE AND CONGESTIVE HEART FAILURE

2.1. Pathophysiology of Ischemic Heart Disease

The narrowing of the coronary arteries which provide the cardiac muscle with oxygenated blood is referred to as Ischemic Heart Disease (IHD), Coronary Artery Disease (CAD), or Coronary Heart Disease (CHD). This narrowing leads to ischemic damage of the myocardium. Although CAD can be asymptomatic in some cases, myocardial ischemia usually causes chest pain and/or discomfort known as angina pectoris (Hereafter discussed) due to an imbalance between local oxygen supply to the myocardial tissue and its oxygen demand.

The primary cause of coronary artery narrowing is the process known as atherosclerosis (Hereafter discussed in more detail in section 5). This process involves the pathological deposition of oxidized cholesterol in the arterial wall. In the early course of the disease, coronary endothelial cells become dysfunctional with a reduction in the production of important mediators like nitric oxide and prostacyclin. This can lead to vasospasms and impaired relaxation of the coronaries. As the disease progresses, leukocytes infiltrate the coronary artery wall causing inflammation, plaque formation and eventually thickening and hardening of the vessel wall; as well as narrowing of the lumen which restricts blood flow [7].

Severe and/or prolonged, myocardial ischemia eventually causes regional necrosis of cardiac tissue (myocardial infarction). Depending on the location and size of the necrotic area, disturbance of ventricular contraction happens. Myocardial necrosis with more than 20% trans-mural involvement can cause permanent cardiac wall motion abnormality [8]. Percutaneous Coronary Intervention (PCI) or coronary artery bypass surgery (CABG) may be applied in severe cases [9]. If blood flow is restored in a timely fashion, wall motion abnormalities might recover within a few days [10]. In addition, ventricular remodeling also occurs and can take several forms such as ventricular dilation or even aneurysm. The greater the degree of left ventricular dysfunction, the greater the likelihood of developing heart failure, arrhythmias, and even death may occur [11]. Ischemic Heart Disease (IHD) remains among the major causes of mortality worldwide [12].

Risk factors include hypertension, diabetes mellitus, obesity, lack of exercise, high serum cholesterol levels, family history of a heart attack before the age of 60 years, smoking, depression and alcohol consumption [13, 14]. A healthy lifestyle is the best way to reduce the risk of developing CAD, including healthy dieting, steady exercise, keeping a healthy body mass index and avoiding smoking.

2.2. Pathophysiology of Congestive Heart Failure (CHF)

Heart failure (HF) is a pathophysiological case that occurs when the heart cannot pump enough blood to satisfy the requirements of the metabolizing tissues. With a few exceptions, HF is usually due to defective myocardial contraction. Heart failure, however, should be distinguished from circulatory failure, which is due to decreased blood volume, damage to blood vessels, or decreased concentration of oxygenated hemoglobin [7]. Although heart failure, by definition, results in circulatory failure, the opposite is not necessarily true.

The underlying pathogenesis of the defective myocardium involves ischemic damage, hemodynamic overload, ischemic damage, excessive neuro-humoral stimulation, silent inflammatory responses, bacterial or viral infections, calcium cycling abnormalities, extracellular matrix proliferation as well as ventricular remodeling [15 - 17].

However, uncontrolled diabetes and long-standing hypertension are considered the strongest risk factors of CHF in patients with coronary heart disease [18]. Age is also a major risk factor for developing heart failure due to increased incidence of atherosclerosis, myocardial wall stiffness, and hypertension, which promotes an increased end-diastolic pressure in a rigid ventricle causing pulmonary edema [19, 20]. With increased life expectancy, the incidence of CHF is projected to more than double over the next two decades and its prevalence will rise ten times between the age of 60 and 80 [21, 22].

Decreased myocardial contractility results in reduced ejection fraction (the percent blood pumped out of the ventricle with respect to the end diastolic volume). At the early stages of heart failure, the cardiac output might show normal levels while resting but fails to increase proportionally with exertion. Consequently, one of the most common symptoms and early signs of heart failure is exercise-intolerance and rapid fatigue. As a result of decreased ejection fraction and increased ventricle filling pressure (increased preload), blood accumulates in the systemic venous bed and pulmonary circulation causing pulmonary and/or peripheral edema depending on the type of heart failure being left-sided, right-sided or both [7]. Hence, a major goal of heart failure treatment is to increase myocardial contractility and ejection fraction.

The cardiac output reduction has a number of short-term circulatory and hemodynamic consequences which are triggered by two main compensatory mechanisms. First, a fast-nervous mechanism: Reduced volume of blood delivered into the major arteries results in changes in baroreceptor signaling which will trigger an increase in sympathetic activity [7, 23]. The increase in sympathetic activity results in tachycardia (elevated heart rate) and increased vascular tone. The increase of arterial tone is better causes increased peripheral resistance (afterload), while higher venous tone causes an increase in venous return (preload). Second, a slower renal mechanism: Decreased arterial blood flow causes a reduction in renal perfusion and Renin-Angiotensin-Aldosterone System (RAAS) activation [24]. The increased RAAS activity eventually causes increased vascular tone (increased preload and afterload), retention of sodium and water in the intravascular and interstitial compartments (increased preload), and long-term changes in the myocardium. The excessive retention of fluid is responsible for many of the clinical manifestations of heart failure including pulmonary congestion, dyspnea, and peripheral edema, hence the name *congestive* heart failure. Thus, alleviation of fluid retention and edema is another major goal of treatment [7].

While the increase in sympathetic tone and activation of RAAS help maintain the blood pressure and augment preload to maintain the perfusion to vital organs *e.g.* heart and brain, they also result in maladaptive responses like pulmonary and peripheral congestion, afterload mismatch, decreased energy efficiency, and cardiac dilatation and remodeling. The gradual exacerbation of heart failure symptoms is clinically described as chronic decompensated heart failure [20, 25]. The patients are usually assigned to one of four different stages of CHF based on the severity of the symptoms, with earlier stages having no or mild symptoms and the end-stage involving failure to do daily activities.

Congestive heart failure generally has a poor prognosis with about a year mortality of 33 - 35% [26, 27]. Regardless of the developments in medicine, the treatment of heart failure still represents a challenge to healthcare providers due to the high rate of hospital readmissions besides mortality and morbidity increase. The key targets of heart failure treatment are to alleviate symptoms, improve prognosis and decrease mortality, and prevent organ system damage [28, 29].

2.3. Natural Products for Management of Congestive Heart Failure and Ischemic Heart Disease

Nutraceuticals are getting more popular all over the world as an adjunct to conventional therapy for cardiovascular diseases [30]. Through multiple mechanisms, natural products can provide several benefits to treatment regimens.

First, products with antioxidant activity might delay the onset and slow the progression of CAD by preventing the oxidation of the LDL cholesterol [31]. In addition, antioxidant compounds prevent oxidative damage that occurs due to ischemia / reperfusion in patients with advanced CAD [32]. They also improve vascular and endothelial function through increased levels of nitric oxide [33]. Second, their anti-inflammatory effects help thwart atherosclerosis, vascular plaque formation, myocardial remodeling, and reperfusion damage. Third, some natural products have potent anti-atherogenic effects due to their ability to improve the blood lipid profile. In addition to antioxidant and anti-inflammatory actions, nature may play other beneficial roles such as anti-apoptotic effects, anticoagulant activity, vasodilation, diuretic, and others. Here, we briefly discuss some of the recent advances in using natural products to manage and protect against CAD and CHF.

2.3.1. Flavonoids

A large class of secondary plant metabolites (flavones, flavonols, flavanones, isoflavones and anthocyanidins) found in onions, citrus fruits, berries, tea and cocoa [34, 35]. They are known for their antioxidant activity which can avert the oxidative stress caused by Reactive Oxygen Species (ROS) [36, 37]. This effect protects against low density lipoprotein (LDL) cholesterol oxidation (an early step of atherosclerosis), decreases platelet aggregation, lessens the ischemic damage, and improves blood vessel function [38, 39]. Flavonoids have been also shown to also have anti-inflammatory activity [40, 41].

The role of flavonoids to protect against cardiovascular diseases is, however, controversial [30]. Several studies have shown a reduction in the incidence and mortality of CAD in cases those consuming flavonoid rich diets [42, 43]. Other studies showed no relationship between flavonoid consumption and the incidence of CAD [44 - 46]. Nonetheless, in one of these studies, flavonoids reduced subsequent coronary events in patients diagnosed with CHD [44]. A meta-analysis that included several studies (including ones that showed no benefits), suggested that consumption of flavonoid rich tea reduces the risk of cardiovascular diseases by more than 10% [47].

2.3.2. Resveratrol

Resveratrol is produced by plants due to injury or fungal infection; it is a naturally occurring phytoalexin [48]. High amount of resveratrol is present in the seeds and skin of grapes and in peanuts [49, 50]. It is currently available in the market as a nutritional supplement. There is strong experimental and clinical evidence that resveratrol exerts cardio protective effects [51].

The cardio protective effects of resveratrol are due to its antioxidant, antithrombotic, antiplatelet, anti-apoptotic and anti-atherosclerotic activities, in addition to improved vascular and endothelial function [52 - 54].

2.3.3. Lycopene

Lycopene is a natural red pigment synthesized by some photosynthetic organisms *e.g.* plants and algae aiming at absorbing light for photosynthesis and also to protect against sunlight. Lycopene and other carotenoids give the bright orange and red colors to many fruits and vegetables. The major source of lycopene in the diet is tomato-based products.

Dietary intake of tomato and its products has shown a negative correlation with CAD and myocardial infarction [55, 56]. The ideal daily intake of lycopene is not yet defined; however, 8 mg / day has been recommended by some studies [57].

The cardiovascular benefits of lycopene include its antioxidant and free radical scavenging activities [58], improved endothelial functions, and LDL reduction [59].

2.3.4. Omega-3 Fatty Acids

The major dietary sources of omega-3 Fatty acids are fish oil, soya beans, canola oil, and flaxseed oil. Omega-3 Fatty acids are regarded as essential dietary components which belong to the polyunsaturated fatty acids (PUFAs) class. PUFAs are known to possess a multiplicity of beneficial cardio protective actions and play an important role in both prevention and management of cardiovascular diseases [30]. Clinical and epidemiological data suggest that omega-3 fatty acids decrease both the incidence of CAD in healthy humans and complications in cardiovascular patients [60 - 62].

The mechanisms of the cardiovascular benefits of omega-3 fatty acids include thromboxane-A2 reduction, decreasing platelet aggregation, improving vascular and endothelial function through increased nitric oxide production, calcium entry into vascular smooth muscles inhibition and plasma nor-epinephrine levels reduction [63].

2.3.5. Olive Oil

In the Mediterranean diet, olive oil is the major fats source; this diet is related to the lower cardiovascular disease mortality [64, 65].

Although its beneficial cardiovascular effects are usually linked to monounsaturated fatty acids (MUFA) high levels, olive oil contains a long list of natural compounds *e.g.* phenolic compounds, hydrocarbons, tocopherols, fatty alcohols, sterols and polar pigments (chlorophylls and pheophytins). Some of these compounds isolated from olive oil have been shown to improve lipoprotein metabolism and LDL/HDL ratio [66, 67], ameliorate endothelial function and nitric oxide production [68], decrease monocyte adhesion [69 - 71], and decrease oxidative damage and inflammation [72, 73].

2.3.6. Soy

For centuries, soybeans have been employed as food and medicine in Asia [74]. In a number of epidemiological studies, a cardiovascular protective action of soy foods has been reported. Soy products reduce the risk of CAD in both men and women [75 - 77].

The cardio protective actions of soy have been linked to isoflavones, however, soy contains several classes of bioactive compounds [76, 78]. Isoflavones are phytoestrogens that protect against atherosclerosis, 38 clinical studies meta-analysis showed that soy proteins consumption significantly improves the blood lipid profile [79].

2.3.7. Cardiac Glycosides

Cardiac glycosides are produced by several plant species and also found in some animal venoms. Digoxin and digitoxin, the most well-characterized and clinically-used cardiac glycosides, have been used for decades as inotropic agents to treat congestive heart failure.

Digoxin acts by inhibiting the activity of the myocardial Na^+/K^+ ATPase pump which leads to Na^+ accumulation inside the myocardial cells with subsequent inhibition of Ca^{2+} extrusion through the Na^+/Ca^{2+} exchanger [7].

Cardiac glycosides are known for their complex pharmacokinetic profile and low therapeutic index. In fact, some of the plants containing cardiac glycosides have been historically used as poisons. Toxicity manifests as ventricular arrhythmias, heart block, gastrointestinal symptoms [80]. Because these glycosides compete for the potassium binding site of the Na^+/K^+ pump, plasma levels of K^+ can be a major determinant of toxicity. A specific fab antibody is now available for treatment of digoxin toxicity [81].

3. HYPERTENSION

Hypertension (HTN) is an important risk factor denoting CVD. Globally, about 970 million people are estimated to be suffering from the disease that can significantly result in morbidity, mortality as well as financial burden. Regardless to the current developments in pharmaceutical therapy, 53% only reached the targeted blood pressure [82].

3.1. Pathophysiology of Hypertension

Hypertensive patients are categorized according to the hypertension type whether primary or essential HTN (95%) or secondary HTN (5%) of hypertensive patients [83]. The major cause of essential HTN is not yet known, however commences mostly at the age of 50 - 60 and frequently correlated with high salt consumption and obesity, in addition to family history, underlining the genetic predisposition possibility for the disease [83]. On the other hand, secondary hypertension etiology includes renal artery stenosis, chronic renal disorders and sleep apnea [83]. Both disorders (primary & secondary) are the import of numerous mechanisms which are responsible for maintaining normal blood pressures which are:

3.1.1. Sympathetic Nervous System

Sympathetic nervous system SNS hyperactivity leads to the promotion, maintenance and development of hypertension HTN. Adrenergic hyperactivity has been correlated with numerous forms of HTN; systolic-diastolic and isolated systolic hypertension [84, 85] white- coat hypertension and masked hypertension [86] as well as dipping, extreme dipping, non-dipping and reverse dipping cases [87, 88], in addition to, gestational hypertension [89]. Accordingly, sympathetic nervous system is aggravated in correlation with hypertension conditions [90]. Numerous reports evidenced that hyperactivity of SNS, demonstrated by norepinephrine increase, extends to patients with HTN approving that the overactive SNS is one of the major reasons in the pathophysiology of hypertension. On the other hand, renal sympathetic nervous system is crucial in the progress and preservation of HTN. It has an impact on blood pressure through two pathways; the efferent and afferent pathways [82].

3.1.2. Endothelial Function

There is a solid basis of a clear relation between the endothelial dysfunction grade and the hypertension severity. The decrease in the nitric oxide level which results from oxidative stress could be the primary mechanism for endothelial dysfunction recognized in hypertension. This impaired nitric oxide production could be resorted by antihypertensive drugs; however, endothelium dependent vaso-relaxation alteration may last directly after hypertension is established. Therefore, endothelium-derived nitric oxide synthase inhibition leads to hypertension in humans [82]. There are other vaso-relaxing factors alongside with nitric oxide (NO) for instance, ROS, arachidonic acid metabolites, vaso-active peptides and endothelial originated micro-particles that are involved in preservation of vascular tone. The aforementioned factors cause extreme vascular oxidative stress and inflammation leading to endothelial dysfunction [91, 92]. Thus endothelial dysfunction could be recognized as massive modifications in the vascular environment that contributes to structural and functional changes inside the arteries. Improvement of vascular function by treatments those targeting key pathways decrease cardiovascular risk.

3.1.3. Renin-Angiotensin-Aldosterone System (RAAS)

The RAAS is crucial in maintaining normal blood pressures. There are two mechanisms controlling RAAS; stimulation of the sympathetic nervous system and glomerular under perfusion [93]. The result of these stimulations is the renin release from the juxtaglomerular apparatus that alters angiotensinogen into inactive angiotensin I. Angiotensin I is then converted by endothelium bound angiotensin converting enzyme (ACE) into angiotensin II, the latter is a potent vasoconstrictor [94]. Conversion of angiotensin I into angiotensin II occurs in all tissue and mainly in the lungs. Furthermore, low intake of salt leads to aldosterone release through RAAS from the adrenal glands which results in reabsorption of salt and retention of water leading to elevation in blood pressure. Studies revealed that only 15% of the patients have shown an increase in the plasma renin level, and it remained normal in 60% and reduced in 25%. Therefore, there is an acquiescent for the occurrence of local renin systems that regulates the blood flow that might be correlated to the pathophysiology of HTN [95].

3.1.4. Obesity

Severity of hypertension is extremely conjugated with obesity. Patients recording 30 kg/m2 BMI are liable to uncontrolled systolic blood pressure (SBP) with increase 1.5 folds as compared with those less than 25 kg/m2. Another report evidenced that obese patients recorded high blood pressure as regards to normal cases. The famous mechanism explaining this phenomenon involved in obesity-induced hypertension is neuro-adrenergic hypothesis in addition to sodium excretion impairment, fluid retention and the RAAS activation [96].

3.1.5. Vascular Smooth Muscles

The vascular smooth muscle cell invades vascular lumen which initiates increase in peripheral vascular resistance and consequently development of hypertension [97]. The whole procedure depends on the interaction between many modulating factors by either stimulating or inhibiting vascular smooth muscle cell (VSMC) progression. The fibroblast growth factor (FGF), platelet-derived growth factor (PDGF), the endothelin-1, the Angiotensin II (Ang II), and the Ca^{2+}- calmodulin interaction are the prominent causes involved in the vascular remodeling. These factors control the cross-bridge cycling actin and myosin (Contractile proteins) [98].

3.1.6. Reactive Oxygen Species

Pathogenesis of hypertension and other vascular complications are clinically evidenced by excessive production of reactive oxygen species ROS through different pathologic states. ROS such as hydrogen peroxide (H_2O_2), superoxide (O_2^-) and hydroxyl (OH^-) anions, normalize many cellular processes [99, 100].

3.2. Natural Products and Hypertension

Nowadays, herbal drugs have drawn attention for treatment of several ailments as cardiovascular disorders including hypertension. Due to their safety and effectiveness herbs and naturals are regarded as an important complement to conventional therapy. Nevertheless, there are some concerns regarding the use of herbs, because of the lack of continuous supervision, serious complications and interactions with other traditional medicines [98].

3.2.1. Nigella Sativa (Black Cumin, Black Seed)

Thymoquinone, the key ingredient of the volatile oil of *Nigella sativa* seeds, evidenced a decreasing action on BP in humans, as well as, animals [101] studied the activity of *N. sativa* seeds oil on lowering blood pressure applying controlled clinical trial, in seventy healthy subjects of age ranging from 34 - 63 years. The protocol was designed that randomized subjects were given 2.5 ml seed oil or placebo twice daily for two months. Results revealed that the oil decreased the SBP. Another similar clinical study dealt with *N. sativa* extract at two dose (100 and 200 ml) levels; two times / day for two months, there was also a reduction in blood pressure [102]. Nigella seed extract exerted also significant reduction in the total and LDL-cholesterol levels. Interestingly, there were no complications due to the chronic administration of nigella seeds. Therefore, it was established that the daily use of nigella seed extract for about two months could lower blood pressure effect in patients suffering from mild hypertension. The suggested mechanism for the antihypertensive effects of *Nigella sativa* was its antioxidant activity by reducing oxidative stress and also by blocking Ca^{2+} channels gate leading to vaso-relaxation.

3.2.2. Beta Vulgaris (Red Beet, Table Beet or Golden Beet)

Beet root is a rich source of dietary NO_3^- [103] several reports have studied its potential for regulating blood pressure in humans which was more prominent in men. A randomized, placebo-controlled study [104], examined the impact of dietary supplementation of beetroot juice on 68 hypertensive subjects, 34 patients were treated as control, and 34 treated with age ranging from 18 - 85 years for one month. Results evidenced that Beetroot intake reduced the blood pressure and enhanced the endothelial function, together with a reduction in arterial stiffness. It was also concluded that beetroot supplements were well tolerated with no tachyphylaxis evidence throughout the treatment. Another crossover study was conducted on fifteen women and fifteen men. The volunteers received 500 g of beetroot juice or placebo juice (PL) randomly. The blood pressure was measured at baseline and each one hour for 24 hours after juice intake using an ambulatory blood pressure monitor (ABPM). The process was repeated two weeks later. Results revealed a decrease in the SBP at the sixth hour by 4 - 5 mmHg after consuming Beetroot juice as compared to placebo juice [105]. The high amount of inorganic nitrates supplement and the endothelial nitric oxide generation account for the antihypertensive actions of beetroot juice.

3.2.3. viz Coptis Chinensis (Goldthread)

Bebeerine alkaloid (a quaternary ammonium salt) is the major active ingredient of *Coptis chinensis*. Bebeerine is reported for the treatment of CVD [106]. The antihypertensive effects of berberine was reviewed on 228 hypertensive patients. The hypertensive volunteering patients were randomized to receive bebeerine at a dose 0.6 g/day in addition to their conventional antihypertensive medications (n = 116) or to control groups receiving antihypertensive medications solely (n = 112).

Results evidenced that concomitant treatment of bebeerine along with the antihypertensive medications reduced blood pressure as regards to control group. The proposed mechanism for bebeerine was claimed to be due to the increased generation of nitric oxide *via* NO synthase (eNOS) stimulation and the catecholamine levels reduction causing peripheral vasodilation and consequently decreasing blood pressure [107]. Another hypothetical mechanism for the hypotensive mechanism of bebeerine that the prostaglandin I2 (PGI2) levels are increased, opening the KATP and blocking the iCa^{2+}voltage gated channels, hence blocking the Ca^{2+} cell influx [108].

3.2.4. Hibiscus Sabdariffa L.

The blood lowering pressure of *Hibiscus sabdariffa* L. has been previously reported and studied on BP-lowering effects have been anthocyanins (polyphenolic compound) and hibiscus acid is the major constituent in *Hibiscus* calyxes and epicalyces are considered the phyto constituents responsible for the antihypertensive studied in both animals and man [109]. There were no signs of hepatic or renal toxicity associated with the consumption of *Hibiscus* extract, except for probable hepatic side effects at higher doses [110].

A trial [111] was conducted on 65 untreated pre-hypertensive and mildly hypertensive cases of ages that ranged from 30– 70 years. The protocol involved randomizing cases to three consumptions daily of 240 ml of either *Hibiscus* or placebo for one and a half months. Results evidenced that *H. sabdariffa* intake lowered the SBP, however the DBP. Participants recording higher baseline blood pressure showed more reductions in BP. Furthermore, there was no evidence of adverse clinical or metabolic effects. It was concluded that Hibiscus tea consumption may decrease the BP of hypertensive patients due to the NO increased production, Ca^{2+} channels inhibition and the KATP channels opening [112].

3.2.5. Crataegus Monogyna (Hawthorn)

Hawthorn berries are rich in oligomeric procyanidins (leucoanthocyanidins) and flavonoids that have been employed traditionally for the management of CVD. Hawthorn extracts evidenced moderate decrease in blood pressure in hypertensive patients [113]. A cross-over study was performed to investigate Hawthorn extract's impact on lowering blood pressure and in flow-mediated vasodilation. Results showed that there was no significant change from baseline in ABP or in flow-mediated vasodilation by hawthorn extracts [114]. It was suggested that Hawthorn extract constitutes bioactive metabolites; procyanidins and flavonoids that might increase nitric oxide level and improve endothelial function and hence exert hypotensive action. Moreover, about 90.5% of the participants recommended the use of Hawthorn extract in combination with their conventional antihypertensive drugs.

3.2.6. Allium Sativum L. (Garlic)

Garlic is an underground stem (bulb) rich in sulfur compound known as allicin, it is present in several preparations whether powder or extract. It has been employed for the management of hyperlipidemia, the prevention of CVD in addition to its hypotensive effect. A randomized, double-blind, placebo-controlled study [115] the aged garlic action on uncontrolled was established. In that study eighty-eight patients suffering from uncontrolled blood pressure received either aged garlic extract at a dose 1200 mg / day or placebo and Bo was monitored for twelve. Results evidenced that the blood pressure was significantly reduced with garlic compared to placebo. Other parameters (central hemodynamic) were measured indicating an improvement in central BP, central pulse pressure (PP), pulse wave velocity (PWV), and arterial stiffness as regards to placebo. It was concluded that garlic significantly reduced the brachial BP and enhanced central hemodynamics, in addition to its tolerance and acceptance by the patients. Another study comprising 482 hypertensive subjects was accomplished to track the effect of garlic on hypertension [116]. The study was conducted from 12 - 26 weeks where patients consumed garlic preparations at different doses. Results revealed that the average decrease in BP was significantly lower than placebo [117]. examined the impact of garlic administration in eighteen trials involving 799 normotensive and hypertensive subjects. The follow–up was from 3 - 6 months at different dose levels of garlic administration 300 - 2400 mg/day. It was reported that the BP was reduced in the hypertensive but not in the normotensive subjects and was better than that of placebo treatment. The mechanism anticipated for the BP lowering effect of garlic was correlated the sulfur compounds- allicin the most important- which are reputed for modulating endothelium-relaxing factors; stimulation for No production and hydrogen sulfide (H2S), also allicin causes ACE inhibition and hence BP was reduced [115].

3.2.7. Crocus Sativus L. (Saffron)

Saffron is rich in interesting bioactive metabolites as safranal, crocetin, crocin and picrocrocin, flavonoids and anthocyanins that exert antihypertensive and vasodilatory effects [118]. A randomized, placebo-controlled study was performed in thirty volunteers to clinically prove the BP-lowering effects of *Crocus sativus* [119]. Study design was achieved by dividing the subjects into three groups (10 per group) and blood pressure was monitored for one week. Results evidenced significant decrease in SBP 11 mmHg and lowering arterial pressure 5 mmHg at dose level 400-mg of the herb. The mechanism of action for the antihypertensive and vasodilatory action of *C. sativus* suggested in this study was mediated *via* Ca^{2+} channels blockade, K^+ channels opening and β-adrenoceptor antagonism.

3.2.8. Panax Ginseng (Ginseng)

Panax ginseng (F. Araliacea) roots have been reputed in folk medicine for different disorders including cardiovascular disorders and hypertension. Triterpenoidal and steroidal saponins are the major bioactive ingredients of ginseng responsible for its CV effects. Clinical trials evidenced a significant decrease in blood pressure. American ginseng (AG) effects on arterial stiffness and BP reduction was revised in a randomized study [120]. The study was pursued in 64 hypertensive diabetic patients aging 63 ± 9.3 years for 12 weeks. Results revealed a reduction in BP, the augmentation index (AIx)and the pulse pressure (PP). Another randomized, double-blind, cross-over [121] investigated the Korean red ginseng effects on BP and arterial stiffness in twenty three normotensive samples aging 25 ± 2 years. The extract exhibited statistically-significant reductions in AIx, central SBP, central DBP and brachial BP, three hours after intervention as compared to the control. The effects of *P. ginseng* extracton BP was further studied in ninety subjects with the age range of 55.2 ± 11.8 years and BP range of 120 - 159/80 - 99 mmHg and the follow-up was for two months [122]. Results showed that the seated SBP (sSBP) and DBP (sDBP) levels were decreased only upon the administration of high dose at the fourth week. Unlikely, at the eighth week, there was a decline in the differences between the groups. Moreover, no significant metabolic or clinical side effects were reported. The effects of *P. ginseng*on BP reduction were mainly accredited to its vascular effects intermediated by a massive eNOS expression increase and NO production increase, in addition to, Ca^{2+} channels blockade [120, 123].

3.2.9. Camelia Sinensis L. (Tea Plant, Tea Shrub)

Camellia sinensis L. (Family Theaeceae) (leaves and leaf buds) is the most commonly consumed beverage worldwide and are the most frequently consumed beverages worldwide. Tea leaves have diverse biological activities; anti-inflammatory, antidiabetic, and antihypertensive actions. Many studies have demonstrated significant antihypertensive action. In a trial by [124], where 95 hypertensive patients in the age ranging from 35 to 75 years under took the study. The BP follow-up duration was for six months. Results were in good agreement where the arterial blood pressure (ABP)measured through 24 hours was reduced in the group receiving tea as compared to the placebo group. Another report on the effect of black and green tea to reduce blood pressure [125]. Eleven trials were revised; 7 consumed green tea and 4 received black tea in 821 subjects for 6 months. It was deduced that the green tea caused more reduction in BP compared to black tea. There were no adverse reactions and was well tolerated treatment as well. On analyzing the mechanism of action of both black and green tea in reducing blood pressure, the major action is supposed to be due to its polyphenolic content mainly catechins. Catechin is a flavan-3-ol with powerful antioxidant activity that stimulates nitric oxide production and reduces endothelin-1concentrations in the plasma. These actions collectively lead to a decrease in vascular tonicity leading to vasodilatation and peripheral vascular resistance reduction and BP reduction.

3.2.10. Cymbopogon Citratus (Lemongrass)

Citral the active ingredient of the volatile oil of Lemongrass has been used in the management of hypertension due its vasodilating action. Lemon grass proved in a hypertensive rat model its effect to reduce blood pressure [126]. This was correlated to its vaso-relaxant and antioxidant effect [127].

3.2.10. Peumus Boldus (Family Monimiaceae)

is an aromatic and evergreen shrub, where the leaves are the most common part used due to its boldine content. Boldine is an alkaloid of the aporphine class with potent antioxidant activity. The effects of boldine on endothelial dysfunction were evaluated in spontaneously hypertensive rats (SHR). The study used SHR *versus* their age-equivalent normotensive rat for one week. Results revealed that control group of SHR demonstrated SBP elevation, endothelium-dependent aortic relaxation to acetylcholine reduction, endothelium-independent aortic relaxation to sodium nitroprusside attenuation, aortic superoxide increase and peroxynitrite production, and p47 protein expression enhancement as regards to control rats. In conclusion, boldine possesses endothelial protective action in hypertension *via* NADPH-mediated superoxide production inhibition [128, 129].

4. ANGINA PECTORIS

Angina, known as angina pectoris/angina cordis / angor pectoris / Rougnon-Heberden disease, is a well-known cardiovascular disorder which is frequently associated with coronary heart diseases. The term "angina pectoris" was first introduced in 1772 by William Heberden [130]. It occurs due to the failure of the coronary blood supply to meet the myocardial oxygen demands. Basically, this failure is a result of coronary obstructions in which the atherosclerosis restricts the blood flow to the heart muscle forming a fixed obstruction. Sometimes this obstruction is dynamic due to coronary spasms or even patients with mixed angina may have both kinds of obstruction. Other causes extend to include anemia, arrhythmia and heart failure [131 - 133].

Globally, CAD is the major cause of mortality, accounting for about 7.2 million deaths annually [134]. The prognosis of angina depends predominantly on the quantity of obstructed vessels and the obstruction extent. The risk of vasospasm and thrombosis is significantly increased in cases of 80% or more vessels obstruction. A twelve-year survival rate is estimated to be 88%, 74%, 59%, and 40% for subjects having zero, one, two, and three-vessel disease respectively. This estimated survival rate could be affected by other factors such as congestive heart failure, ejection fraction, previous myocardial infarction, diabetes, age and smoking history. It could be concluded that, patient prognosis remarkably varies by up to 10 folds according to several parameters as clinical, anatomical and functional factors [135, 136].

The diagnostic tools employed for angina are clinical manifestations, laboratory tests and other invasive and non-invasive cardiac investigations. These tools are usually used for both diagnostic and prognostic evaluations which are done randomly. The history of the patient is considered the foundation of angina diagnosis; hence, confident diagnosis could be based solely on it [136].

Angina patients suffer from paroxysmal thoracic pain with a heavy strangulation or pressure-like sensation that radiates to the left arm, jaw, epigastrium, back and shoulder as explained by referred pain. This pain is usually accompanied by suffocation feeling, shortness of breath, tiredness, sweating, dizziness, sometimes nausea, tachycardia and hypertension [137].

The chest pain in angina patients should be described in regards to its location, duration, character and its relation to exertion to prevent any confusion with other cardiovascular diseases [136]. Angina should not be confused with heart attacks, where in case of angina the blood flow restrictions are related to physical exercise, temporary and does not cause damage or destruction to the heart muscles. However, angina patients are at higher risk of having heart attacks and its complications [133].

Laboratory tests for angina includes tests undertaken to (a) Determine the causes of ischemia, such as hemoglobin and thyroid hormones (if susceptible thyroid disorder), also, markers of myocardial injuries as Creatinine Kinase Myocardial Band (CKMB) could be used to exclude myocardial damage if required clinically.

(b) Evaluate cardiovascular risk factors, for example, fasting blood glucose, glycated hemoglobin, serum creatinine and total lipid profile and furthermore, cholesterol subfractions (Apo A and Apo B), homocysteine, lipoprotein a (Lpa), and hemostatic abnormalities, inflammatory markers (hs-C-reactive protein) and NT-BNP are used as predictors of long-term risk factors. (c) Evaluate the prognosis, such as complete blood count including WBCs count. However, the laboratory tests used for initial diagnosis and routine reassessment are controversial and variable according to the case evaluated [136].

Non-invasive investigations include the regular resting Electrocardiography (ECG); ECG stress testing, stress testing (with imaging), echocardiography (at rest) and ambulatory ECG monitoring. In addition, coronary calcification and coronary anatomy assessments such as computed tomography (CT) scans and Magnetic Resonance (MR) arteriography may be used as non-invasive diagnostic tools for angina. Invasive investigations are used to ascertain the diagnosis or treatment options [136].

There are four major classes of angina;

(a) Stable angina: It is characterized by chest pain and associated symptoms that are precipitated by physical activity, cold weather, heavy metals, excitement or emotional stress. These symptoms subside at rest or upon treatment with nitroglycerin. Hence, this type of angina is the classical type and referred to as effort angina [138]. Stable angina is regarded as the most common manifestation of myocardial infarction [139].

(b) Unstable angina: It is defined as the worsening of angina, in which the chest pain occurs with sudden-onset at rest or minimal exercise and lasts for more than ten minutes, becomes more severe and more frequent. This type of angina is referred to as crescendo angina as it occurs with a crescendo pattern *i.e.* prolonged, more severe and more frequent [131].

(c) Prinzmetal angina: It is similar to the unstable angina in which the patients suffer from severe pain that usually occurs while resting or sleeping; however, it arises from transient increase in coronary vascular tone (vasospasm). It is also known as variant or vasospastic angina [140].

(d) Microvascular angina: It was historically known as cardiac syndrome X, characterized by angina-like chest pain [141]. Studies consider this type of angina a part of the pathophysiology of ischaemic heart disease that is more common in women [142, 143]. It does not show major arterial blockages however it is suggested to result from endothelial dysfunction and reduced flow in the micro-blood vessels of the heart [144].

The major risk factors of angina are the age factor (men over forty-five years and women over 55 years), smoking, Diabetes mellitus, hypercholesterolemia, hypertension, renal diseases, obesity (body mass index exceeding 30), family history of premature cardiovascular diseases, sedentary lifestyle and emotional stress [145].

The patient age is paramount to the prevalence of angina, as it increases from 0.1 - 1% to 10 - 15% as for 45-54 years old women to 65 - 74 years old women respectively, similarly, it increases form 2 - 5% to 10 - 20% as for 45 - 54 years old men to 65 - 74 years old men respectively. Fortunately, there is a pragmatic decline in the incidence rate of angina in the recent decades [136].

4.1. Pathophysiology of Angina Pectoris

The imbalance between the oxygen supply to the heart and its demand will evoke angina. This imbalance could arise from exercise, for example, in which there is an increase in the demand for oxygen and in cases of atherosclerosis or coronary arteries obstruction there will not be a sufficient oxygen supply. The myocardial oxygen demands vary according to the heart rate, heart muscle contractility and most importantly, the intra-myocardial wall tension. The myocardial oxygen supply is affected by the difference of arteriovenous oxygen pressure and the coronary blood flow [139]. This blood flow may be radically altered by atherosclerotic plaque which will result in an imbalance in case of increased myocardial oxygen demand. In most cases, the pathophysiological substrate of angina is atheromatous, nevertheless, it varies according to the patient's gender, whereas; women usually suffer from non-obstructive coronary disease type of angina [136, 146, 147].

Conventional treatment of angina is primarily aiming to relieve its symptoms, slow its progression and prevent its long-term complications as decreasing the risks of its development to heart attacks or even mortality. Different treatment pathways are depicted in Fig. (**1**). These treatments comprise the use of vasodilators, mainly nitroglycerin (used sublingual for acute cases with short duration, oral for intermediate duration cases and transdermal for longer durations) [148]. Caution should be taken with patients taking a phosphodiesterase (PDE5) inhibitor, as sildenafil, as it is contraindicated with any form of nitrates causing sudden decrease in the blood pressure. Other vasodilators used for treatment of angina include Ca^{2+} channel blockers, β- blockers and ACE inhibitors in which their mechanisms of action involve decreasing the heart work load which will decrease the myocardial oxygen demand or increase the coronary blood flow resulting in myocardial oxygen supply increase. Both mechanisms will in turn reverse the case of imbalance between the oxygen supply and demand

[136, 149]. Cyto-protective medications such as trimetazidine, are usually used as antianginal agents to increase the cell tolerance to ischemia by maintaining cellular homeostasis [150]. Recently, new classes has been used in the treatment of angina, for example If inhibitors (Ivabradine), which act by decreasing the heart rate with major anti-ischaemic and antianginal efficacy [151] and potassium channel openers (Nicorandil).

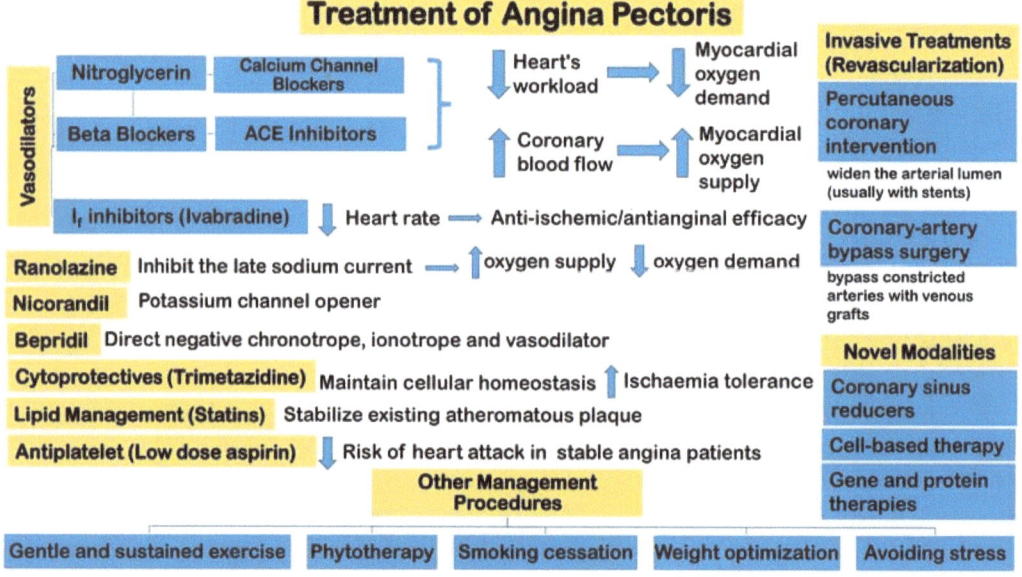

Fig. (1). Different treatments for angina pectoris [136, 148 - 158].

In 1990, the FDA approved bepridil as an antianginal agent having direct negative chronotropic, ionotropic and vasodilator effects. It differs from calcium channel blockers in which it causes the inhibition of receptor-operated, voltage-gated Ca^{2+} channels as well as K^+ currents and intracellular Ca^{2+}/calmodulin complexes [152]. Also, ranolazine was recently approved as a treatment of angina either as a replacement of beta blockers or as a complementary therapy with them. It acts by inhibiting the late sodium current, therefore reducing intracellular Na^+ and Ca^{2+} accumulation which in turn increases oxygen supply and reduces oxygen demand [153]. In addition, anti-hypercholesterolimics as statins, could be used to stabilize the atheromatous plaque and reduce the regression of coronary atherosclerosis [154]. Although, classically the administration of antiplatelets such as low doses of aspirin was a standard treatment for angina along with the vasodilators, it is now restricted to cases of high risk of myocardial infarction as it was found to cause hemorrhagic stroke and gastrointestinal bleeding [155].

Invasive treatment of angina (Revascularization) includes Percutaneous Coronary

Intervention (PCI), where a catheter enclosing a balloon enters to the arterial lumen then inflates to cause lumen widening; it is usually accompanied with stents to maintain the widening effect. Also, coronary-artery bypass surgeries (CABG) may be employed where venous grafts are used to bypass the constricted arteries. Revascularization is basically performed to relieve the angina symptoms yet it also has a prognostic benefit for patients who are at high risk [156].

Cell-based therapies for ischemic cardiomyopathy are still in its preclinical phases questioning its efficacy and feasibility. Experimentally, it was found that induced pluripotent stem cells and embryonic stem cells have regenerative abilities and cause cardiac function improvement after ischemia [152]. However, novel treatment modalities, for example coronary sinus reducers, cell-based therapies, gene and protein therapies, are still under evaluation [157].

Other management procedures could be used for the control of angina such as; gentle long-term exercise aiming to improve the blood pressure and promote the collateralization of the coronary arteries. In addition to, the control of lipid profile, blood pressure, diabetes and weight, quitting smoking and avoiding psychological stress [158].

4.2. Natural Products and Angina Pectoris

The evidence-based therapy of cardiovascular diseases by natural products is controversial. In fact, the use of botanicals in the treatment of angina is questionable as it may not cause relieving of the angina symptoms directly, which is the chief goal of the treatment as fore-mentioned. However, these natural products may be employed as secondary treatments for cardiovascular diseases [159]. Table **1** represents the key individual botanicals employed in the management of angina pectoris, it includes parts used, major active ingredients, the designs of different experiments that reported their activity and their mechanisms of action.

Key botanicals used in the treatment of angina includes Hawthorn (*Crataegus oxyacantha, C. monogyna, C. laevigata, and C. pinnatifida*) [159, 160], Danshen (*Salvia miltiorrhizae*) [159], San qi (*Panax notoginseng*) [159], Garlic (*Allium sativum*) [159], *Gingko biloba* [159, 161], Arjuna (*Terminalia arjuna*) [159, 160], Pushkarmoola (*Inula racemose*) [159, 160, 162], Turmeric (*Curcuma longa*) [159], *Ligusticum chuanxiong* Hort [159]. Guggul (*Commiphora mukul*) [160], Gualoupi (*Trichosanthis kirilowii or T. rosthornii*) [163].

Other natural products that could be used as antianginal agents are; grapes, as it has been proposed that resveratrol is an antiaging metabolite and prevents the decline in cardiovascular function caused by aging through the expression of several longevity genes [164]. Coleus contains the alkaloid forskolin, exhibits hypotensive, positive inotrophic, vasodilator, anti-platelet aggregation activities [165]. Khellin, from khella, was reported to have more potent action than many of the common coronary vasodilators [166]. Also, Alfalfa leaves, sprouts, ginger, green tea, lingzhi and brindle berry were found to possess hypolipidimic activities, through which they have potential antiatherosclerotic effects [167].

A step further was undertaken to evaluate the beneficial effects of single compounds in the treatment of angina. However, most of these compounds were assessed as an approach to avert its long-term complications, with exception to puerarin, a well-established antianginal agent. It is an isoflavone purified from Pueraria genus, which significantly reduces the frequency of angina events and myocardial oxygen consumption, increases the duration of exercise and reverses the abnormal rest ECG in a clinical study involving unstable angina patients [168].

Table 1. Key botanicals used in the treatment of stable angina pectoris.

Plant	Part Used	Main Active Constituents	Experimental Design	Mechanism of Action
Hawthorn *(Crataegus oxyacantha),* *(C. monogyna),* *(C. laevigata),* and *(C. pinnatifida)*	Leaves, flowers, and berries	Oligomeric proanthocyanidin	Randomized controlled trials, observational cohort study, multicenter, placebo-controlled, double-blind study and *In vitro* studies	• Increases the force of myocardial contraction • Enhances coronary blood flow and coronary perfusion • Improves oxygen utilization by cardiomyocytes • Prolonges the refractory period and action-potential duration in heart and papillary muscles • Has a mild hypotensive effect • Antagonizes atherogenesis with a negative chronotropic effect and a positive inotropic effect on the contraction amplitude of cardiac myocytes • Inhibits 3′,5′-cyclic adenosine monophosphate phosphodiesterase • Lowers arrhythmogenic risk as it prolongs the effective refractory period

(Table 1) cont.....

Plant	Part Used	Main Active Constituents	Experimental Design	Mechanism of Action
Danshen *Salvia miltiorrhizae*	Root	Tanshinone (I, IIA, and IIB) and salvianolic acids (A, B)	Animal studies, *In vitro* studies and randomized controlled trials	• Enhances the recovery of contractile force upon reoxygenation following myocardial ischemia • Reduces ischemic symptoms and improves the pathological electrocardiogram (ECG) pattern • Has a negative inotropic effect and increases the coronary flow rate • Can reduce the infarct size caused by myocardial ischemia • Reduces the risk of myocardial tissue necrosis. • Upregulates the expression of vascular endothelial growth factors • Improves microcirculation, causes endothelium-dependent vasodilation in aortic strips, causes general vasodilation (low dose) and vasoconstriction in noncoronary arteries (high dose) • Inhibits angiotensin-converting enzyme • Increases nitric oxide production by endothelial cells. • Inhibits thrombosis, thromboxane B2 formation, and platelet aggregration • Antioxidant activity

(Table 1) cont.....

Plant	Part Used	Main Active Constituents	Experimental Design	Mechanism of Action
San qi *Panax notoginseng*	Root	Saponines (ginsenosides) and notoginsenosides	Animal studies, *In vitro* studies	• Reduces myocardial oxygen consumption and protects the myocardium • Increase coronary blood flow • Enhances blood fibrinolytic parameters • Dilates coronary arteries (dose dependent) • Inhibits atherosclerosis by inhibiting the proliferation of aortic smooth muscle cells • Reduces thrombogenicity and increases erythrocyte deformability. • Suppresses cardiac arrhythmias during oxygen-deprivation ischemia and reperfusion • Calcium ion channel antagonist in vascular tissues, resulting in hypotension • Lipid-lowering effects and antioxidant activity
Garlic *Allium sativum*	Bulbs	Garlicin	Randomized controlled trials, double-blind, crossover study and *In vitro* studies	• Inhibits platelet aggregation • Hypolipidemic action • Enhances the fibrinolytic activity • Protects the elastic properties of the aorta • Hypoglycemic action
Maidenhair *Gingko biloba*	Leaves	Ginkgolides, flavonoid glycosides, terpene lactones and ginkgolic acid	Animal models, and clinical trials	• Inhibits the platelet-activating factor • Antioxidant activity • Increases the blood flow *via* release of nitric oxide and prostaglandins
Arjuna *Terminalia arjuna*	Stem bark	Triterpinoids, flavonoids, and minerals	Animal models, double-blind crossover study, open-label studies and randomized controlled trials	• Positive inotropic • Vasodilator effect on coronary arteries • Reverses smoking-related endothelial dysfunction • Lipid-lowering effects and antioxidant activity

(Table 1) cont.....

Plant	Part Used	Main Active Constituents	Experimental Design	Mechanism of Action
Pushkarmoola *Inula racemosa*	Root	Sesquiterpene lactones (alantolactone and isoalantolactone)	Animal studies, preliminary clinical study, open-label clinical study	• Negative ionotropic and negative chronotropic effect • Blocks the action of adrenaline • Act as an agonist for propranolol • Improves hemodynamic function and left-ventricular function • Antioxidant activity
Turmeric *Curcuma longa*	Rhizome	Curcuminoids demethoxycurcumin (curcumin II), bisdemethoxycurcumin (curcumin III), and cyclocurcumin	Animal studies, randomized controlled trials	• Antioxidant effects that attenuate adriamycin-induced cardiotoxicity • Prevents cardiovascular complications associated with diabetes • Inhibit p300-HAT and thus can ameloriate the development of cardiac hypertrophy and heart failure • Antiinflammatory effects may prevent atrial arrhythmias • Lipid lowering effects
Ligusticum *chuanxiong* Hort .	Root	Phalides (senkyunolide, Z-ligustilide, ligustiliden, ligustilide dimers, ligustrazine neocnidilide, 3-butylphthalide, Butylidenephthalide, and Tetramethylpyrazine)	*In vitro* studies, controlled and self-crossover clinical trial	• Relaxes the vascular rings and inhibits against contractions induced by phenylephrine; the potentiation of relaxation is postulated to be related to nitric oxide • Increases coronary blood flow and decreases myocardial contractile force • Inhibits the TNF-alpha production and TNF-alpha bioactivity in human monocytic cell lines
Guggul *Commiphora mukul*	Oleo-gum-resin	Guggulipid and guggulsterones	Animal studies, double-blind placebo control study	• It is an antagonist ligand for the bile acid receptor (farnesoid X receptor) which causes hypolipidemia • Increases the plasma fibrinolytic activity

(Table 1) cont.....

Plant	Part Used	Main Active Constituents	Experimental Design	Mechanism of Action
Gualoupi *Trichosanthis kirilowii* or *T. rosthornii*	Pericarp of ripe fruits	Lignan, trichobenzolignan and trichosanthin	Animal studies, randomized controlled trials	• Regulates lipid metabolism, exerts antiatherosclerotic effects and protects the vascular endothelium. • Protects against ischemia reperfusion, injury, hypoxia, and calcium antagonism

Its mechanism of action involves the preservation of the mitochondrial structure and decreasing the myocardial lactate production and creatine phosphokinase release following a myocardial injury in a dog model [169]. Another clinical study proved that puerarinis involved in regulating endothelin, rennin, and angiotensin II imbalance in acute myocardial infarction patients [170]. Nevertheless, another clinical study suggested an alternative mechanism of action of puerarin involving platelet activating factors in patients with unstable angia pectoris [171].

Tetrahydropalmatine, an isoquinoline alkaloid isolated from *Corydalis* genus and *Stephania rotunda,* was reported to treat the increase of creatine kinase and aspartate aminotransferase in a rat model [172]. Magnesium tanshinoate B isolated from *Salvia miltiorrhizae* was found to stimulate NO release, enhance the cellular activities of NO synthase and associated increase the levels of constitutive NO in human endothelial cells *in vitro* [173]. Scutellarin, the major constituent of *Erigeron breviscapus,* decreased the degree of MI induced by isoprenaline in rats as proved recently by Huang *et al.* [174] Similarly, Baicalin from the genus Scutellaria, possesses protective actions on MI in rats. The probable mechanisms may involve its resistance to oxidative stress, and up-regulation of B-cell lymphoma-2 (Bcl-2) protein expression and down-regulation of Bcl-2 associated X (Bax) protein expression in myocardial tissue [175]. Also, the benzylisoquinoline alkaloid, berberine, significantly reduced the release of creatine phosphokinase and reversed the ultrastructural damage in isolated rat hearts [176], berberine's positive inotropic effect and mild vasodilation action helps its amelioration of the impaired left ventricular function and the decreased cardiac output in dogs [177, 178].

In conclusion, the mechanisms of action of most of these natural products need further clarifications and there is insufficient basis of their effectiveness in the treatment of various CVD. Hence, it is a need rather than an interest, to pay more attention to confirm the traditional claims of their use as antianginal agents. Multidisciplinary research is very important to evaluate the therapeutic potential of these natural plants and point out the active constituent(s) responsible for the activity and its/their effective dose, through biologically guided studies. In addition to, their possible synergistic interactions with each other or other antianginal drugs and their adverse side effects. This will aid in their establishment as antianginal agents and their addition to the mainstream of cardiovascular remedies.

5. ATHEROSCLEROSIS

5.1. Pathophysiology of Atherosclerosis

Atherosclerosis is the key cause for the development of various CVD such as angina, myocardial infarction and ischemic heart failure. Atherosclerosis is characterized by endothelial dysfunction, inflammatory responses, extracellular matrix alteration, Smooth Muscle Cell (SMC) proliferation and thrombosis [179]. Atherosclerosis development may lead to blood supply reduction to the coronary arteries which can cause MI, which is the main pathological factor for coronary heart diseases [180].

Large and middle-sized arteries intima are particularly the sites of arterial bifurcations and they are highly influenced by atherosclerosis. Vascular SMCs, WBCs and modified lipids are accumulated in the intima. The accumulated SMCs at the tunica intima layer of the arteries can then migrate to form atheroma plaque through their proliferation. Pro-inflammatory activation of vascular SMCs causes a change to synthetic from contractile phenotype, leading to cell proliferation and migration. This migration of the activated vascular SMCs from the media to the intima leads to pro-atherosclerotic vascular remodelling [181].

The matrix metalloproteinases (MMPs), are involved in the process of proliferation and migration of vascular SMCs as it has a proteolytic activity that allows it to cause elastic lamina barrier of extracellular matrix degradation leading to various pathological conditions [182, 183].

In addition, these arterial regions suffer a turbulent shear stress that promotes endothelial cells (ECs) pro-inflammatory activation [184]. This activation is stimulated by the modified LDL, especially the oxidized LDL (oxLDL). The activated ECs express intercellular adhesion molecule-1 (ICAM-1) and vascular cell adhesion molecule (VCAM-1) which attract monocytes and lymphocytes binding the endothelium and infiltrate the intima. Also accumulation of oxLDL takes place in the sub-endothelial level developing the atheorosclerotic plaque. In the intima, monocytes differentiate to macrophages which engulf oxLDL deposits and transform into foam cells [185]. Other immune cells are present in the lesion and are involved in the intraplaque inflammation [186]. During the progression of atherosclerosis, immune and non-immune vascular cells release a variety of pro-inflammatory messengers that preserve and improve the local inflammation and atherosclerotic lesions development) Fig. (**2**). Also, the concomitant up-regulation of pro-inflammatory signalling pathways in both vascular and blood cells stimulates atherogenesis [187].

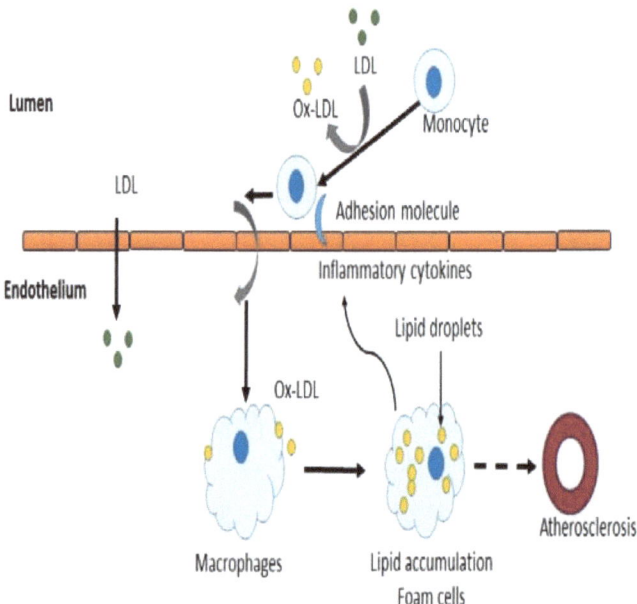

Fig. (2). Schematic representation of the mechanism of atherosclerosis.

There is increasing evidence that NO and NO synthase (NOS) systems in vascular SMCs can regulate the local vascular injury accompanying atherosclerosis. In healthy vessels, endothelial isoform of NOS (eNOS) produces NO in the endothelium and acts as an endothelium-derived relaxing factor essential for maintenance of vascular homeostasis. In atherosclerotic vessels, the endothelium-dependent relaxation impaired and represents the reduced eNOS-derived NO bioavailability that promotes atherosclerosis development [187]. In case of atherosclerosis, the inducible isoform of NOS (iNOS) is unable to recompense for the lost functional endothelium and eNOS [188]. Increased expression of iNOS has been linked to stimulating the pathogenesis of atherosclerosis [189]. In the advanced atherosclerotic plaques, iNOS may constantly indorse a pathogenic environment *via* oxidative and nitrosative stress enhancements [190]. There are much evidences that foresees the NO and NOS system as a potential target for atherosclerosis management.

5.2. Natural Products and Atherosclerosis

5.2.1. Ginkgetin

Medicinal plants have proven great efficacy as therapeutic agents for atherosclerosis. *G. biloba* is a plant of family Ginkgocea whose leaves have high content of acylatedflavonols, bioflavonoids and terpenoids [191]. Among Ginkgo biflavones, ginkgetin **3)** Fig. **(3)** has been shown to possess anti-inflammatory, neuroprotective, and anti-cancer activities [192]. Ginkgetin has been reported to down-regulate the expression of the matrix metalloproteinase (MMP-2 and MMP-9) in thoracic aortas of atherosclerotic rats [193]. As mentioned before, MMPs have a primary role in enhancing vascular remodeling and SMC migration [194]. Various matrix cells and macrophages produce MMP-9 which contributes in the degradation process of active substance in extracellular matrix of various tissues [195]. Thus, reduction in MMPs expression helps the remodeling of vascular extracellular matrices and reduces the migration of SMCs, thus contributes to the improvement of atherosclerotic rats.

Fig. (3). Structure of Ginkgetin.

NO can suppress the progression of atherosclerosis by decreasing monocyte-endothelial cell interaction, hindering the adherence and aggregation of the platelets, and thus prevent SMC proliferation. Moreover, in the atherosclerotic rats, the expression of eNOS in serum and thoracic aortas was notably reduced, indicating that absence of NO promotes the pathogenesis of atherosclerosis [193]. Ginkgetin could increase the levels of NO in atherosclerotic rats. Ginkgetin was also found to up-regulate the levels of eNOS expression and down-regulate the levels of iNOS expression which were elevated atherosclerotic rats [193]. The increased expression and activity of iNOS was linked to the progression of atherosclerosis that was induced in vascular SMCs by pro-inflammatory cytokines released from injured cells [190]. Thus that ginkgetin can be said to ameliorate atherosclerosis through modulation of NO/NOS system.

5.2.2. Colchicine

Colchicine as shown in Fig. (**4**) is a tropolone alkaloid isolated from the seeds and corms of genus Colchicum. Now, Colchicine is used for relieving the pain resulting from gout or familial Mediterranean fever, and under research to be used for treatment of pericarditis, and Behçet's disease due to its anti-inflammatory activity but its clinical applications is still limited due to its toxicity [196 - 198]. Anti-inflammatory activity of colchicine through which it inhibits inflammation in patients with acute coronary syndrome (ACS) or after acute MI is mediated by its anti-tubulin action and neutrophil function inhibition [199].

In a clinical trial, administration of oral dose (1 mg) of colchicine daily for 4 weeks has caused reduction in CRP levels in patients suffering from CAD [200]. In another clinical trial conducted on larger sample (532 of CAD patients), a daily dose of colchicine (0.5 mg) for 30 days caused a three-fold reduction of incidence cardiac arrest and non-embolic stroke and this effect last during the median three-year follow-up period [201].

In a prospective non-randomized pilot study conducted on 80 subjects with recent post-acute coronary syndrome (ACS) that last for less than one month, patients received either 0.5 mg/day colchicine plus optimal medical therapy (OMT) or OMT alone and with a followed up over a year. The results of this pilot study showed that colchicine at low dose caused modification of the coronary plaque, independent of high-dose statin combined therapy and significantly reduced the low-density lipoprotein (LDL). Colchicine also improved the plaque morphology through its anti-inflammatory effect which also helped in the reduction of high-sensitivity C-reactive protein (hsCRP), rather than changes in lipoproteins [202].

A review of 4992 patients in thirty nine trials of any clinical setting involving long-term colchicine compared to control showed that colchicine proved no effect on heart failure and stroke, however it showed efficacy in populations suffering Myocardial Infarction (MI) at high-risk [203]. Administration of colchicine for more than 6 months showed potential efficacy in minimizing MI risk and cardiovascular mortality [204].

A study was conducted on 1288 subjects having gout, and at high cardiovascular risk, in which the administration of colchicine caused a fifty four percent reduction in relative risk of MI [205]. Another retrospective cohort study investigated 501 gout patients and similar protective effects of colchicine were observed [206].

Another trial was performed on 196 patients suffering from diabetes mellitus who had percutaneous coronary intervention with a bare metal stent. Administration of Colchicine for six months exerted a decrease in in-stent restenosis relative to placebo as shown in the follow-up angiography and intravascular ultrasound [207]. However, another double blinded, placebo-controlled study of 145 patients using the same dose of colchicine did not show improvement in the rate of angiographic restenosis in elective coronary angioplasty of 393 lesions without stent placement [208].

Furthermore, the role of colchicine was assessed specifically in a randomized trial conducted on 151 patients with ST-segment elevation MI (STEMI) who received colchicine for five days. Colchicine treated group showed a significant lower infarct size, as evaluated by creatine kinase-muscle/brain (CK-MB) concentration when compared to the placebo group. The cardiac magnetic resonance imaging of 60 of these patients confirmed that colchicine could significantly reduce the infarct size when compared to the left ventricular myocardial volume [209].

Fig. (4). Structure of Colchicine.

5.2.3. Garlic

Garlic (*Allium sativum*) contains active ingredients which exert prophylactic and treating effects against atherosclerosis [210].

A garlic-based herbal preparation was prepared and named Allicor. This preparation was tested in a pilot study which included 28 healthy men with the age range of 46–58 (52.0 ± 9.0). Anti-atherosclerotic activity of the preparation was indicated by the carotid intima-media thickness (cIMT), the subjects received Allicor daily for total duration of a year, however, ultrasound examination of the carotid arteries were held every 3 months. The product was well-tolerated that was deduced from the absence of the adverse effects during the follow-up period. Allicor significantly reduced the tendency to cIMT [210].

In a clinical study, the effect of Allicor on the cIMT progression in 211 asymptomatic men aged 40 - 74 was studied. By the end of the first year follow-up period, a significant reduction of cIMT was observed in the Allicor-treated group, when compared to the placebo group [211]. After the 2-years follow-up period, the mean rate of cIMT was significantly reduced in the Allicor-treated group, relative to the placebo group [212, 213]. Consequently, it was recorded that long-term treatment with Allicor possessed an anti-atherosclerotic effect which was attributable to the improvement of serum atherogenicity [212, 213].

5.2.4. Anti-Inflammatory Herbs

Inflammation has a crucial role in all the development stages of atherosclerosis [214, 215]. Many anti-inflammatory plants of the Mediterranean region can be used for the protection against atherosclerosis. Therefore, Calendula (*Calendula officinalis*), elder (*Sambucus nigra*) and violet (*Viola tricolor*) have been reported to have both anti-inflammatory and anti-atherogenic effects [216, 217]. Inflaminat is a combination of the three above mentioned plants, its effect was evaluated on cIMT in a pilot phase of a study designed on 67 asymptomatic men for a year [213, 218, 219]. In subclinical atherosclerosis, inflaminat could induce cIMT regression, which was significant relative to the placebo group. Thus, Inflaminat demonstrated anti-inflammatory and anti-atherosclerotic effects on cellular levels and induced regression of subclinical atherosclerosis in asymptomatic men.

5.2.5. Phytoestrogen-Rich Herbs

Several natural herbs that are rich in phytoestrogen, showed promising *in vitro* and *ex vivo* anti-atherogenic activity were incorporated into an herbal preparation named Karinat [220 - 222]. These herbs are garlic powder, extract of grape seeds (*Vitis vinifera*), green tea leaves (*Camellia sinensis*) and hops (*Humulus lupulus*). Additionally, Karinat was rich in biologically active polyphenols including resveratrol, genistein and daidzein, thus it could improve phytoestrogen profile. Karinat was tested for anti-atherosclerotic effect in a pilot clinical study on 157 asymptomatic postmenopausal women for a year [223, 224]. At the end, an increase in the mean cIMT was detected in the placebo group, with a 40% growth in the atherosclerotic plaque in postmenopausal women. Inversely, the mean cIMT remained stable in the Karinat-treated group. The studied phytoestrogen complex suppressed the formation of new atherosclerotic lesions in postmenopausal women [213, 225].

6. HERBAL TREATMENT OF CEREBROVASCULAR DISORDERS

Cerebrovascular disorders involve different kinds of diseases, such as stroke, cerebral edema, vascular dementia, and transient ischemic attack, in addition to age-associated memory impairment which is experienced by elderly people, as dizziness, depression, and tinnitus [226]. Regrettably, the mortality data conveyed to the WHO by different countries are inconsistent [227]. However, these diseases, especially stroke, represent the third leading cause of death in the United States after heart diseases and cancer [226].

This category of diseases is considered as a type of peripheral vascular diseases. They occur as a consequence of the brain cells dysfunction, which happens due to free radicals including superoxide, hydrogen peroxide and hydroxylation radicals or decreased oxygenation level. This part of the chapter will focus mainly on the second point; major causes of decreased oxygen level supplied to brain neuronal cells and its possible herbal treatment.

Cerebral tissues consume approx. 20% of the total body requirement from oxygen to live and work properly. Deficiency of oxygen supply in cerebral tissues has many reasons, which could be classified into abnormalities of the vessels supplying the blood to the brain due to atherosclerosis or arthritis or abnormalities in the blood flow itself. Diseases in blood vessels provoke secretion of platelet-activating factor (PAF) and thrombus formation. Thrombosis or embolism reduces the oxygen supply to the cerebral tissues significantly and results in tissue hypoxia or ischemia affecting the blood flow and tissue oxygenation as well.

Major developments in treating ischemic stroke have been performed over the last decade. However, stroke is still a serious concern for which effective drug therapy is not yet available [228]. To date, the FDA only approved Recombinant plasminogen activator (rt-PA) for the treatment of stroke. However, thrombolysis lessens stroke morbidity but is only relevant to a small percentage of stroke patients [229].

6.1. Physiology and Pathophysiology of Blood Coagulation

Physiologically, blood coagulation systems or hemostasis functions through extrinsic and intrinsic pathways that are promoted differently *via* tissue injury or abnormal pathological conditions. However, they joined in a common pathway at the conversion step of thrombin from prothrombin.

Coagulation cascades are monitored through a number of clinical laboratory tests, such as APTT for the intrinsic pathway, PT for extrinsic pathway, and TT for common pathway. In addition, International Normalized Ratio (INR) or standardized prothrombin time is sometimes required especially for patients taking anti-clotting medicines, such as warfarin.

6.2. Natural Treatments of Coagulation Abnormalities

Natural herbal antioxidants are out of scope of this part. Therefore, a number of herbal treatments that could be used to alleviate symptoms of thrombosis and resulting cerebrovascular disorders will be covered in the following section.

6.2.1 Ginkolides and Bilobalides

Ginko tree (*Ginko biloba* L., Ginkoaceae) is always described by the "living fossil". Additionally, it has a long history, some 2000 years especially in China, in treating many diseases. *Ginkgo biloba* is amongst the best seller medicinal plants with 4.5 to 5.1 million pounds annual consumption in 2001 of the dried leaves. Currently there are about 142 *G. biloba* products on the market worldwide and its utilization is estimated to grow threefold in the upcoming five years [230].

Standardized leaf extracts of *G. biloba* (SGB extracts) have neuroprotective activities. In addition, it may be useful in preventing and treating CVD, mainly ischemic cardiac syndrome [231, 232].

These bioactivities owe to its mixture contents from flavonol and biflavone glycosides, such as quercetin and kaempferol, in addition to sesquiterpene and diterpene lactones, including bilobalide and ginkolides, respectively. Flavonoid contents enhance the capillary integrity in addition to its function as free-radical scavengers as well [233]. While terpene lactones work as platelet-activating factor inhibitors produced by different tissues. This function prevents platelet aggregation and its subsequent thrombus formation.

6.2.2. Sulphated Polysaccharides

Marine macroalgae produce sulphated and non-sulphated polysaccharides possessing a wide-range of interesting medical applications making them promising pharmaceutical products [234]. Among them are Phaeophytes or brown algae polysaccharides, *e.g.*, fucoidan, alginate and laminarin. Several reports investigated the potential anticoagulant activity of the sulphated polysaccharide fucoidan [235 - 237]. They reported that it acts in a heparin-like manner and interfered mainly with the intrinsic pathway of the coagulation system [238, 239]. In addition, the negative charge distribution of its structure together with its long polysaccharide chain, high molecular weight, and structure comfort ability contributed to inhibition of thrombin and discontinuation of the fibrinogen conversion to fibrin [240].

6.2.3. Garlic Thiosulphinates

Chemistry and biology of garlic (*Allium sativum* L., family Alliaceae) have been intensively investigated as one of the most investigated medicinal plants. More than 3000 research articles were published in the last few decades during 1960 to 2007. Most of these studies focused on the possible indication of garlic in treatment of CVD [241]. Garlic contains over a hundred 100 sulfur-containing metabolites. Allicin represents 70-80% of the total thiosulphinates. The anti-platelet activity of garlic has been attributed to adenosine, allicin and other thiosulfinates [242].

6.2.4. Extract of Antrodia Camphora

A. camphorate is a fungal parasite that lives and grows on *Cinnamomum kanehirae* (Bull camphor tree) Hayata (Lauraceae) [243]. Polysaccharides, terpenoids, lignans, benzenoids, benzoquinone derivatives have been identified.

Pharmacologically, it is used in Traditional Chinese Medicine (TCM) for the treatment of viral hepatitis and cancer, yet, it has shown neuroprotective effects in embolic rats, recently [228]. It is useful in reestablishing blood flow to the ischemic brain through the reduction of perfusion deficits following ischemia and without causing any hemorrhagic incidence when used in conjunction with aspirin therapy [244].

6.2.5. Alpha-lipois Acid

Alpha-lipoic acid or ALA is found in various foods. It shows a significant part in metabolic processes. It functions as a cofactor for several key enzymes. It has been known as the "perfect" antioxidant [245]. It protects against oxidation, thus prevents Ischemia-reperfusion injury [245]. It attenuates middle cerebral artery occlusion-induced cerebral ischemia and reperfusion injury. It acts *via* insulin receptor-dependent and PI3K/Akt-dependent inhibition of NADPH oxidase. Moreover, an interesting study established the effects of Tetra Methyl Pyrazine (TMP) on functional recovery and neuronal dendritic plasticity after experimental stroke. In that study, the authors have demonstrated that enhanced dendritic plasticity contributes to TMP-elicited functional recovery after ischemic stroke [246].

CONCLUDING REMARKS

The increase in the popularity of the use of natural products has raised the interest in natural remedies that can be beneficial in the treatment of cardiovascular diseases. This chapter highlights the cardiovascular effects of natural products and their metabolites in controlling cardiovascular diseases especially those subjected to sub-clinical or clinical trials. Although most of the mentioned plants have a long history in treating heart diseases, recent research strategies show how efficient they are in the treatment of different cardiovascular diseases including ischemic heart disease, congestive heart failure, and hypertension by unique mechanisms. In addition, we also discussed the chemical constituents of these plant species which provide beneficial effects by various modes of action that can improve the quality of life in patients with heart disease and potentially save their lives.

CONSENT FOR PUBLICATION

Not applicable.

CONFLICT OF INTEREST

The author confirms that this chapter contents have no conflict of interest.

ACKNOWLEDGEMENTS

Declared none.

REFERENCES

[1]   W.H.O. Hearts. technical package for cardiovascular disease management in primary health care WHO Press, 20 Avenue Appia, 1211 Geneva 27, Switzerland.

[2]   Kulczyński B, Gramza-Michałowska A, Kobus-Cisowska J, Kmiecik D. The role of carotenoids in the prevention and treatment of cardiovascular disease – Current state of knowledge. J Funct Foods 2017; 38: 45-65.
        [http://dx.doi.org/10.1016/j.jff.2017.09.001]

[3]   Piepoli MF, Hoes AW, Agewall S, *et al.* 2016 European Guidelines on cardiovascular disease prevention in clinical practice. Atherosclerosis 2016; 252: 207-74.
        [http://dx.doi.org/10.1016/j.atherosclerosis.2016.05.037] [PMID: 27664503]

[4]   Chomistek AK, Manson JE, Stefanick ML, *et al.* Relationship of sedentary behavior and physical activity to incident cardiovascular disease: results from the Women's Health Initiative. J Am Coll Cardiol 2013; 61(23): 2346-54.
        [http://dx.doi.org/10.1016/j.jacc.2013.03.031] [PMID: 23583242]

[5]   Chistiakov DA, Orekhov AN, Bobryshev YV. Treatment of cardiovascular pathology with epigenetically active agents: Focus on natural and synthetic inhibitors of DNA methylation and histone deacetylation. Int J Cardiol 2017; 227: 66-82.
        [http://dx.doi.org/10.1016/j.ijcard.2016.11.204] [PMID: 27852009]

[6]   W.H.O. World health statistics 2018. monitoring health for the SDGs, sustainable development goals Geneva: World Health Organization; Licence. 2018. CC BY-NC-SA 3.0 IGO.

[7]   Mann D, Zipes D, Libby P, Bonow R. Braunwald's Heart Disease: A Textbook of Cardiovascular Medicine. Saunders 2014; p. 2040.

[8]   Homans DC, Asinger R, Elsperger KJ, *et al.* Regional function and perfusion at the lateral border of ischemic myocardium. Circulation 1985; 71(5): 1038-47.
        [http://dx.doi.org/10.1161/01.CIR.71.5.1038] [PMID: 3986974]

[9]   Deb S, Wijeysundera HC, Ko DT, Tsubota H, Hill S, Fremes SE. Coronary artery bypass graft surgery *vs* percutaneous interventions in coronary revascularization: a systematic review. JAMA 2013; 310(19): 2086-95.
        [http://dx.doi.org/10.1001/jama.2013.281718] [PMID: 24240936]

[10]   Nidorf SM, Siu SC, Galambos G, Weyman AE, Picard MH. Benefit of late coronary reperfusion on ventricular morphology and function after myocardial infarction. J Am Coll Cardiol 1993; 21(3): 683-91.
        [http://dx.doi.org/10.1016/0735-1097(93)90101-6] [PMID: 8436750]

[11]   Sabia P, Abbott RD, Afrookteh A, Keller MW, Touchstone DA, Kaul S. Importance of two-dimensional echocardiographic assessment of left ventricular systolic function in patients presenting to the emergency room with cardiac-related symptoms. Circulation 1991; 84(4): 1615-24.
        [http://dx.doi.org/10.1161/01.CIR.84.4.1615] [PMID: 1914101]

[12]   Cassar A, Holmes DR Jr, Rihal CS, Gersh BJ. Chronic coronary artery disease: diagnosis and management. Mayo Clin Proc 2009; 84(12): 1130-46.
        [http://dx.doi.org/10.4065/mcp.2009.0391] [PMID: 19955250]

[13]   Charlson FJ, Moran AE, Freedman G, *et al.* The contribution of major depression to the global burden of ischemic heart disease: a comparative risk assessment. BMC Med 2013; 11: 250.
        [http://dx.doi.org/10.1186/1741-7015-11-250] [PMID: 24274053]

[14]   Mehta PK, Wei J, Wenger NK. Ischemic heart disease in women: a focus on risk factors. Trends Cardiovasc Med 2015; 25(2): 140-51.
        [http://dx.doi.org/10.1016/j.tcm.2014.10.005] [PMID: 25453985]

[15]   Anker SD, von Haehling S. Inflammatory mediators in chronic heart failure: an overview. Heart 2004; 90(4): 464-70.
        [http://dx.doi.org/10.1136/hrt.2002.007005] [PMID: 15020532]

[16]   Dassanayaka S, Jones SP. Recent developments in heart failure. Circ Res 2015; 117(7): e58-63.
        [http://dx.doi.org/10.1161/CIRCRESAHA.115.305765] [PMID: 26358111]

[17]   Hofmann U, Frantz S. How can we cure a heart "in flame"? A translational view on inflammation in heart failure. Basic Res Cardiol 2013; 108(4): 356.
        [http://dx.doi.org/10.1007/s00395-013-0356-y] [PMID: 23740214]

[18]   Bibbins-Domingo K, Lin F, Vittinghoff E, *et al.* Predictors of heart failure among women with coronary disease. Circulation 2004; 110(11): 1424-30.
        [http://dx.doi.org/10.1161/01.CIR.0000141726.01302.83] [PMID: 15353499]

[19]   Stein GY, Kremer A, Shochat T, *et al.* The diversity of heart failure in a hospitalized population: the role of age. J Card Fail 2012; 18(8): 645-53.
        [http://dx.doi.org/10.1016/j.cardfail.2012.05.007] [PMID: 22858081]

[20]   Lazzarini V, Mentz RJ, Fiuzat M, Metra M, O'Connor CM. Heart failure in elderly patients:

distinctive features and unresolved issues. Eur J Heart Fail 2013; 15(7): 717-23.
[http://dx.doi.org/10.1093/eurjhf/hft028] [PMID: 23429975]

[21]   Roger VL, Go AS, Lloyd-Jones DM, *et al.* Heart disease and stroke statistics-2011 update: a report from the American Heart Association. Circulation 2011; 123(4): e18-e209.
[http://dx.doi.org/10.1161/CIR.0b013e3182009701] [PMID: 21160056]

[22]   Lloyd-Jones D, Adams RJ, Brown TM, *et al.* Heart disease and stroke statistics-2010 update: a report from the American Heart Association. Circulation 2010; 121(7): e46-e215.
[http://dx.doi.org/10.1161/CIRCULATIONAHA.109.192667] [PMID: 20019324]

[23]   Floras JS. Sympathetic nervous system activation in human heart failure: clinical implications of an updated model. J Am Coll Cardiol 2009; 54(5): 375-85.
[http://dx.doi.org/10.1016/j.jacc.2009.03.061] [PMID: 19628111]

[24]   Zucker IH, Xiao L, Haack KK. The central renin-angiotensin system and sympathetic nerve activity in chronic heart failure. Clin Sci (Lond) 2014; 126(10): 695-706.
[http://dx.doi.org/10.1042/CS20130294] [PMID: 24490814]

[25]   Mangini S, Pires PV, Braga FG, Bacal F. Decompensated heart failure. Einstein (Sao Paulo) 2013; 11(3): 383-91.
[http://dx.doi.org/10.1590/S1679-45082013000300022] [PMID: 24136770]

[26]   Johansen H, Strauss B, Arnold JM, Moe G, Liu P. On the rise: The current and projected future burden of congestive heart failure hospitalization in Canada. Can J Cardiol 2003; 19(4): 430-5.
[PMID: 12704491]

[27]   Azad N, Lemay G. Management of chronic heart failure in the older population. J Geriatr Cardiol 2014; 11(4): 329-37.
[http://dx.doi.org/10.11909/j.issn.1671-5411.2014.04.008] [PMID: 25593582]

[28]   Tamargo J, López-Sendón J. Novel therapeutic targets for the treatment of heart failure. Nat Rev Drug Discov 2011; 10(7): 536-55.
[http://dx.doi.org/10.1038/nrd3431] [PMID: 21701502]

[29]   Inamdar AA, Inamdar AC. Heart Failure: Diagnosis, Management and Utilization. J Clin Med 2016; 5(7)E62
[http://dx.doi.org/10.3390/jcm5070062] [PMID: 27367736]

[30]   Shukla SK, Gupta S, Ojha SK, Sharma SB. Cardiovascular friendly natural products: a promising approach in the management of CVD. Nat Prod Res 2010; 24(9): 873-98.
[http://dx.doi.org/10.1080/14786410903417378] [PMID: 20461632]

[31]   Esterbauer H, Waeg G, Puhl H, Dieber-Rotheneder M, Tatzber F. Inhibition of LDL oxidation by antioxidants. EXS 1992; 62: 145-57.
[PMID: 1450582]

[32]   Janero DR. Ischemic heart disease and antioxidants: mechanistic aspects of oxidative injury and its prevention. Crit Rev Food Sci Nutr 1995; 35(1-2): 65-81.
[http://dx.doi.org/10.1080/10408399509527688] [PMID: 7748481]

[33]   Weseler AR, Bast A. Oxidative stress and vascular function: implications for pharmacologic treatments. Curr Hypertens Rep 2010; 12(3): 154-61.
[http://dx.doi.org/10.1007/s11906-010-0103-9] [PMID: 20424954]

[34]   Arai Y, Watanabe S, Kimira M, Shimoi K, Mochizuki R, Kinae N. Dietary intakes of flavonols, flavones and isoflavones by Japanese women and the inverse correlation between quercetin intake and plasma LDL cholesterol concentration. J Nutr 2000; 130(9): 2243-50.
[http://dx.doi.org/10.1093/jn/130.9.2243] [PMID: 10958819]

[35]   Arima H, Ashida H, Danno G. Rutin-enhanced antibacterial activities of flavonoids against *Bacillus cereus* and *Salmonella enteritidis*. Biosci Biotechnol Biochem 2002; 66(5): 1009-14.
[http://dx.doi.org/10.1271/bbb.66.1009] [PMID: 12092809]

[36] Binsack R, Boersma BJ, Patel RP, *et al.* Enhanced antioxidant activity after chlorination of quercetin by hypochlorous acid. Alcohol Clin Exp Res 2001; 25(3): 434-43.
[http://dx.doi.org/10.1111/j.1530-0277.2001.tb02232.x] [PMID: 11290856]

[37] Kähkönen MP, Heinonen M. Antioxidant activity of anthocyanins and their aglycons. J Agric Food Chem 2003; 51(3): 628-33.
[http://dx.doi.org/10.1021/jf025551i] [PMID: 12537433]

[38] de Whalley CV, Rankin SM, Hoult JR, Jessup W, Leake DS. Flavonoids inhibit the oxidative modification of low density lipoproteins by macrophages. Biochem Pharmacol 1990; 39(11): 1743-50.
[http://dx.doi.org/10.1016/0006-2952(90)90120-A] [PMID: 2344371]

[39] Duffy SJ, Keaney JF Jr, Holbrook M, *et al.* Short- and long-term black tea consumption reverses endothelial dysfunction in patients with coronary artery disease. Circulation 2001; 104(2): 151-6.
[http://dx.doi.org/10.1161/01.CIR.104.2.151] [PMID: 11447078]

[40] Guardia T, Rotelli AE, Juarez AO, Pelzer LE. Anti-inflammatory properties of plant flavonoids. Effects of rutin, quercetin and hesperidin on adjuvant arthritis in rat. Farmaco 2001; 56(9): 683-7.
[http://dx.doi.org/10.1016/S0014-827X(01)01111-9] [PMID: 11680812]

[41] Choi JH, Chang HW, Rhee SJ. Effect of green tea catechin on arachidonic acid cascade in chronic cadmium-poisoned rats. Asia Pac J Clin Nutr 2002; 11(4): 292-7.
[http://dx.doi.org/10.1046/j.1440-6047.2002.00305.x] [PMID: 12495261]

[42] Hollman PC, Hertog MG, Katan MB. Role of dietary flavonoids in protection against cancer and coronary heart disease. Biochem Soc Trans 1996; 24(3): 785-9.
[http://dx.doi.org/10.1042/bst0240785] [PMID: 8878848]

[43] Hollman PC, Katan MB. Dietary flavonoids: intake, health effects and bioavailability. Food Chem Toxicol 1999; 37(9-10): 937-42.
[http://dx.doi.org/10.1016/S0278-6915(99)00079-4] [PMID: 10541448]

[44] Rimm EB, Katan MB, Ascherio A, Stampfer MJ, Willett WC. Relation between intake of flavonoids and risk for coronary heart disease in male health professionals. Ann Intern Med 1996; 125(5): 384-9.
[http://dx.doi.org/10.7326/0003-4819-125-5-199609010-00005] [PMID: 8702089]

[45] Brown CA, Bolton-Smith C, Woodward M, Tunstall-Pedoe H. Coffee and tea consumption and the prevalence of coronary heart disease in men and women: results from the Scottish Heart Health Study. J Epidemiol Community Health 1993; 47(3): 171-5.
[http://dx.doi.org/10.1136/jech.47.3.171] [PMID: 8350026]

[46] Hertog MG, Sweetnam PM, Fehily AM, Elwood PC, Kromhout D. Antioxidant flavonols and ischemic heart disease in a Welsh population of men: the Caerphilly Study. Am J Clin Nutr 1997; 65(5): 1489-94.
[http://dx.doi.org/10.1093/ajcn/65.5.1489] [PMID: 9129481]

[47] Peters U, Poole C, Arab L. Does tea affect cardiovascular disease? A meta-analysis. Am J Epidemiol 2001; 154(6): 495-503.
[http://dx.doi.org/10.1093/aje/154.6.495] [PMID: 11549554]

[48] Frémont L. Biological effects of resveratrol. Life Sci 2000; 66(8): 663-73.
[http://dx.doi.org/10.1016/S0024-3205(99)00410-5] [PMID: 10680575]

[49] Wang L, Xu M, Liu C, *et al.* Resveratrols in grape berry skins and leaves in vitis germplasm. PLoS One 2013; 8(4)e61642
[http://dx.doi.org/10.1371/journal.pone.0061642] [PMID: 23637874]

[50] Sales JM, Resurreccion AV. Resveratrol in peanuts. Crit Rev Food Sci Nutr 2014; 54(6): 734-70.
[http://dx.doi.org/10.1080/10408398.2011.606928] [PMID: 24345046]

[51] Magyar K, Halmosi R, Palfi A, *et al.* Cardioprotection by resveratrol: A human clinical trial in patients with stable coronary artery disease. Clin Hemorheol Microcirc 2012; 50(3): 179-87.

[http://dx.doi.org/10.3233/CH-2011-1424] [PMID: 22240353]

[52]   Frankel EN, Waterhouse AL, Kinsella JE. Inhibition of human LDL oxidation by resveratrol. Lancet 1993; 341(8852): 1103-4.
[http://dx.doi.org/10.1016/0140-6736(93)92472-6] [PMID: 8097009]

[53]   Pendurthi UR, Williams JT, Rao LV. Resveratrol, a polyphenolic compound found in wine, inhibits tissue factor expression in vascular cells : A possible mechanism for the cardiovascular benefits associated with moderate consumption of wine. Arterioscler Thromb Vasc Biol 1999; 19(2): 419-26.
[http://dx.doi.org/10.1161/01.ATV.19.2.419] [PMID: 9974427]

[54]   Rotondo S, Rajtar G, Manarini S, *et al.* Effect of trans-resveratrol, a natural polyphenolic compound, on human polymorphonuclear leukocyte function. Br J Pharmacol 1998; 123(8): 1691-9.
[http://dx.doi.org/10.1038/sj.bjp.0701784] [PMID: 9605577]

[55]   Kohlmeier L, Kark JD, Gomez-Gracia E, *et al.* Lycopene and myocardial infarction risk in the EURAMIC Study. Am J Epidemiol 1997; 146(8): 618-26.
[http://dx.doi.org/10.1093/oxfordjournals.aje.a009327] [PMID: 9345115]

[56]   Sesso HD, Buring JE, Norkus EP, Gaziano JM. Plasma lycopene, other carotenoids, and retinol and the risk of cardiovascular disease in women. Am J Clin Nutr 2004; 79(1): 47-53.
[http://dx.doi.org/10.1093/ajcn/79.1.47] [PMID: 14684396]

[57]   Matulka RA, Hood AM, Griffiths JC. Safety evaluation of a natural tomato oleoresin extract derived from food-processing tomatoes. Regul Toxicol Pharmacol 2004; 39(3): 390-402.
[http://dx.doi.org/10.1016/j.yrtph.2004.03.005] [PMID: 15135216]

[58]   Miller NJ, Sampson J, Candeias LP, Bramley PM, Rice-Evans CA. Antioxidant activities of carotenes and xanthophylls. FEBS Lett 1996; 384(3): 240-2.
[http://dx.doi.org/10.1016/0014-5793(96)00323-7] [PMID: 8617362]

[59]   Iribarren C, Folsom AR, Jacobs DR Jr, Gross MD, Belcher JD, Eckfeldt JH. Association of serum vitamin levels, LDL susceptibility to oxidation, and autoantibodies against MDA-LDL with carotid atherosclerosis. A case-control study. The ARIC Study Investigators. Atherosclerosis Risk in Communities. Arterioscler Thromb Vasc Biol 1997; 17(6): 1171-7.
[http://dx.doi.org/10.1161/01.ATV.17.6.1171] [PMID: 9194770]

[60]   Djoussé L, Folsom AR, Province MA, Hunt SC, Ellison RC. Dietary linolenic acid and carotid atherosclerosis: the National Heart, Lung, and Blood Institute Family Heart Study. Am J Clin Nutr 2003; 77(4): 819-25.
[http://dx.doi.org/10.1093/ajcn/77.4.819] [PMID: 12663278]

[61]   Albert CM, Campos H, Stampfer MJ, *et al.* Blood levels of long-chain n-3 fatty acids and the risk of sudden death. N Engl J Med 2002; 346(15): 1113-8.
[http://dx.doi.org/10.1056/NEJMoa012918] [PMID: 11948270]

[62]   Salen P, de Lorgeril M. GISSI-Prevenzione trial. Lancet 1999; 354(9189): 1555.
[http://dx.doi.org/10.1016/S0140-6736(05)76583-1] [PMID: 10551520]

[63]   Carroll DN, Roth MT. Evidence for the cardioprotective effects of omega-3 Fatty acids. Ann Pharmacother 2002; 36(12): 1950-6.
[http://dx.doi.org/10.1345/aph.1A314] [PMID: 12452760]

[64]   Knoops KT, de Groot LC, Kromhout D, *et al.* Mediterranean diet, lifestyle factors, and 10-year mortality in elderly European men and women: the HALE project. JAMA 2004; 292(12): 1433-9.
[http://dx.doi.org/10.1001/jama.292.12.1433] [PMID: 15383513]

[65]   Trichopoulou A, Costacou T, Bamia C, Trichopoulos D. Adherence to a Mediterranean diet and survival in a Greek population. N Engl J Med 2003; 348(26): 2599-608.
[http://dx.doi.org/10.1056/NEJMoa025039] [PMID: 12826634]

[66]   Covas MI, Nyyssönen K, Poulsen HE, *et al.* The effect of polyphenols in olive oil on heart disease risk factors: a randomized trial. Ann Intern Med 2006; 145(5): 333-41.

[http://dx.doi.org/10.7326/0003-4819-145-5-200609050-00006] [PMID: 16954359]

[67]   Fitó M, Cladellas M, de la Torre R, *et al.* Antioxidant effect of virgin olive oil in patients with stable coronary heart disease: a randomized, crossover, controlled, clinical trial. Atherosclerosis 2005; 181(1): 149-58.
[http://dx.doi.org/10.1016/j.atherosclerosis.2004.12.036] [PMID: 15939067]

[68]   Rodríguez-Rodríguez R, Herrera MD, Perona JS, Ruiz-Gutiérrez V. Potential vasorelaxant effects of oleanolic acid and erythrodiol, two triterpenoids contained in 'orujo' olive oil, on rat aorta. Br J Nutr 2004; 92(4): 635-42.
[http://dx.doi.org/10.1079/BJN20041231] [PMID: 15522132]

[69]   Carluccio MA, Massaro M, Bonfrate C, *et al.* Oleic acid inhibits endothelial activation : A direct vascular antiatherogenic mechanism of a nutritional component in the mediterranean diet. Arterioscler Thromb Vasc Biol 1999; 19(2): 220-8.
[http://dx.doi.org/10.1161/01.ATV.19.2.220] [PMID: 9974401]

[70]   Yaqoob P, Knapper JA, Webb DH, Williams CM, Newsholme EA, Calder PC. Effect of olive oil on immune function in middle-aged men. Am J Clin Nutr 1998; 67(1): 129-35.
[http://dx.doi.org/10.1093/ajcn/67.1.129] [PMID: 9440387]

[71]   Karantonis HC, Antonopoulou S, Demopoulos CA. Antithrombotic lipid minor constituents from vegetable oils. Comparison between olive oils and others. J Agric Food Chem 2002; 50(5): 1150-60.
[http://dx.doi.org/10.1021/jf010923t] [PMID: 11853496]

[72]   Hillestrøm PR, Covas MI, Poulsen HE. Effect of dietary virgin olive oil on urinary excretion of etheno-DNA adducts. Free Radic Biol Med 2006; 41(7): 1133-8.
[http://dx.doi.org/10.1016/j.freeradbiomed.2006.06.013] [PMID: 16962938]

[73]   Fitó M, Cladellas M, de la Torre R, *et al.* Anti-inflammatory effect of virgin olive oil in stable coronary disease patients: a randomized, crossover, controlled trial. Eur J Clin Nutr 2008; 62(4): 570-4.
[http://dx.doi.org/10.1038/sj.ejcn.1602724] [PMID: 17375118]

[74]   Shurtleff W, Aoyagi A. History of Soybeans and Soyfoods in Southeast Asia (13th Century to 2010). 2010.

[75]   Zhang X, Shu XO, Gao YT, *et al.* Soy food consumption is associated with lower risk of coronary heart disease in Chinese women. J Nutr 2003; 133(9): 2874-8.
[http://dx.doi.org/10.1093/jn/133.9.2874] [PMID: 12949380]

[76]   Jenkins DJ, Kendall CW, Garsetti M, *et al.* Effect of soy protein foods on low-density lipoprotein oxidation and *ex vivo* sex hormone receptor activity--a controlled crossover trial. Metabolism 2000; 49(4): 537-43.
[http://dx.doi.org/10.1016/S0026-0495(00)80022-0] [PMID: 10778882]

[77]   Cavallini DC, Abdalla DS, Vendramini RC, *et al.* Effects of isoflavone-supplemented soy yogurt on lipid parameters and atherosclerosis development in hypercholesterolemic rabbits: a randomized double-blind study. Lipids Health Dis 2009; 8: 40.
[http://dx.doi.org/10.1186/1476-511X-8-40] [PMID: 19814806]

[78]   Anthony MS, Clarkson TB, Williams JK. Effects of soy isoflavones on atherosclerosis: potential mechanisms. Am J Clin Nutr 1998; 68(6) (Suppl.): 1390S-3S.
[http://dx.doi.org/10.1093/ajcn/68.6.1390S] [PMID: 9848505]

[79]   Anderson JW, Johnstone BM, Cook-Newell ME. Meta-analysis of the effects of soy protein intake on serum lipids. N Engl J Med 1995; 333(5): 276-82.
[http://dx.doi.org/10.1056/NEJM199508033330502] [PMID: 7596371]

[80]   Felicilda-Reynaldo RF. Cardiac glycosides, digoxin toxicity, and the antidote. Medsurg Nurs 2013; 22(4): 258-61.
[PMID: 24147325]

[81]   Pincus M. Management of digoxin toxicity. Aust Prescr 2016; 39(1): 18-20.
        [http://dx.doi.org/10.18773/austprescr.2016.006] [PMID: 27041802]

[82]   Delacroix S, Chokka R, Worthley S. Hypertension: pathophysiology and treatment. J Neurol
        Neurophysiol 2014; 5: 2.
        [http://dx.doi.org/10.4172/2155-9562.1000250]

[83]   Weber MA, Schiffrin EL, White WB, *et al.* Clinical practice guidelines for the management of
        hypertension in the community: a statement by the American Society of Hypertension and the
        International Society of Hypertension. J Clin Hypertens (Greenwich) 2014; 16(1): 14-26.
        [http://dx.doi.org/10.1111/jch.12237] [PMID: 24341872]

[84]   Grassi G, Seravalle G, Bertinieri G, *et al.* Sympathetic and reflex alterations in systo-diastolic and
        systolic hypertension of the elderly. J Hypertens 2000; 18(5): 587-93.
        [http://dx.doi.org/10.1097/00004872-200018050-00012] [PMID: 10826562]

[85]   Bavishi C, Goel S, Messerli FH. Isolated systolic hypertension: an update after SPRINT. Am J Med
        2016; 129(12): 1251-8.
        [http://dx.doi.org/10.1016/j.amjmed.2016.08.032] [PMID: 27639873]

[86]   Artom N, Salvo F, Camardella F. White-coat hypertension and masked hypertension: an update. Ital J
        Med 2015; 10: 96-102.
        [http://dx.doi.org/10.4081/itjm.2015.662]

[87]   Yan B, Peng L, Han D, *et al.* Blood pressure reverse-dipping is associated with early formation of
        carotid plaque in senior hypertensive patients. Medicine (Baltimore) 2015; 94(10)e604
        [http://dx.doi.org/10.1097/MD.0000000000000604] [PMID: 25761180]

[88]   Grassi G, Seravalle G, Quarti-Trevano F, *et al.* Adrenergic, metabolic, and reflex abnormalities in
        reverse and extreme dipper hypertensives. Hypertension 2008; 52(5): 925-31.
        [http://dx.doi.org/10.1161/HYPERTENSIONAHA.108.116368] [PMID: 18779438]

[89]   Garovic VD, August P. Preeclampsia and the future risk of hypertension: the pregnant evidence. Curr
        Hypertens Rep 2013; 15(2): 114-21.
        [http://dx.doi.org/10.1007/s11906-013-0329-4] [PMID: 23397213]

[90]   Grassi G. Assessment of sympathetic cardiovascular drive in human hypertension: achievements and
        perspectives. Hypertension 2009; 54(4): 690-7.
        [http://dx.doi.org/10.1161/HYPERTENSIONAHA.108.119883] [PMID: 19720958]

[91]   Coca-Robinot D, Fabregate R, Sanchez-Largo E, *et al.* P-470: Clinical, biochemical and
        cardiovascular implications of endothelial dysfunction in the dermal microcirculation. Am J Hypertens
        2005; 18: 177A.
        [http://dx.doi.org/10.1016/j.amjhyper.2005.03.487]

[92]   Widlansky ME, Gokce N, Keaney JF Jr, Vita JA. The clinical implications of endothelial dysfunction.
        J Am Coll Cardiol 2003; 42(7): 1149-60.
        [http://dx.doi.org/10.1016/S0735-1097(03)00994-X] [PMID: 14522472]

[93]   Sarzani R, Salvi F, Dessi-Fulgheri P, Rappelli A. Renin-angiotensin system, natriuretic peptides,
        obesity, metabolic syndrome, and hypertension: an integrated view in humans. J Hypertens 2008;
        26(5): 831-43.
        [http://dx.doi.org/10.1097/HJH.0b013e3282f624a0] [PMID: 18398321]

[94]   Simões E Silva AC, Flynn JT. The renin-angiotensin-aldosterone system in 2011: role in hypertension
        and chronic kidney disease. Pediatr Nephrol 2012; 27(10): 1835-45.
        [http://dx.doi.org/10.1007/s00467-011-2002-y] [PMID: 21947887]

[95]   Atlas SA. The renin-angiotensin aldosterone system: pathophysiological role and pharmacologic
        inhibition. J Manag Care Pharm 2007; 13(8) (Suppl. B): 9-20.
        [http://dx.doi.org/10.18553/jmcp.2007.13.s8-b.9] [PMID: 17970613]

[96]   Tsioufis C, Kordalis A, Flessas D, *et al.* Pathophysiology of resistant hypertension: the role of sympathetic nervous system. International journal of hypertension 2011.
[http://dx.doi.org/10.4061/2011/642416]

[97]   Dzeufiet PDD, Mogueo A, Bilanda DC, *et al.* Antihypertensive potential of the aqueous extract which combine leaf of *Perseaamericana Mill.* (Lauraceae), stems and leaf of *Cymbopogon citratus* (D.C) Stapf. (Poaceae), fruits of *Citrus medical L.* (Rutaceae) as well as honey in ethanol and sucrose experimental model. BMC Complement Altern Med 2014; 14: 507.
[http://dx.doi.org/10.1186/1472-6882-14-507] [PMID: 25519078]

[98]   Chrysant SG, Chrysant GS. Herbs used for the treatment of hypertension and their mechanism of action. Curr Hypertens Rep 2017; 19(9): 77.
[http://dx.doi.org/10.1007/s11906-017-0775-5] [PMID: 28921053]

[99]   Virdis A, Duranti E, Taddei S. Oxidative stress and vascular damage in hypertension: role of angiotensin II. International journal of hypertension 2011.
[http://dx.doi.org/10.4061/2011/916310]

[100]   Montezano AC, Tsiropoulou S, Dulak-Lis M, Harvey A, Camargo LdeL, Touyz RM. Redox signaling, Nox5 and vascular remodeling in hypertension. Curr Opin Nephrol Hypertens 2015; 24(5): 425-33.
[http://dx.doi.org/10.1097/MNH.0000000000000153] [PMID: 26197203]

[101]   Fallah Huseini H, Amini M, Mohtashami R, *et al.* Blood pressure lowering effect of *Nigella sativa* L. seed oil in healthy volunteers: a randomized, double-blind, placebo-controlled clinical trial. Phytother Res 2013; 27(12): 1849-53.
[http://dx.doi.org/10.1002/ptr.4944] [PMID: 23436437]

[102]   Dehkordi FR, Kamkhah AF. Antihypertensive effect of Nigella sativa seed extract in patients with mild hypertension. Fundam Clin Pharmacol 2008; 22(4): 447-52.
[http://dx.doi.org/10.1111/j.1472-8206.2008.00607.x] [PMID: 18705755]

[103]   Webb AJ, Patel N, Loukogeorgakis S, *et al.* Acute blood pressure lowering, vasoprotective, and antiplatelet properties of dietary nitrate *via* bioconversion to nitrite. Hypertension 2008; 51(3): 784-90.
[http://dx.doi.org/10.1161/HYPERTENSIONAHA.107.103523] [PMID: 18250365]

[104]   Kapil V, Khambata RS, Robertson A, Caulfield MJ, Ahluwalia A. Dietary nitrate provides sustained blood pressure lowering in hypertensive patients: a randomized, phase 2, double-blind, placebo-controlled study. Hypertension 2014; 65(2): 320-7.
[http://dx.doi.org/https://dx.doi.org/10.1161%2FHYPERTENSIONAHA.114.04675]
[PMID: 25421976]

[105]   Coles LT, Clifton PM. Effect of beetroot juice on lowering blood pressure in free-living, disease-free adults: a randomized, placebo-controlled trial. Nutr J 2012; 11: 106.
[http://dx.doi.org/10.1186/1475-2891-11-106] [PMID: 23231777]

[106]   Affuso F, Mercurio V, Fazio V, Fazio S. Cardiovascular and metabolic effects of Berberine. World J Cardiol 2010; 2(4): 71-7.
[http://dx.doi.org/10.4330/wjc.v2.i4.71] [PMID: 21160701]

[107]   Lan J, Zhao Y, Dong F, *et al.* Meta-analysis of the effect and safety of berberine in the treatment of type 2 diabetes mellitus, hyperlipemia and hypertension. J Ethnopharmacol 2015; 161: 69-81.
[http://dx.doi.org/10.1016/j.jep.2014.09.049] [PMID: 25498346]

[108]   Al Disi SS, Anwar MA, Eid AH. Anti-hypertensive herbs and their mechanisms of action: part I. Front Pharmacol 2016; 6: 323.
[http://dx.doi.org/10.3389/fphar.2015.00323] [PMID: 26834637]

[109]   Inuwa I, Ali BH, Al-Lawati I, Beegam S, Ziada A, Blunden G. Long-term ingestion of *Hibiscus sabdariffa* calyx extract enhances myocardial capillarization in the spontaneously hypertensive rat. Exp Biol Med (Maywood) 2012; 237(5): 563-9.
[http://dx.doi.org/10.1258/ebm.2012.011357] [PMID: 22678012]

[110]   Hopkins AL, Lamm MG, Funk JL, Ritenbaugh C. *Hibiscus sabdariffa* L. in the treatment of hypertension and hyperlipidemia: a comprehensive review of animal and human studies. Fitoterapia 2013; 85: 84-94.
[http://dx.doi.org/10.1016/j.fitote.2013.01.003] [PMID: 23333908]

[111]   McKay DL, Chen CY, Saltzman E, Blumberg JB. *Hibiscus sabdariffa* L. tea (tisane) lowers blood pressure in prehypertensive and mildly hypertensive adults. J Nutr 2010; 140(2): 298-303.
[http://dx.doi.org/10.3945/jn.109.115097] [PMID: 20018807]

[112]   Alarcón-Alonso J, Zamilpa A, Aguilar FA, Herrera-Ruiz M, Tortoriello J, Jimenez-Ferrer E. Pharmacological characterization of the diuretic effect of *Hibiscus sabdariffa* Linn (Malvaceae) extract. J Ethnopharmacol 2012; 139(3): 751-6.
[http://dx.doi.org/10.1016/j.jep.2011.12.005] [PMID: 22178178]

[113]   Tassell MC, Kingston R, Gilroy D, Lehane M, Furey A. Hawthorn (Crataegus spp.) in the treatment of cardiovascular disease. Pharmacogn Rev 2010; 4(7): 32-41.
[http://dx.doi.org/10.4103/0973-7847.65324] [PMID: 22228939]

[114]   Asher GN, Viera AJ, Weaver MA, Dominik R, Caughey M, Hinderliter AL. Effect of hawthorn standardized extract on flow mediated dilation in prehypertensive and mildly hypertensive adults: a randomized, controlled cross-over trial. BMC Complement Altern Med 2012; 12: 26.
[http://dx.doi.org/10.1186/1472-6882-12-26] [PMID: 22458601]

[115]   Ried K, Travica N, Sali A. The effect of aged garlic extract on blood pressure and other cardiovascular risk factors in uncontrolled hypertensives: the AGE at Heart trial. Integr Blood Press Control 2016; 9: 9-21.
[http://dx.doi.org/10.2147/IBPC.S93335] [PMID: 26869811]

[116]   Rohner A, Ried K, Sobenin IA, Bucher HC, Nordmann AJ. A systematic review and metaanalysis on the effects of garlic preparations on blood pressure in individuals with hypertension. Am J Hypertens 2015; 28(3): 414-23.
[http://dx.doi.org/10.1093/ajh/hpu165] [PMID: 25239480]

[117]   Wang HP, Yang J, Qin LQ, Yang XJ. Effect of garlic on blood pressure: a meta-analysis. J Clin Hypertens (Greenwich) 2015; 17(3): 223-31.
[http://dx.doi.org/10.1111/jch.12473] [PMID: 25557383]

[118]   Srivastava R, Ahmed H, Dixit RK, Dharamveer , Saraf SA. Crocus sativus L.: A comprehensive review. Pharmacogn Rev 2010; 4(8): 200-8.
[http://dx.doi.org/10.4103/0973-7847.70919] [PMID: 22228962]

[119]   Modaghegh M-H, Shahabian M, Esmaeili H-A, Rajbai O, Hosseinzadeh H. Safety evaluation of saffron (Crocus sativus) tablets in healthy volunteers. Phytomedicine 2008; 15(12): 1032-7.
[http://dx.doi.org/10.1016/j.phymed.2008.06.003] [PMID: 18693099]

[120]   Mucalo I, Jovanovski E, Rahelić D, Božikov V, Romić Z, Vuksan V. Effect of American ginseng (Panax quinquefolius L.) on arterial stiffness in subjects with type-2 diabetes and concomitant hypertension. J Ethnopharmacol 2013; 150(1): 148-53.
[http://dx.doi.org/10.1016/j.jep.2013.08.015] [PMID: 23973636]

[121]   Jovanovski E, Bateman EA, Bhardwaj J, *et al.* Effect of Rg3-enriched Korean red ginseng (Panax ginseng) on arterial stiffness and blood pressure in healthy individuals: a randomized controlled trial. J Am Soc Hypertens 2014; 8(8): 537-41.
[http://dx.doi.org/10.1016/j.jash.2014.04.004] [PMID: 24997863]

[122]   Rhee M-Y, Cho B, Kim K-I, *et al.* Blood pressure lowering effect of Korea ginseng derived ginseol K-g1. Am J Chin Med 2014; 42(3): 605-18.
[http://dx.doi.org/10.1142/S0192415X14500396] [PMID: 24871654]

[123]   Kim J-H. Cardiovascular diseases and Panax ginseng: a review on molecular mechanisms and medical applications. J Ginseng Res 2012; 36(1): 16-26.

[http://dx.doi.org/10.5142/jgr.2012.36.1.16] [PMID: 23717100]

[124] Hodgson JM, Puddey IB, Woodman RJ, *et al.* Effects of black tea on blood pressure: a randomized controlled trial. Arch Intern Med 2012; 172(2): 186-8.
[http://dx.doi.org/10.1001/archinte.172.2.186] [PMID: 22271130]

[125] Hartley L, Flowers N, Holmes J, *et al.* Green and black tea for the primary prevention of cardiovascular disease. Cochrane Database Syst Rev 2013; 6(6)CD009934
[http://dx.doi.org/10.1002/14651858.CD009934.pub2] [PMID: 23780706]

[126] Devi RC, Sim S, Ismail R. Effect of Cymbopogon citratus and citral on vascular smooth muscle of the isolated thoracic rat aorta. Evidence-Based Complementary and Alternative Medicine 2012; 2012: 8.
[http://dx.doi.org/https://doi.org/10.1155/2012/539475] [PMID: 539475]

[127] Hao P, Jiang F, Cheng J, Ma L, Zhang Y, Zhao Y. Traditional Chinese medicine for cardiovascular disease: evidence and potential mechanisms. J Am Coll Cardiol 2017; 69(24): 2952-66.
[http://dx.doi.org/10.1016/j.jacc.2017.04.041] [PMID: 28619197]

[128] Lau Y-S, Machha A, Achike FI, Murugan D, Mustafa MR. The aporphine alkaloid boldine improves endothelial function in spontaneously hypertensive rats. Exp Biol Med (Maywood) 2012; 237(1): 93-8.
[http://dx.doi.org/10.1258/ebm.2011.011145] [PMID: 22156043]

[129] Lau YS, Ling WC, Murugan D, Mustafa MR. Boldine ameliorates vascular oxidative stress and endothelial dysfunction: Therapeutic implication for hypertension and diabetes. J Cardiovasc Pharmacol 2015; 65(6): 522-31.
[http://dx.doi.org/10.1097/FJC.0000000000000185] [PMID: 25469805]

[130] Heberden W. Some Account of a Disorder of the Breast. Med Transact R Coll Phys Lond 1772; 2: 59.

[131] Dorland D. Dorland's Illustrated Medical Dictionary. 32nd ed., Saunders 2017.

[132] Mosby Mosby's Dictionary of Medicine, Nursing & Health Professions. 10th ed., Elsevier 2017.

[133] Arrebola-Moreno A, Dungu J, Kaski JC. Treatment strategies for chronic stable angina. Expert Opin Pharmacother 2011; 12(18): 2833-44.
[http://dx.doi.org/10.1517/14656566.2011.634799] [PMID: 22098227]

[134] Organization WH. 2004.www.who.int/whr/2004/en/report04_en.pdf

[135] Emond M, Mock MB, Davis KB, *et al.* Long-term survival of medically treated patients in the Coronary Artery Surgery Study (CASS) Registry. Circulation 1994; 90(6): 2645-57.
[http://dx.doi.org/10.1161/01.CIR.90.6.2645] [PMID: 7994804]

[136] Fox K, Garcia MA, Ardissino D, *et al.* Guidelines on the management of stable angina pectoris: executive summary: The task force on the management of stable angina pectoris of the european society of cardiology. Eur Heart J 2006; 27(11): 1341-81.
[http://dx.doi.org/10.1093/eurheartj/ehl001] [PMID: 16735367]

[137] Sun H, Mohri M, Shimokawa H, Usui M, Urakami L, Takeshita A. Coronary microvascular spasm causes myocardial ischemia in patients with vasospastic angina. J Am Coll Cardiol 2002; 39(5): 847-51.
[http://dx.doi.org/10.1016/S0735-1097(02)01690-X] [PMID: 11869851]

[138] Tobin KJ. Stable angina pectoris: what does the current clinical evidence tell us? J Am Osteopath Assoc 2010; 110(7): 364-70.
[PMID: 20693568]

[139] Talbert RL. Ischemic heart disease. Pharmacotherapy: A Pathophysiologic Approach. 8th ed., New York: McGraw-Hill 2011.

[140] Keller KB, Lemberg L. Prinzmetal's angina. *American journal of critical care: an official publication.* American Association of Critical-Care Nurses 2004; 13: 350-4.

[141] Kaski JC. Chest pain with normal coronary angiograms: pathogenesis, diagnosis and management.

Boston: Kluwer 1999; pp. 5-6.
[http://dx.doi.org/10.1007/978-1-4615-5181-2]

[142] Gulati M, Shaw LJ, Bairey Merz CN. Myocardial ischemia in women: lessons from the NHLBI WISE study. Clin Cardiol 2012; 35(3): 141-8.
[http://dx.doi.org/10.1002/clc.21966] [PMID: 22389117]

[143] Shaw LJ, Merz CN, Pepine CJ, *et al.* The economic burden of angina in women with suspected ischemic heart disease: results from the National Institutes of Health--National Heart, Lung, and Blood Institute--sponsored Women's Ischemia Syndrome Evaluation. Circulation 2006; 114(9): 894-904.
[http://dx.doi.org/10.1161/CIRCULATIONAHA.105.609990] [PMID: 16923752]

[144] Guyton A. Textbook of Medical Physiology. 11th ed., Philadelphia: Elsevier 2006.

[145] Linden W, Stossel C, Maurice J. Psychosocial interventions for patients with coronary artery disease: a meta-analysis. Arch Intern Med 1996; 156(7): 745-52.
[http://dx.doi.org/10.1001/archinte.1996.00440070065008] [PMID: 8615707]

[146] Vaccarino V. Ischemic heart disease in women: many questions, few facts. Circ Cardiovasc Qual Outcomes 2010; 3(2): 111-5.
[http://dx.doi.org/10.1161/CIRCOUTCOMES.109.925313] [PMID: 20160161]

[147] Banks K, Lo M, Khera A. Angina in women without obstructive coronary artery disease. Curr Cardiol Rev 2010; 6(1): 71-81.
[http://dx.doi.org/10.2174/157340310790231608] [PMID: 21286281]

[148] Anthony J. Trevor, BGK, Marieke Knuidering-Hall Katzung & Trevor's Pharmacology Examination and Board Review. 11th ed., McGraw-Hill Education 2015.

[149] Sneader W. Drug discovery: a history. 1st ed., 2005.
[http://dx.doi.org/10.1002/0470015535]

[150] McClellan KJ, Plosker GL. Trimetazidine. A review of its use in stable angina pectoris and other coronary conditions. Drugs 1999; 58(1): 143-57.
[http://dx.doi.org/10.2165/00003495-199958010-00016] [PMID: 10439934]

[151] Sulfi S, Timmis AD. Ivabradine -- the first selective sinus node I(f) channel inhibitor in the treatment of stable angina. Int J Clin Pract 2006; 60(2): 222-8.
[http://dx.doi.org/10.1111/j.1742-1241.2006.00817.x] [PMID: 16451297]

[152] Gupta AK, Winchester D, Pepine CJ. Antagonist molecules in the treatment of angina. Expert Opin Pharmacother 2013; 14(17): 2323-42.
[http://dx.doi.org/10.1517/14656566.2013.834329] [PMID: 24047238]

[153] Fihn SD, Gardin JM, Abrams J, *et al.* 2012 ACCF/AHA/ACP/AATS/PCNA/SCAI/STS guideline for the diagnosis and management of patients with stable ischemic heart disease: executive summary: a report of the American College of Cardiology Foundation/American Heart Association task force on practice guidelines, and the American College of Physicians, American Association for Thoracic Surgery, Preventive Cardiovascular Nurses Association, Society for Cardiovascular Angiography and Interventions, and Society of Thoracic Surgeons. Circulation 2012; 126(25): 3097-137.
[http://dx.doi.org/10.1161/CIR.0b013e3182776f83] [PMID: 23166210]

[154] Nissen SE, Nicholls SJ, Sipahi I, *et al.* Effect of very high-intensity statin therapy on regression of coronary atherosclerosis: the ASTEROID trial. JAMA 2006; 295(13): 1556-65.
[http://dx.doi.org/10.1001/jama.295.13.jpc60002] [PMID: 16533939]

[155] Barnett H, Burrill P, Iheanacho I. Don't use aspirin for primary prevention of cardiovascular disease. BMJ 2010; 340: c1805.
[http://dx.doi.org/10.1136/bmj.c1805] [PMID: 20410163]

[156] Pfisterer ME, Zellweger MJ, Gersh BJ. Management of stable coronary artery disease. Lancet 2010; 375(9716): 763-72.
[http://dx.doi.org/10.1016/S0140-6736(10)60168-7] [PMID: 20189028]

[157] Kocyigit D, Gurses KM, Yalcin MU, Tokgozoglu L. Traditional and Alternative Therapies for Refractory Angina. Curr Pharm Des 2017; 23(7): 1098-111.
[http://dx.doi.org/10.2174/1381612823666161123145148] [PMID: 27881061]

[158] Ades PA, Waldmann ML, Poehlman ET, *et al.* Exercise conditioning in older coronary patients. Submaximal lactate response and endurance capacity. Circulation 1993; 88(2): 572-7.
[http://dx.doi.org/10.1161/01.CIR.88.2.572] [PMID: 8339420]

[159] O'Brien K, Vitetta L. The potential role of herbal medicines in the treatment of chronic stable angina pectoris: A review of key herbs, and as illustration, exploration of the Chinese herbal medicine approach. Botanics 2012; 3: 1.
[http://dx.doi.org/10.2147/BTAT.S28866]

[160] Mahmood ZA, Sualeh M, Mahmood SB, Karim MA. Herbal treatment for cardiovascular disease the evidence based therapy. Pak J Pharm Sci 2010; 23(1): 119-24.
[PMID: 20067878]

[161] Koch E. Inhibition of platelet activating factor (PAF)-induced aggregation of human thrombocytes by ginkgolides: considerations on possible bleeding complications after oral intake of *Ginkgo biloba* extracts Phytomedicine : international journal of phytotherapy and phytopharmacology 2005; 12: 10-16.
[http://dx.doi.org/10.1016/j.phymed.2004.02.002.]

[162] Singh J, Pandey A. A review: An impact of *inula racemosa* (puskarmula) on dyslipidemia and obesity. World journal of scientific research 2016; 5: 528-38.

[163] Zhu Y, Xia W, Liu W, Xu C, Gu N. Gualoupi (Pericarpium Trichosanthis) injection in combination with convention therapy for the treatment of angina pectoris: a Meta- analysis. Journal of traditional Chinese medicine = Chung i tsa chih ying wen pan 2017; 37: 1- 11.

[164] Das DK, Mukherjee S, Ray D. Resveratrol and red wine, healthy heart and longevity. Heart Fail Rev 2010; 15(5): 467-77.
[http://dx.doi.org/10.1007/s10741-010-9163-9] [PMID: 20238161]

[165] Jagtap M, Chandola HM, Ravishankar B. Clinical efficacy of *Coleus forskohlii* (Willd.) Briq. (Makandi) in hypertension of geriatric population. Ayu 2011; 32(1): 59-65.
[http://dx.doi.org/10.4103/0974-8520.85729] [PMID: 22131759]

[166] Conn JJ, Kissane RW, Koons RA, Clark TE. The treatment of angina pectoris with khellin. Ann Intern Med 1952; 36(5): 1173-8.
[http://dx.doi.org/10.7326/0003-4819-36-5-1173] [PMID: 14924454]

[167] Lokhande D, Jagdale S, Chabuksawar AR. Natural remedies for heart diseases. Indian J Tradit Knowl 2006; 5: 420-7.

[168] Zhao Z, Yang X, Zhang Y. Clinical study of puerarin in treatment of patients with unstable angina Chinese journal of integrated traditional and Western medicine 1998; 18: 282-284.

[169] Fan LL, Sun LH, Li J, *et al.* Protective effect of puerarin against myocardial reperfusion injury. Myocardial metabolism and ultrastructure. Chin Med J (Engl) 1992; 105(6): 451-6.
[PMID: 1451545]

[170] Li SM, Liu B, Chen HF. Beneficial effects of berberine on hemodynamics during acute ischemic left ventricular failure in dogs Chinese medical journal 1992; 105: 1014-9.

[171] Luo ZR, Zheng B. Effect of Puerarin on platelet activating factors CD63 and CD62P, plasminogen activator inhibitor and C-reactive protein in patients with unstable angia pectoris. Chinese journal of integrated traditional and Western medicine 2001; 21: 31-33.

[172] Xuan B, Li DX, Wang W. Protective effects of tetrahydroprotoberberines on experimental myocardial infarction in rats. Zhongguo Yao Li Xue Bao 1992; 13(2): 167-71.
[PMID: 1598835]

[173] O K, Cheung F, Sung FL, Zhu DY, Siow YL. Effect of magnesium tanshinoate B on the production of nitric oxide in endothelial cells. Mol Cell Biochem 2000; 207(1-2): 35-9.
[http://dx.doi.org/10.1023/A:1007081911734] [PMID: 10888224]

[174] Huang H, Geng Q, Yao H, *et al.* Protective effect of scutellarin on myocardial infarction induced by isoprenaline in rats. Iran J Basic Med Sci 2018; 21(3): 267-76.
[http://dx.doi.org/10.22038/ijbms.2018.26110.6415] [PMID: 29511493]

[175] Wang L, Li Y, Lin S, Pu Z, Li H, Tang Z. Protective effects of baicalin on experimental myocardial infarction in rats. Rev Bras Cir Cardiovasc 2018; 33(4): 384-90.
[http://dx.doi.org/10.21470/1678-9741-2018-0059] [PMID: 30184036]

[176] Huang Z, Chen S, Zhang G, *et al.* Protective effects of berberine and phentolamine on myocardial reoxygenation damage. Chinese Med Sci J 1992; 7: 221-225.

[177] Huang WM, Wu ZD, Gan YQ. Effects of berberine on ischemic ventricular arrhythmia. Zhonghua Xin Xue Guan Bing Za Zhi 1989; 17(5): 300-301, 319.
[PMID: 2483987]

[178] Huang WM, Yan H, Jin JM, Yu C, Zhang H. Beneficial effects of berberine on hemodynamics during acute ischemic left ventricular failure in dogs. Chin Med J (Engl) 1992; 105(12)· 1014-9.
[PMID: 1299549]

[179] Bennett MR, Sinha S, Owens GK. Vascular smooth muscle cells in atherosclerosis. Circ Res 2016; 118(4): 692-702.
[http://dx.doi.org/10.1161/CIRCRESAHA.115.306361] [PMID: 26892967]

[180] Yurdagul A Jr, Finney AC, Woolard MD, Orr AW. The arterial microenvironment: the where and why of atherosclerosis. Biochem J 2016; 473(10): 1281-95.
[http://dx.doi.org/10.1042/BJ20150844] [PMID: 27208212]

[181] Lim S, Park S. Role of vascular smooth muscle cell in the inflammation of atherosclerosis. BMB Rep 2014; 47(1): 1-7.
[http://dx.doi.org/10.5483/BMBRep.2014.47.1.285] [PMID: 24388105]

[182] George SJ. Therapeutic potential of matrix metalloproteinase inhibitors in atherosclerosis. Expert Opin Investig Drugs 2000; 9(5): 993-1007.
[http://dx.doi.org/10.1517/13543784.9.5.993] [PMID: 11060722]

[183] Visse R, Nagase H. Matrix metalloproteinases and tissue inhibitors of metalloproteinases: structure, function, and biochemistry. Circ Res 2003; 92(8): 827-39.
[http://dx.doi.org/10.1161/01.RES.0000070112.80711.3D] [PMID: 12730128]

[184] Koch M, Zernecke A. The hemostatic system as a regulator of inflammation in atherosclerosis. IUBMB Life 2014; 66(11): 735-44.
[http://dx.doi.org/10.1002/iub.1333] [PMID: 25491152]

[185] Pirillo A, Norata GD, Catapano AL. LOX-1, OxLDL, and atherosclerosis. Mediators of inflammation 2013; 12.
[http://dx.doi.org/https://doi.org/10.1155/2013/152786]

[186] Tabas I, Lichtman AH. Monocyte-macrophages and T cells in atherosclerosis. Immunity 2017; 47(4): 621-34.
[http://dx.doi.org/10.1016/j.immuni.2017.09.008] [PMID: 29045897]

[187] Chistiakov DA, Melnichenko AA, Grechko AV, Myasoedova VA, Orekhov AN. Potential of anti-inflammatory agents for treatment of atherosclerosis. Exp Mol Pathol 2018; 104(2): 114-24.
[http://dx.doi.org/10.1016/j.yexmp.2018.01.008] [PMID: 29378168]

[188] Ginnan R, Guikema BJ, Halligan KE, Singer HA, Jourd'heuil D. Regulation of smooth muscle by inducible nitric oxide synthase and NADPH oxidase in vascular proliferative diseases. Free Radic Biol

Med 2008; 44(7): 1232-45.
[http://dx.doi.org/10.1016/j.freeradbiomed.2007.12.025] [PMID: 18211830]

[189] Luoma JS, Ylä-Herttuala S. Expression of inducible nitric oxide synthase in macrophages and smooth muscle cells in various types of human atherosclerotic lesions. Virchows Arch 1999; 434(6): 561-8.
[http://dx.doi.org/10.1007/s004280050384] [PMID: 10394893]

[190] Ikeda U, Maeda Y, Shimada K. Inducible nitric oxide synthase and atherosclerosis. Clin Cardiol 1998; 21(7): 473-6.
[http://dx.doi.org/10.1002/clc.4960210705] [PMID: 9669055]

[191] Ahmed HH, Shousha WG, El-Mezayen HA, El-Toumy SA, Sayed AH, Ramadan AR. Biochemical and molecular evidences for the antitumor potential of *Ginkgo biloba* leaves extract in rodents. Acta Biochim Pol 2017; 64(1): 25-33.
[PMID: 27741326]

[192] Baek SH, Lee JH, Ko JH, *et al.* Ginkgetin blocks constitutive STAT3 activation and induces apoptosis through induction of SHP-1 and PTEN tyrosine phosphatases. Phytother Res 2016; 30(4): 567-76.
[http://dx.doi.org/10.1002/ptr.5557] [PMID: 27059688]

[193] Lian N, Tong J, Li W, Wu J, Li Y. Ginkgetin ameliorates experimental atherosclerosis in rats. Biomed Pharmacother 2018; 102: 510-6.
[http://dx.doi.org/10.1016/j.biopha.2018.03.107] [PMID: 29579712]

[194] Fan W-H, Karnovsky MJ. Increased MMP-2 expression in connective tissue growth factor over-expression vascular smooth muscle cells. J Biol Chem 2002; 277(12): 9800-5.
[http://dx.doi.org/10.1074/jbc.M111213200] [PMID: 11773059]

[195] Gliesche DG, Hussner J, Witzigmann D, *et al.* Secreted matrix metalloproteinase-9 of proliferating smooth muscle cells as a trigger for drug release from stent surface polymers in coronary arteries. Mol Pharm 2016; 13(7): 2290-300.
[http://dx.doi.org/10.1021/acs.molpharmaceut.6b00033] [PMID: 27241028]

[196] Ozen S, Kone-Paut I, Gül A. Colchicine resistance and intolerance in familial Mediterranean fever: definition, causes, and alternative treatments. Proceedings of Seminars in arthritis and rheumatism. 115-20.
[http://dx.doi.org/10.1016/j.semarthrit.2017.03.006]

[197] Nava F, Ghilotti F, Maggi L, *et al.* Biologics, colchicine, corticosteroids, immunosuppressants and interferon-alpha for Neuro-Behçet's Syndrome. Cochrane Database Syst Rev 2014; (12): CD010729
[http://dx.doi.org/10.1002/14651858.CD010729.pub2] [PMID: 25521793]

[198] Raval J, Nagaraja V, Eslick GD, Denniss AR. The role of colchicine in pericarditis–a systematic review and meta-analysis of randomised trials. Heart Lung Circ 2015; 24(7): 660-6.
[http://dx.doi.org/10.1016/j.hlc.2015.01.010] [PMID: 25766664]

[199] Dziezanowski MA, DeStefano MJ, Rabinovitch M. Effect of antitubulins on spontaneous and chemotactic migration of neutrophils under agarose. J Cell Sci 1980; 42: 379-88.
[PMID: 7400242]

[200] Nidorf M, Thompson PL. Effect of colchicine (0.5 mg twice daily) on high-sensitivity C-reactive protein independent of aspirin and atorvastatin in patients with stable coronary artery disease. Am J Cardiol 2007; 99(6): 805-7.
[http://dx.doi.org/10.1016/j.amjcard.2006.10.039] [PMID: 17350370]

[201] Nidorf SM, Eikelboom JW, Budgeon CA, Thompson PL. Low-dose colchicine for secondary prevention of cardiovascular disease. J Am Coll Cardiol 2013; 61(4): 404-10.
[http://dx.doi.org/10.1016/j.jacc.2012.10.027] [PMID: 23265346]

[202] Vaidya K, Arnott C, Martínez GJ, *et al.* Colchicine therapy and plaque stabilization in patients with acute coronary syndrome: A CT coronary angiography study. JACC Cardiovasc Imaging 2018; 11(2 Pt 2): 305-16.

[http://dx.doi.org/10.1016/j.jcmg.2017.08.013] [PMID: 29055633]

[203] Hemkens LG, Ewald H, Gloy VL, *et al.* Colchicine for prevention of cardiovascular events. Cochrane Database Syst Rev 2016; (1): CD011047
[PMID: 26816301]

[204] Hemkens LG, Ewald H, Gloy VL, *et al.* M. Cardiovascular effects and safety of long-term colchicine treatment: Cochrane review and meta-analysis. Heart , heartjnl-2015-308542 Natural Products and Metabolic Syndrome 2016.

[205] Crittenden DB, Lehmann RA, Schneck L, *et al.* Colchicine use is associated with decreased prevalence of myocardial infarction in patients with gout. J Rheumatol 2012 Jul; 39(7): 1458-1464.
[http://dx.doi.org/10.3899/jrheum.111533]

[206] Solomon DH, Liu C-C, Kuo I-H, Zak A, Kim SC. Effects of colchicine on risk of cardiovascular events and mortality among patients with gout: a cohort study using electronic medical records linked with Medicare claims. Ann Rheum Dis 2016; 75(9): 1674-9.
[http://dx.doi.org/10.1136/annrheumdis-2015-207984] [PMID: 26582823]

[207] Deftereos S, Giannopoulos G, Raisakis K, *et al.* Colchicine treatment for the prevention of bare-metal stent restenosis in diabetic patients. J Am Coll Cardiol 2013; 61(16): 1679-85.
[http://dx.doi.org/10.1016/j.jacc.2013.01.055] [PMID: 23500260]

[208] O'Keefe JH Jr, McCallister BD, Bateman TM, Kuhnlein DL, Ligon RW, Hartzler GO. Ineffectiveness of colchicine for the prevention of restenosis after coronary angioplasty. J Am Coll Cardiol 1992; 19(7): 1597-600.
[http://dx.doi.org/10.1016/0735-1097(92)90624-V] [PMID: 1593057]

[209] Deftereos S, Giannopoulos G, Angelidis C, *et al.* Anti-inflammatory treatment with colchicine in acute myocardial infarction: a pilot study. Circulation 2015; 132(15): 1395-403.
[http://dx.doi.org/10.1161/CIRCULATIONAHA.115.017611] [PMID: 26265659]

[210] Koscielny J, Klüssendorf D, Latza R, *et al.* The antiatherosclerotic effect of *Allium sativum.* Atherosclerosis 1999; 144(1): 237-49.
[http://dx.doi.org/10.1016/S0021-9150(99)00060-X] [PMID: 10381297]

[211] Sobenin IA, Salonen JT, Zhelankin AV, *et al.* Low density lipoprotein-containing circulating immune complexes: role in atherosclerosis and diagnostic value. BioMed Res Int 2014; 2014205697
[http://dx.doi.org/10.1155/2014/205697] [PMID: 25054132]

[212] Sobenin IA, Chistiakov DA, Bobryshev YV, Orekhov AN. Blood atherogenicity as a target for anti-atherosclerotic therapy. Curr Pharm Des 2013; 19(33): 5954-62.
[http://dx.doi.org/10.2174/1381612811319330014] [PMID: 23438956]

[213] Orekhov AN, Sobenin IA, Korneev NV, *et al.* Anti-atherosclerotic therapy based on botanicals. Recent Pat Cardiovasc Drug Discov 2013; 8(1): 56-66.
[http://dx.doi.org/10.2174/18722083113079990008] [PMID: 23176379]

[214] Libby P, Okamoto Y, Rocha VZ, Folco E. Inflammation in atherosclerosis: transition from theory to practice. Circ J 2010; 74(2): 213-20.
[http://dx.doi.org/10.1253/circj.CJ-09-0706] [PMID: 20065609]

[215] Wolf D, Stachon P, Bode C, Zirlik A. Inflammatory mechanisms in atherosclerosis. Hamostaseologie 2014; 34(1): 63-71.
[http://dx.doi.org/10.5482/HAMO-13-09-0050] [PMID: 24343521]

[216] Gorchakova TV, Suprun IV, Sobenin IA, Orekhov AN. Use of natural products in anticytokine therapy. Bull Exp Biol Med 2007; 143(3): 316-9.
[http://dx.doi.org/10.1007/s10517-007-0099-6] [PMID: 18225751]

[217] Gorchakova T, Sobenin I, Orekhov A. The reduction of proinflammatory cytokine expression by natural components: a new approach to the prevention and treatment of atherosclerosis at the cellular level. J Clin Lipidol 2007; 1: 492.

[218] Gorchakova T, Suprun I, Sobenin I, Orekhov A. YI-844 Combined anti-inflammatory and anti-atherogenic activity of natural drug i nflaminat - a perspective for long-term atherosclerosis prevention and treatment. Atheroscler Suppl 2007; 8: 224.
[http://dx.doi.org/10.1016/S1567-5688(07)71854-8]

[219] Gorchakova T, Myasoedova V, Sobenin I, Orekhov A. P387 atherosclerosis prevention with the anti-inflammatory dietary supplement Inflaminat. Atheroscler Suppl 2009; 10e697
[http://dx.doi.org/10.1016/S1567-5688(09)70682-8]

[220] Sobenin L, Nikitina N, Myasoedova V, Korenmaya V, Khalilov E, *et al.* 4P-1202 Antiatherogenic properties of isoflavones from phytoesrogen-rich botanicals. Atheroscler Suppl 2003; 4: 339.
[http://dx.doi.org/10.1016/S1567-5688(03)91458-9]

[221] Korennaya V, Mysoedova V, Nikitina N, Sobenin I, Orekhov A. We-P14: 442 Bioflavonoid-rich botanicals reduce blood serum atherogenicity in perimenopausal women. Atheroscler Suppl 2006; 7: 444.
[http://dx.doi.org/10.1016/S1567-5688(06)81795-2]

[222] Nikitina NA, Sobenin IA, Myasoedova VA, *et al.* Antiatherogenic effect of grape flavonoids in an *ex vivo* model. Bull Exp Biol Med 2006; 141(6): 712-5.
[http://dx.doi.org/10.1007/s10517-006-0260-7] [PMID: 17364057]

[223] Sobenin I, Myasoedova V, Orekhov A. Antiatherogenic action of isoflavonoid-rich botanicals: an implementation for atherosclerosis prevention in postmenopausal women. J Clin Lipidol 2007; 1: 491-1.

[224] Myasoedova V, Sobenin I. Background, rationale and design of clinical study of the effect of isoflavonoid-rich botanicals on natural history of atherosclerosis in women. Atheroscler Suppl 2008; 9: 171.
[http://dx.doi.org/10.1016/S1567-5688(08)70689-5]

[225] Sobenin I, Myasoedova V, Orekhov A. Atherosclerosis prevention in postmenopausal women with the isoflavonoid-rich dietary supplement Karinat. J Clin Lipidol 2008; 2: S26-7.
[http://dx.doi.org/10.1016/j.jacl.2008.08.059]

[226] Awang DVC. Tyler's Herbs of Choice: The Therapeutic Use of Phytomedicinals In Cardiovascular system problems. 3rded., Boca Raton: CRC Taylor & Francis Group, LLC 2009.
[http://dx.doi.org/10.1136/aim.18.1.84-bpp 91-114]

[227] Thrift AG, Howard G, Cadilhac DA, *et al.* Global stroke statistics: An update of mortality data from countries using a broad code of "cerebrovascular diseases". Int J Stroke 2017; 12(8): 796-801.
[http://dx.doi.org/10.1177/1747493017730782] [PMID: 28895807]

[228] Sheu J-R, Geraldine P, Yen M-H. Bioactives and traditional herbal medicine for the treatment of cardiovascular/Cerebrovascular diseases 2015. Evid Based Complement Alternat Med 2015; 2015320545
[http://dx.doi.org/10.1155/2015/320545] [PMID: 26379742]

[229] Gupta YK, Briyal S, Gulati A. Therapeutic potential of herbal drugs in cerebral ischemia. Indian J Physiol Pharmacol 2010; 54(2): 99-122.
[PMID: 21090528]

[230] Singh B, Kaur P, Gopichand, Singh RD, Ahuja PS. Biology and chemistry of *Ginkgo biloba.* Fitoterapia 2008; 79(6): 401-18.
[http://dx.doi.org/10.1016/j.fitote.2008.05.007] [PMID: 18639617]

[231] Le Bars PL, Kastelan J. Efficacy and safety of a *Ginkgo biloba* extract. Public Health Nutr 2000; 3(4A): 495-9.
[http://dx.doi.org/10.1017/S1368980000000574] [PMID: 11276297]

[232] Mahady GB. *Ginkgo biloba* for the prevention and treatment of cardiovascular disease: a review of the literature. J Cardiovasc Nurs 2002; 16(4): 21-32.
[http://dx.doi.org/10.1097/00005082-200207000-00004] [PMID: 12597260]

[233] Gattuso G, Barreca D, Gargiulli C, *et al.* Flavonoid composition of Citrus juices. Molecules 2007; 12(8): 1641-73.
[http://dx.doi.org/10.3390/12081641] [PMID: 17960080]

[234] de Jesus Raposo MF, de Morais AMB, de Morais RMSC. Marine polysaccharides from algae with potential biomedical applications. Mar Drugs 2015; 13(5): 2967-3028.
[http://dx.doi.org/10.3390/md13052967] [PMID: 25988519]

[235] Chandía NP, Matsuhiro B. Characterization of a fucoidan from *Lessonia vadosa* (Phaeophyta) and its anticoagulant and elicitor properties. Int J Biol Macromol 2008; 42(3): 235-40.
[http://dx.doi.org/10.1016/j.ijbiomac.2007.10.023] [PMID: 18054382]

[236] Dürig J, Bruhn T, Zurborn KH, Gutensohn K, Bruhn HD, Béress L. Anticoagulant fucoidan fractions from Fucus vesiculosus induce platelet activation *in vitro*. Thromb Res 1997; 85(6): 479-91.
[http://dx.doi.org/10.1016/S0049-3848(97)00037-6] [PMID: 9101640]

[237] Irhimeh MR, Fitton JH, Lowenthal RM. Pilot clinical study to evaluate the anticoagulant activity of fucoidan. Blood Coagul Fibrinolysis 2009; 20(7): 607-10.
[http://dx.doi.org/10.1097/MBC.0b013e32833135fe] [PMID: 19696660]

[238] Zayed A, Dienemann C, Giese C, Krämer R, Ulber R. An immobilized perylene diimide derivative for fucoidan purification from a crude brown algae extract. Process Biochem 2018; 65: 233-8.
[http://dx.doi.org/10.1016/j.procbio.2017.10.012]

[239] Zayed A, Muffler K, Hahn T, *et al.* Physicochemical and biological characterization of fucoidan from fucus vesiculosus purified by dye affinity chromatography. Mar Drugs 2016; 14(4): 1-15.
[http://dx.doi.org/10.3390/md14040079] [PMID: 27092514]

[240] Li B, Lu F, Wei X, Zhao R. Fucoidan: structure and bioactivity. Molecules 2008; 13(8): 1671-95.
[http://dx.doi.org/10.3390/molecules13081671] [PMID: 18794778]

[241] Singh VK, Singh DK. Pharmacological effects of garlic (*Allium sativum* L.). Annual Review of Biomedical Sciences 2008; 10: 6-26.
[http://dx.doi.org/10.5016/1806-8774.2008.v10p6]

[242] Srivastava K, Mustafa T. Pharmacological effects of spices : eicosanoid modula-ting activities and their significance in human health. Biomedical Reviews 2 1993; 29: 15-29.

[243] Levin RM, Juan Y-S, Schuler C, Leggett RE, Lin AD. Medicinal properties of antrodia camphorata - a review. Curr Top Nutraceutical Res 2012; 10: 53-60.
[http://dx.doi.org/10.5455/spatula.201604130153531]

[244] Lee YM, Chang CY, Yen TL, *et al.* Extract of Antrodia camphorata exerts neuroprotection against embolic stroke in rats without causing the risk of hemorrhagic incidence. Sci World J 2014; 2014686109
[http://dx.doi.org/10.1155/2014/686109] [PMID: 25140341]

[245] Majeed M, Praksh L. Alpha-Lipoic Acid : An Efficient Antioxidant Sabinsa corporation 2014.

[246] Dong Y, Wang H, Chen Z. Alpha-lipoic acid attenuates cerebral ischemia and reperfusion injury *via* insulin receptor and PI3K/Akt-Dependent inhibition of NADPH oxidase. Int J Endocrinol 2015; 2015903186
[http://dx.doi.org/10.1155/2015/903186] [PMID: 26294909]

CHAPTER 5

Implication of Natural Compounds for the Prevention of Ocular Diseases

Kaid Johar SR[1,*], Pooja Rathaur[2], Shraddha Bhadada[3] and A.R Vasavada[4]

[1] *Department of Zoology, Biomedical Technology and Human Genetics, Gujarat University, Ahmedabad, India*

[2] *Department of Life Science, Gujarat University, Ahmedabad, India*

[3] *Institute of Pharmacy, Nirma University, Ahmedabad, India*

[4] *Iladevi Cataract and IOL Research Centre, Gurukul road, Memnagar, Ahmedabad, India*

Abstract: Our eyes are a window to this world and like other parts of our body are affected by various diseases and injuries. Prevalence of various ocular diseases is although very high, very few remedies are available. Diseases affecting eye and vision are on the rise particularly those associated with potentially blinding conditions such as diabetic retinopathy, age-related macular degeneration, and glaucoma. Prevention appears to be a better modality for most of the ocular diseases compared to that of the treatment options. Natural compounds have found its use in the prevention and treatment of many ocular diseases. Several natural compounds with properties such as anti-oxidative, anti-proliferative, immunomodulatory have been implicated in the prevention of various ocular diseases. However, there are many avenues left for the application of natural compounds for the prevention and treatment of various ocular diseases. Understanding of the probable mechanism responsible for the disease formation, identification of targets, evaluation of candidate molecules by *in silico*, *in vitro* and *in vivo* assays can strengthen the application of natural compounds for the prevention of ocular diseases. Besides disease prevention, natural compounds have also found its use in various ocular surgical procedures.

Keywords: Age-related macular degeneration, Anti-aging, Anti-inflammatory, Antioxidants, Anti-proliferative, Apoptosis, Cataract, Diabetic retinopathy, Dry eye, Eye disorders, Eye injuries, Glaucoma, Immunomodulatory, Intraocular pressure, Natural compounds, Ocular surgeries, Ocular viscoelastic devices, Phytochemicals, Phacoemulsification, Viscoelastic substance.

---

* **Corresponding author Dr. Kaid Johar SR:** Department of Zoology, Biomedical Technology and Human Genetics, School of Sciences, Gujarat University, Ahmedabad 380009, India; E-mails: kaidjohar@gujaratuniversity.ac.in; qaidjohar110@gmail.com

Atta-ur-Rahman, Shazia Anjum and Hesham Al-Seedi (Eds.)

INTRODUCTION

Natural compounds have been used widely for years for the prevention and treatment of many diseases but, lack of scientific pieces of evidence is limiting their use. Several compounds have succeeded to be considered as drugs for chronic debilitating disorders due to systematic scientific studies on it. Most of the compounds isolated from natural sources have anti-oxidative, anti-inflammatory, immunomodulatory and anti-proliferative activities. Eye disorders like cataract, age-related degeneration (AMD), glaucoma, and diabetic retinopathy "(DR)". are generally occurring or progressing due to similar mechanisms. Natural products can thus be molecules of consideration to develop into novel drugs. This is also supported by history which shows that several modern drugs developed have their origin in natural compounds. Also, the WHO (World Health Organization) states that probably 80% of the world's population depends on traditional medicines which includes plant extracts or active molecules of the plant [1]. This indicates that developing molecules for the prevention or treatment of disorders can have a wide market for the future. Many plants or plant extracts have been tested for different ocular diseases. Some of them have shown promising results in animal studies or *in vitro* studies. However, active molecules need to be identified and developed as drugs.

Majority of the ocular disorders include (AMD), glaucoma, cataract, and DR. All these disorders, even though quite prevalent, have very few or no treatments available except surgery. As well as, potentially blinding diseases that can affect eye and vision are on the rise. Thus, prevention always remains a better solution for these disorders. Natural compounds, either in the diet or as pills or powders are used as functional foods that have proven to be effective in the prevention or delaying the progression of the disease. Several of the natural compounds or crude plant extracts are been used for ocular disorders. This chapter summarizes the evidence of the therapeutic benefits provided by several natural compounds obtained from different plants and other natural resources.

MAJOR OCULAR DISORDERS

According to WHO, 80% of the world population relies on traditional medicine and hence increasing the awareness and steps to prevent such disorders by dietary supplements or nutraceuticals can be instrumental in reducing the prevalence [2, 3]. Major pathogenesis for these disorders includes oxidation of proteins, inflammation, and angiogenesis.

Age-related Macular Degeneration

AMD is a common retinal disorder of the aging eye. It slowly develops bilaterally and hence is responsible for blindness. It progresses by reducing the visual acuity and thus the quality of life [4]. Age is the foremost risk factor associated with AMD however; other major risk factors include cigarette smoking, cardiovascular diseases, diet, and genetic history. These risk factors are mainly involving angiogenesis, oxidative pathway or inflammation, and extracellular matrix pathways. It has been reported that dietary antioxidant supplementation may help in slow down the progression of the disease [5, 6]. The current treatment for AMD involves intraocular or intravitreal injections of anti-vascular endothelial growth factor (anti-VEGF) agents and sometimes combined with other modalities [6]. The newer therapies are utilizing gene therapy but yet to be fully investigated [7]. Some clinical studies have shown that dietary supplements like antioxidants, zinc, and carotenoids help in the reduction of progression to advanced AMD in some patients [8, 9].

Glaucoma

Glaucoma, both open-angle or closed-angle, is a multifactorial disease involving several mechanisms including oxidative stress or inflammation leading to vision loss [10]. There is an increased intraocular pressure (IOP) in the eye which finally damages the optic nerve through apoptosis of retinal cells [11]. The current therapy involves the use of eye drops or oral drugs to lower IOP and finally the surgery. Since it is mainly occurring due to apoptosis of cells and damage to optic nerve, several studies have been done for the implication of neuroprotection in glaucoma patients [12]. Many natural compounds do show potent neuroprotection and thus may be promising in the prevention of glaucoma.

Cataract

Cataract, an opacity of eye lens, is due to several metabolic, environmental, nutritional and genetic factors. It is a leading cause of blindness worldwide according to WHO (WHO-Prevention of Blindness and Deafness Program). The major pathogenesis includes an aggregation of proteins due to genetic mutations or molecular mechanisms leading to opacity in the eye lens [13]. Various risk factors are known to propagate cataracts like age, diabetes, smoking, exposure to UV radiation and family history [14]. The only treatment currently available is surgery which removes the opacified lens and replaces with an artificial intraocular lens. It is generally said that if the development of cataracts can be delayed by 10 years, it can reduce the possibility of surgery by 50% [15]. Studies have shown that the incorporation of anti-oxidants in the diet may help in delaying the progression by preventing the aggregation or degradation of the lens proteins [16, 17].

Diabetic Retinopathy

Diabetic retinopathy (DR) is a common complication associated with type I and type II diabetes mellitus and is a leading cause of blindness among diabetics. It is a progressive disease mainly affecting the retinal microvasculature [18]. DR can be broadly classified as non-proliferative diabetic retinopathy and an advanced stage of proliferative diabetic retinopathy. An additional category of DR is diabetic macular edema which is the most common cause of vision loss. Currently, no treatment is employed for non-proliferative DR whereas several modalities like laser photocoagulation, vitreoretinal surgery or intra-vitreous administration of anti-VEGF or steroid agents are available for proliferative DR or diabetic macular edema [19]. Even then, there are still unmet needs for the prevention of vision loss which can prevent the progression of non-proliferative DR to proliferative DR.

NATURAL COMPOUNDS EMPLOYED IN OCULAR DISORDERS

Several natural compounds such as polyphenols, terpenes, omega-3-fatty acids, vitamins, carotenoids have shown a beneficial effect in the prevention and treatment of ocular diseases. Table 1 enlist the natural compounds which were used for the prevention and treatment of ocular diseases.

Table 1. Natural compounds used against ocular diseases.

Plant	Family	Active Compound	Mechanism of Action	Treated Eye Disease
Curcuma longa (Turmeric)	Zingiberaceae	Curcumin	Blocks NF-κB activation, suppresses TNF-α synthesis, inhibits the release cytokines such as IL-1, IL-6, IL-8, decreases VEGF and increases the levels of antioxidant enzymes SOD and catalase [20].	Cataract [21, 22]; DR [23]; Conjunctivitis [24]; Glaucoma [25]; Chronic anterior uveitis [26]
Green tea (*Camellia sinensis*)	Theaceae	Catechin	Modulation of nitric oxide synthase isoforms [27]	Dry eye [28]; cataract [29]
Eupatorium ballotaefolium (boneset)	Asteraceae	Nepetin	Decrease the nuclear translocation of p65 [30]	AMD [30]; DR [30]

(Table 1) cont.....

Plant	Family	Active Compound	Mechanism of Action	Treated Eye Disease
Vitis vinifera (Grapes)	Vitaceae	Resveratrol	Increases expression of SIRT1, inhibition of ERK1/2 and MAPK signaling cascade [31].	Glaucoma [32]; AMD [33]; DR [34]
Andrographis paniculata (green chireta)	Acanthaceae	Andrographolide	Inhibited p38 MAPK/HO'-NF--B-ERK2 cascade [35]	Posterior capsular opacification [97]
Boswellia serrata (Salai guggul)	Burseraceae	Acetyl-11-keto-b-boswellic acid	Reduction of VEGF expression and VEGFR-2 phosphorylation [36].	DR [36, 37]
Foeniculum vulgare (Fennel)	Apiaceae	Trans-anethole	Reduction of glutathione, catalase and SOD activity [38]	Cataract [38]
Coffea (Coffee)	Rubiaceae	Caffeine	Prevent oxidative stress and apoptosis [39]	Diabetic cataract [39] (Varma *et al.*, 2010)

Polyphenols

Polyphenols are phytochemicals with at least one aromatic ring connected with a hydroxyl group (phenolic group). Polyphenols may have several other groups attached to the ring and can be accordingly classified into flavonoids, stilbenes, coumarins, phenolic acids, and tannins. Polyphenols are commonly present in plants like red wine, turmeric and green tea [3]. Many natural compounds such as curcumin, quercetin, catechin, nepetin and resveratrol are shown to be effective in preventing various ocular ailments.

Curcumin

Curcumin is the main water-insoluble curcuminoid isolated from the rhizome of the popular Indian spice, turmeric (*Curcuma longa*). This plant belongs to the *Zingiberaceae* family. Turmeric has been very widely used as a therapeutic agent in Ayurveda since ancient times for several disorders and is widely available throughout South Asia. The main active compound isolated from the rhizome *i.e.* curcumin has been tested in several disorders to date showing potential benefits in most of them [40, 41]. However, it still faces the problems of solubility and bioavailability due to which liposomes and nanoparticles are being studied for its biomedical potential [42]. Curcumin has been reported to possess benefits in several disorders due to its anti-inflammatory and anti-oxidant properties [43].

Recently, the pharmacological effects of curcumin are also attributed to its ability to modulate the expression of several pathogenic miRs in non-cancer disorders like brain, ocular, renal and liver disorders [44]. Several molecular targets have been identified for its action like cyclooxygenase-2 (COX-2), lipoxygenase, nitric oxide synthase, nuclear factor kappa-beta (NF-κB) and tumor necrosis factor-alpha (TNF-α) [45, 46]. Curcumin also targets some cell signalling pathways (Fig. **1**). Several studies have been done in ocular disorders to evaluate the efficacy and mechanism of curcumin [47, 48]. Curcumin has been tested for retinal neuroprotection desired for preventive therapy of AMD by studying light-induced retinal degeneration (LIRD) in rats and effect on retina-derived cell lines. It was supplemented with the diet and showed significant improvement which was proposed to be due to inhibition of NF-κB and down-regulation of certain inflammatory genes [49]. Another study has also suggested it as a therapeutic strategy for AMD suppression as they have shown suppression of choroidal neovascularization in addition to the NF-κB inhibition and HIF-α activation [50]. Also, Lu *et al.* (2015) concluded in their study on aging RPE cells that curcumin can regulate oxidative stress, proliferation, and apoptosis. Thus, curcumin can be suggested as a novel therapeutic adjuvant for AMD [51].

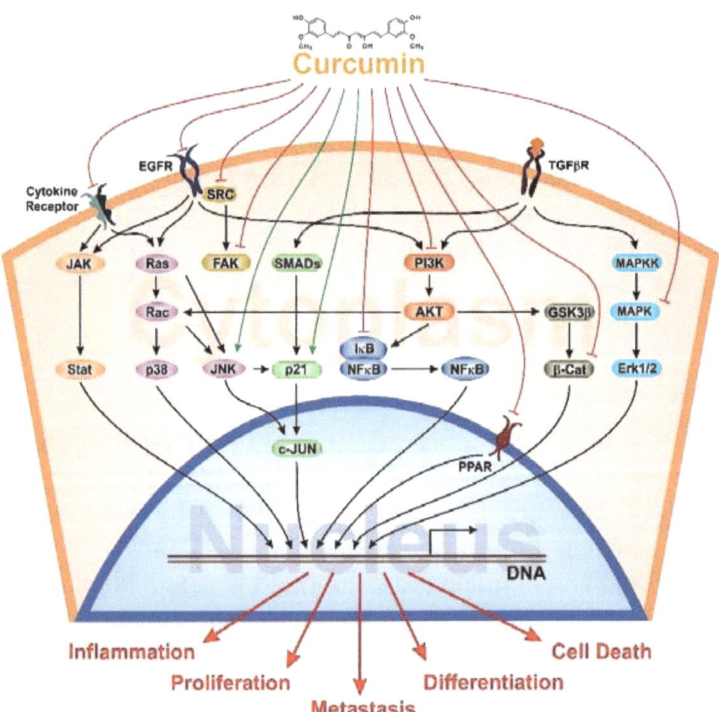

Fig. (1). Effect of curcumin on various cell signaling pathways.

Curcumin is a potent antioxidant and anti-inflammatory (5-hydroxy-eicosatetraenoic acid, cyclooxygenase and lipoxygenase inhibition) has been shown to have a beneficial effect in DR [52]. Curcumin significantly reduced the expression of angiogenic factors like VEGF, iNOS and ICAM-1 in a rat model of streptozotocin diabetes which may suggest its beneficial role in the management of DR [53].

Curcumin is also suggested to be an adjunct therapy for glaucoma. Glaucoma is known to cause loss of retinal ganglion cells and hence leading to progressive vision loss. Curcumin administration has shown significant neuroprotective effects in ischemic reperfusion-induced retinal injury in rats which is related to glaucoma suggesting its vaso-protective effects primarily due to inhibition of anti-inflammatory pathways [54]. Besides, curcumin has shown protective effects in *N*-methyl-D-aspartate (NMDA) mediated excitotoxicity in primary mixed retinal neuronal/glial cultures [55]. In a chronic high intraocular pressure rat model, curcumin pretreatment could prevent loss of retinal ganglion cells as well as inhibit the oxidative damage to microglia [56]. These studies suggest curcumin to be an effective strategy for the treatment of glaucoma.

Several studies have been done on the delaying of cataract by curcumin using various models like the diabetic cataract model, selenite induced model or even cell cultures [47, 57]. Most of the studies have reported the anti-oxidative effect of curcumin to be mainly responsible for its beneficial effect in cataract [58]. Curcumin pre-treatment may improve antioxidant enzymes like glutathione peroxidase (GPx), glucose-6- phosphate dehydrogenase (G6PD) as well as protein carbonyls whereas significantly reduced GSH levels in an animal model of diabetic cataract [59]. Curcumin administration was found to increase vitamin C and vitamin E levels indicating a preventing role in cataract [60]. Furthermore, it has been indicated to be effective against osmotic stress by inhibiting aldose reductase [59, 61]. There is severe cross-linking of proteins and high molecular weight aggregate formations causing protein modifications, precipitation and degradation and hence cataract progression [62, 63]. Curcumin could alleviate these protein changes in rat models of diabetic and selenite cataract seen as suppression of heat shock protein 70 (Hsp 70), αA-crystalline and αB-crystallin [64, 65]. Also, curcumin could increase the Ca-ATPase activity thus lowering the Ca^{+2} levels which can mediate degradation of the crystallins in the lens through calpain and other enzymes [66]. *In vitro*, curcumin could inhibit the proliferation of human lens epithelial B3 (hLEB3) cells and induce apoptosis in bovine lens epithelial cells showing potential for the prevention of progression of cataract [67, 68].

Quercetin

Quercetin (3,3',4',5,7-pentahydroxyflavone) is found in more than 20 plants such as onions, grapes, berries, cherries, broccoli and citrus fruits [69]. The name is derived from the Latin word "Quercetum" an oak forest, it is a flavonol that can be obtained from various fruits and vegetables. It is broadly used in the treatment of metabolic disorders and as anti-inflammatory, anti-oxidant, in neuro-degenerative diseases, in cancer and apoptosis, in the prevention of cardiovascular diseases, ulcer, and gastritis [70]. The effect of dietary quercetin was studied for its protective effect against oxidative stress on RPE (retinal pigment epithelial) [71]. It is commonly present in *Ginkgo biloba* and red wine and inhibits the initiation of glaucomatous damage through the suppression of nitric oxide and TNFα [3, 72].

Catechin

Catechin is a polyphenolic antioxidant, which is present in the green tea. Epigallocatechin gallate (EGCG) is the most abundant catechin of green tea. In ischemia-reperfusion injury, catechins reduced mitochondrial damage [73]. Catechin is also present in apples, berries, grape seeds, kiwi, red wine, chocolate, and cocoa [74]. Intraocular injection of EGCG with sodium nitroprusside exhibited a protective effect on the retinal photoreceptors, demonstrating that EGCG may benefit patients suffering from oxidative stress involved in the development of ocular diseases [75]. In *in vivo* rat models, oral administration of EGCG reduced light-induced retinal neuronal death, indicating that EGCG may be used in preventing photoreceptor cell death [76, 77]. In the same way, supplementation of catechin on N-methyl-N-nitrosourea induced cataracts in Sprague-Dawley rats displayed inhibition of cataract-induced apoptosis in the lens epithelium, suggesting that catechin may prove beneficial in the treatment or prevention of cataract [78]. Also, EGCG has the potential to inhibit RPE cell migration and adhesion [79] and hence can be implemented in the prevention of retinopathies involving RPE cells.

Nepetin

Nepetin is known as eupafolin or 6-methoxyluteolin [80]. Nepetin generally presents in plants such as *Eupatorium arnottianum* Griseb, *Clerodendrum petasites,* and *Lippia nodiflora* [81 - 83]. Nepetin exhibits anti-inflammatory properties. Nepetin can significantly decrease the inflammatory mediators in a dose-dependent manner at both the protein and mRNA levels. Nepetin eliminates IL-1β (Interleukin 1 beta) induced IL-6 (Interleukin 6), IL-8 (Interleukin 8) and MCP-1 (Monocyte chemoattractant protein-1) secretion in ARPE-19 cells (retinal pigment epithelial cells) [84]. Nepetin can reduce p65 nuclear localization by suppressing phosphorylation of inhibitor of nuclear factor kappa B (IκB) and also suppress the phosphorylation of extracellular signal-regulated kinases (ERK) 1/2, c-Jun N-terminal kinase (JNK) and p38 MAPK (*P38* mitogen-activated protein kinases) [84].

Resveratrol

Resveratrol (3,5,41-trihydroxy-trans-stilbene) is a naturally occurring plant polyphenol and a phytoalexin by various plants in response to injury or pathogen attack [85]. The skin of grapes, blueberries, raspberries, and mulberries are the food sources of resveratrol [86]. Attention on resveratrol for medical research began with the "French Paradox" describing the cardiovascular health benefits of red wine, which contains a high concentration of resveratrol [87]. Since then, researchers focused more on resveratrol due to its potent anti-oxidative and anti-inflammatory properties and found that resveratrol can be cardio-protective [88], neuroprotective [89], chemotherapeutic [90], and exhibit anti-aging effects [91]. The proliferation of RPE cells has been reduced due to the treatment of resveratrol through the inhibition of ERK1/2 and MAPK signaling cascade [92]. Luna *et al.* (2009) investigated the therapeutic effects of chronic administration of the dietary supplement resveratrol on the expression of inflammation, oxidative stress and cellular senescence markers in primary trabecular meshwork cells of open-angle glaucoma [93]. The study proved that resveratrol treatment effectively prevented increased production of intracellular reactive oxygen species (iROS) and inflammatory markers and reduced expression of the senescence markers. These results suggest that resveratrol has a great role in preventing the trabecular meshwork tissue abnormalities observed in open-angle glaucoma. Analogue of resveratrol is also useful in ophthalmic diseases. Pinosylvin (3,5-dihydroxy-tras-s-stilbene) is a stilbenoid polyphenol and resveratrol analog, commonly found at higher concentrations in bark waste of *Pinus* species. Due to its antioxidant potential, it possesses a protective effect against several diseases such as AMD [94]. Koskela *et al.*, (2014) suggested that pinosylvin shows antioxidant protection against heme oxygenase-1 induced oxidative stress in the human retinal pigment epithelial cell line, ARPE-19 cells [95].

Terpenes

Terpenes are characterized by a combination of isoprene units (C5H8). Their classification is based on the number of isoprene units such as hemiterpenes (one isoprene unit), monoterpenes (two isoprene unit), sesquiterpenes (three isoprene unit), diterpenes (four isoprene unit), *etc*. The volatility of terpenes decreases with an increasing number of isoprene units. Terpenes have various properties such as anti-inflammatory, wound healing and anti-neoplastic. Andrographolide and acetyl-11-keto-b-boswellic acid are related to this class of natural compounds and shown to be useful in the prevention of ocular diseases.

Andrographolide

Andrographolide is a labdane diterpenoid and it is the main bioactive component of the medicinal plant, *Andrographis paniculata*. Andrographolide has shown various pharmacological effects such as anti-proliferative, anti-migratory, anti-fibrotic, anti-inflammatory and anti-cancerous. Posterior capsular opacification (PCO), which is also known as secondary cataract, develops after cataract surgery due to the proliferation and abnormal differentiation in a form of epithelial-mesenchymal transition (EMT) [96]. Kayastha *et al.* (2015) studied the effect of andrographolide on EMT, which was induced by some growth factors (Transforming growth factor-beta 2 and basic fibroblast growth factor) in the fetal human lens epithelial cell line (FHL 124) [97]. They showed significantly increased protein and mRNA levels of epithelial markers, pax6 and E-cadherin while EMT markers α-smooth muscle actin, fibronectin, and collagen significantly decreased after the treatment of andrographolide. They also demonstrated that the treatment of andrographolide can also cause inhibition phosphorylation of ERK and JNK. Andrographolide also reduces proliferation, migration, and phosphorylation of Akt in lens epithelial cells. Thus, andrographolide may be used for the prevention of PCO by affecting various signalling pathways (Fig. **2**) [98].

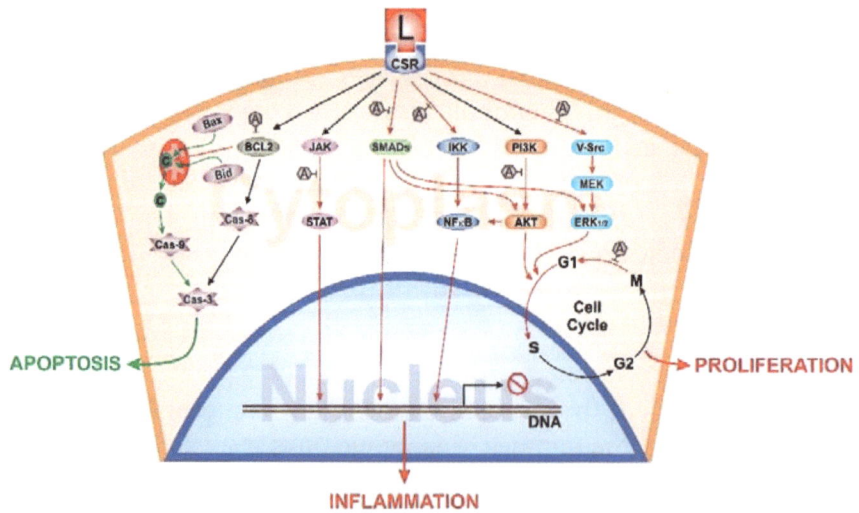

Fig. (2). Effects of andrographolide on various cell signaling pathways.

Acetyl-11-keto-b-boswellic Acid

Acetyl-11-keto-b-boswellic acid (AKBA) is a boswellic acid, which is derived from plant *Boswellia serrata* [99, 100]. Recently, it has been reported that AKBA may increase the expression of Src homology region 2 containing phosphatase 1 and reduced the expression of VEGF, VEGF receptor-2 (VEGF-2) phosphorylation and transcription factor signal transducer and activator of transcription 3 (STAT3) phosphorylation [101, 102]. AKBA reduced proliferation, migration and tube formation of exogenous VEGF stimulated human retinal microvascular endothelial cells (HRMECs), while it also decreases the migration and tube formation of untreated HRDMECs of oxygen-induced retinopathy (OIR) model [101]. Thus, AKBA has a great potential of anti-angiogenesis which can prevent microvasculature associated conditions.

Vitamins

Vitamins are made by living organisms and they are essential for life. They are also useful for the management of various disease conditions such as hyperhomocysteinemia, cataract formation, *etc*. Vitamins are usually anti-oxidant in nature. Some vitamins such as folic acid, α-tocopherol, and methylcobalamin are very useful in eye-related diseases.

Folic Acid

Folate is essential for the maintenance of the cells and the breakdown of homocysteine in the body [103]. Hyperhomocysteinemia is responsible for the damage of coronary arteries, the development of exfoliation syndrome (XFS) and central retinal vein occlusion [104]. In glaucoma patients, homocysteine can alter extracellular matrix and neuronal cell death [105]. Folate reduces hyperhomocysteinemia [106]. In patients with XFS both with and without glaucoma, elevated plasma homocysteine level was detected [107]. Thus, hyperhomocysteinemia may be a risk factor for XFS. In the primary, open-angle glaucoma homocysteine level and the frequency of heterozygous methylenetetrahydrofolate reductase C677T mutation are increased [108].

α-Tocopherol

α- tocopherol or vitamin E is a potent anti-oxidant that neutralizes reactive oxygen species (ROS) in our body including various parts of the eye [109]. The AREDS study (Age-Related Eye Disease Study) stated that vitamin E along with other nutrients is beneficial for people having moderate AMD. The Baltimore Longitudinal Study of Aging suggested a protective effect for AMD in patients with high plasma levels of a-tocopherol [110]. The Blue Mountain Eye study concluded no protective association between a-tocopherol and age-related maculopathy [111]. Besides, a large-scale randomized trial of female health professionals also concluded that α-tocopherol had no large beneficial or harmful effects on the risk of AMD [112]. A preclinical study done using a mouse model of severe vitamin E deficiency showed increased lipid peroxidation in the retina and accelerated the degenerative damage of the retina with age [113]. A case-control study done is in Japan also demonstrated that a high dietary intake of α-tocopherol and vitamin C was associated with a reduced risk of neovascular AMD [114]. A recent study done in rabbits evaluated the effect of UV irradiation on the ocular structures and demonstrated the protective effect of topical application of antioxidants including vitamin E on the eye from oxidative stress [115].

α-tocopherol acetate and α-tocopherol succinate showed significantly lowered IOP than the control group in a preclinical study suggesting a beneficial role of vitamin- E for glaucoma [116]. Following this, the effect of studied of oral α-tocopherol acetate and found that differences between the pulsatility indexes and resistivity indexes of both ophthalmic arteries and posterior ciliary arteries of patients receiving α-tocopherol. Thus, it was concluded that α-tocopherol may be protecting the retina from glaucomatous damage [117]. Furthermore, vitamin E supplementation was also evaluated for preventing the failure of glaucoma surgery, trabeculectomy, and phaco trabeculectomy in a double-blind randomized placebo-controlled trial. However, supplementation did not show any differences between the α-tocopherol and the placebo group [118]. A large cross-sectional study was carried out to study the effect of supplement intake of vitamin A, C, and E but there was no association found with glaucoma and vitamin E [119]. A recent meta-analysis on the effect of vitamin E on glaucoma concluded no significant association of vitamin E with open-angle glaucoma suggesting further studies to be designed to confirm its protective role [120].

Several preclinical studies have shown the beneficial effect of vitamin E supplementation for delaying the progression of cataract. But a study evaluating long term supplementation with α-tocopherol for 5 to 8 years does not influence the cataract prevalence among middle-aged, smoking men [121]. A 2-year double-blind placebo-controlled study showed no improvement in the visual function of patients with age-related cataract [122]. Furthermore, review analysis of vitamin E supplementation encourages the use of low dose vitamin E supplementation which may be beneficial in cataract [123]. A clinical study on a small population concluded that low levels of α-tocopherol were associated with delayed cataract formation [124]. A preclinical study on rats showed dose-dependent protection of oral vitamin E supplementation against UV radiation-induced cataract [125]. Also, a study on 599 elderly participants indicated that high daily intakes of fruits and vegetables and vitamin C and E were associated with reduced prevalence of cataract or cataract surgery [126].

Several studies have evaluated the efficacy of α-tocopherol in preventing DR. Millen *et al.* (2003) carried out an epidemiologic survey to study the association of vitamin E with DR [127]. But no associations were found between the serum levels of vitamin E and DR [128]. They suggested no association between dietary intake or plasma levels of vitamin E and DR. Another study in rats suggested its beneficial effect to be mediated by normalization of the hyperglycemia-induced activation of the diacylglycerol-protein kinase C pathway which leads to improvement in the retinal blood flow [129]. However, none of the clinical studies showed any beneficial effect.

Methylcobalamin

Methylcobalamin is a homolog of vitamin B12. It is involved in nucleic acid synthesis, protein synthesis and metabolism of phospholipids [129]. Methylcobalamin also provides methyl groups to the myelin sheath that protects nerve fibers and regenerates damaged neurons [129]. Several studies have shown possible improvement or stabilization in visual field performance with oral vitamin B12 supplementation in glaucoma patients [130]. Kikuchi *et al.* (1997) showed that methylcobalamin can also protect cultured retinal ganglion cells against glutamate-induced neurotoxicity [131].

Amino Acids and their Derivatives

Amino acids are organic compounds; they are the building blocks of protein. They have two terminals; amine terminal (-NH2) and carboxyl-terminal (-COOH). Amino acids and their derivative both are helpful in various eye-related diseases such as diabetes, retinitis pigmentosa, and glaucoma.

Taurine

Taurine is a free amino acid commonly present in the retina [132]. Taurine deficiency has a major role in visual dysfunction in both humans as well as in animals, which can be reversed by nutritional supplementation [133]. Taurine distribution is tightly regulated during the development of the retina [133]. The exact function of taurine in the retina is still unresolved. Nevertheless, release and uptake of taurine have been found to play distinct regulatory mechanisms in the retina [133]. In diabetic rats, supplementation of taurine significantly decreased lipid peroxidation and preserved ATPase activity [134]. In the study of neuritic outgrowth from post crush goldfish retinal explants, the maximum neuritic outgrowth was supported by the presence of fetal calf serum, under the same conditions, taurine increased the length and density of neurites [135]. In patients with retinitis pigmentosa, the combination of taurine, diltiazem, and vitamin E treatment showed the beneficial effect of reducing the rate of visual field loss, likely through a protective action against free radical reactions in affected photoreceptors [136].

L- Glutathione

Glutathione is composed of three amino acids (cysteine, glutamic acid, and glycine) and it is naturally occurring antioxidant [137]. Oxidative DNA damage and glutathione-S-transferase M1 (GSTM1) gene deletion both are responsible for glaucoma development and they are also associated with an increased risk of cancer of various sites [130]. GSTM1 positive patients have a higher risk of glaucoma development [138]. A study was conducted by Yang *et al.* (2001) to identify the role of retinal proteins, which are the target of serum autoantibodies in glaucoma patients [139]. To counter glutathione-S- transferase (GST) antigen, serum antibodies were recognized by 52% of patients of glaucoma and 20% age-matched controls [139]. This finding indicates that GST can be targeted in glaucoma patients by serum autoantibodies. Reduced level of glutathione can induce EMT by wnt/β-catenin pathway in lens epithelial cells [140].

N-acetyl-L-cysteine

The N-acetyl-L-cysteine (NAC) is derived from L-cysteine and it is a precursor for the biosynthesis of glutathione antioxidant [141]. Increased level of cellular ceramide and diacylglycerol is associated with apoptosis in retinal microvessels in DR and cellular ceramide and diacylglycerol production can be inhibited by NAC [142]. NAC was also responsible for the inhibition of protein carbonylation which is a non-enzymatic modification that occurs in cellular oxidative stress [143]. Furthermore, NAC increased the neuronal cell survival rate of cultured neurons from embryonic mouse cortex and striatum [144]. The higher level of MMP-9 activity in the ocular surface is responsible for the pathogenesis of corneal diseases [145]. In human corneal epithelial cells, MMP-9 production may be inhibited by NAC and it also inhibits cell migration *in vitro* [146]. Thus, NAC may be useful for the management of corneal erosions and related conditions.

Carnitine

Carnitine, (3R)-3-hydroxy-4-(trimethylazaniumyl) butanoate is an amino acid derivative of lysine, plays a key role as an endogenous and exogenous nutrient in the metabolism of lipid [147]. Carnitine in humans is mainly obtained from dietary sources [148]. There are two isomeric forms; L-carnitine which plays an important role in the production of cellular energy, whereas D-carnitine is inactive physiologically as well as toxic in biochemical processes [149]. Requisitely, L-carnitine is involved in the transportation of the fatty acid chains in the mitochondrial matrix which allows the breaking of fat and obtains energy from the stored fats [150].

L-carnitine was studied in a small population of patients with AMD where it had shown its beneficial effect against oxidative damage by reducing the malondialdehyde (MDA) levels and increasing GSH [151]. Another randomized, double-blind, placebo-controlled clinical trial evaluated the efficacy of the combination of acetyl-L-carnitine, omega-3 fatty acids, and coenzyme Q10 on the visual functions and found significant improvement in visual functions as well as fundus alterations in patients affected by early AMD [152]. Acetyl-L-carnitine along with omega-3 fatty acid, H2O2, coenzyme Q10, α-lipoic acid, lutein, and zeaxanthin demonstrated beneficial effects in retinal gangliar cell function in patients with AMD [153].

It has been suggested that carnitine may have a role for secondary neuroprotection in glaucoma [154]. Administration of acetyl-L-carnitine in the anterior chamber had an anti-apoptotic effect on astrocytes and improvement in optic nerve morphology may be due to alterations in the mitochondrial membrane permeability [153]. Calandrella *et al.* (2010) have shown in an experiment on rats that L-carnitine reduces the expression of the glial fibrillary acidic protein, inducible nitric oxide synthase, ubiquitin and caspase 3 in ocular hypertension [154]. Also, the optic nerve morphology was improved. The proposed mechanism suggested for the protective effect was a reduction in lipid peroxidation by L-carnitine [154].

Carnitine levels in human ocular structures are yet unknown, however, several studies in rabbits have shown it to be higher in ocular tissue where muscular cells are present [155]. Carnitine levels were evaluated in the human lens and cataract [156]. The significant difference was found in the total and free carnitine levels between the lenses with mature cataract and with partial cataract [156]. This suggested the beneficial role of supplementation of carnitine in patients with older age. Kocer *et al.* (2007) studied the antioxidant activity of carnitine supplementation experimentally in Sprague Dawley rats with radiation-induced cataract [157]. The levels of MDA, the end product of lipid peroxidation, was found to be significantly lower while the activity of superoxide dismutase and glutathione peroxidase enzymes were improved in the animals treated with carnitine which indicated the protection against the γ-radiation-induced cataracts [157]. The antioxidant activity of acetyl-L-carnitine was also studied in selenite induced cataractogenesis where similar beneficial results were obtained [158, 159]. Besides, calpain activity was measured in selenite induced cataracts in rats. Acetyl-L-carnitine was able to maintain the calpain activity near normal values suggesting it to be a novel drug for the prevention of cataract [160]. Besides, Elanchezhian *et al.* (2010) also investigated the role of acetyl-L-carnitine in regulating the expression of antioxidants and apoptotic genes in selenite induced cataracts of rats [161]. The results suggested that acetyl-L-carnitine may be able to prevent cataractogenesis by preventing the abnormal expression of lenticular genes regulating apoptosis. It was also studied in combination with nifedipine in selenite induced cataract in rats wherein combination was concluded to be having better antioxidative potential than alone acetyl-L-carnitine [162]. These preclinical studies were extended to human LECs treated with homocysteine, responsible for causing cataract. It was observed that carnitine protected the lens epithelial cells against the endoplasmic reticulum induced stress, thus increasing the levels of kelch-like ECH-associated protein 1 (Keap1) and nuclear factor erythroid 2 (Nrf2) genes which in turn improves the antioxidant enzyme status [163]. Besides, studies are required to develop it as an anti-cataract agent.

A cross-sectional study including 33 diabetic patients revealed that free serum L-carnitine levels are very low in patients with complications as compared to diabetic patients without complications [164]. This suggested that supplementation of L-carnitine may be beneficial in patients with diabetic complications. However, another study was done in type 1 and type 2 diabetic patients revealed no significant benefit of supplementing L-carnitine to delay the development of late diabetic complications [165]. *In vitro* studies done in retinal ganglion cells suggested that L-carnitine may protect these cells from high glucose-induced injury may be due to inhibition of oxidative damage, mitochondrial dysfunction and thus cell apoptosis [166]. This beneficial effect on retinal ganglion cells was related to the Nrf2-Keap1 pathway [167]. Nevertheless, clinical studies depicting the beneficial role of L-carnitine in ocular disorders is still lacking and require further research.

Carotenoids

Carotenoids widely occur in plants, microorganisms, algae, and animals [168]. These compounds are responsible for the pigments such as yellow, orange and red [169]. Carotenoids compounds exist in the trans isoform, naturally [170]. They have a long series of conjugated double bonds in the central part of the molecule, which is responsible for maintaining shape, chemical reactivity and light-absorbing properties [171]. Orange vegetables and fruits, including carrots, sweet potatoes, winter squash, pumpkin, papaya, mango, and cantaloupe, are major sources of the β-carotene [172]. Tomatoes, watermelons, apricots, and pink guavas are the rich sources of lycopene [173]. Some carotenoids can function as provitamin A such as β-carotene, α-carotene, and β-cryptoxanthin [174]. They are considered to play an important role in the prevention of various oxidative stress-related diseases such as cardiovascular disease, AMD, and cancer of various organs [175, 176].

Lutein and Zeaxanthin

Lutein and Zeaxanthin are carotenoids found in our daily diet obtained from dark green leafy vegetables, orange and yellow fruits. Both are also known as natural anti-oxidants found in high amounts in the macular region of the retina of human eyes. They protect the eyes by filtering the harmful high energy blue wavelength light [177]. Both the compounds may be effective in eye disorders mainly due to their antioxidant activity. Many of the observational studies suggested that high dietary intake of lutein and zeaxanthin is associated with decreased risk of development of AMD, however, the results of the several studies were variable. Ma *et al*. (2012) conducted a meta-analysis of several observational studies and found that dietary intake of both the compound was not associated with reduced risk of AMD [178]. The primary analysis of the Age-Related Eye Disease Study 2 (AREDS2) randomized clinical trial suggested that the addition of lutein and zeaxanthin into the formulation did not lead to a reduction in the progression to advanced AMD [179]. However, secondary exploratory analyses showed a beneficial effect of lutein/zeaxanthin in reducing this risk and could be more appropriate as a supplement [179]. Also, Wang *et al*. (2014) observed a statistically significant beneficial effect of them in the improvement of macular pigment optical density (MPOD) [180]. The detailed study done by Murray *et al*. (2013) showed that supplementation of these compounds could increase the MPOD suggesting an improvement in progression from early to advanced AMD [181]. Liu *et al*. (2014) also suggested it to be a safe strategy where they studied the dose-response relationship of these compounds for visual acuity, contrast sensitivity and glare recovery time in AMD patients [182]. Functional and morphologic benefits were also reported by lutein/zeaxanthin supplementation in persons with early AMD [183]. Another study also reported that the addition of lutein/zeaxanthin along with other minerals and antioxidants in the diet of patients with low MPOD led to an increase in the MPOD scores [184]. Furthermore, higher intake of these dietary carotenoids is associated with reduced risk of AMD in the long run and hence the incorporation of these carotenoids in the diet may reduce the occurrence of AMD [185]. Eggersdorfer and Wyss reviewed several studies and suggested that the lutein may be implemented for the prevention of AMD [186]. The mechanism of lutein/zeaxanthin effects in the prevention of AMD is still under investigation. It is suggested that they trigger the anti-oxidant cascade and thus protects the macula and the photoreceptor retinal segments [187]. They also absorb the harmful blue light entering the eyes and thus protects the retina [188].

A study done on retinal pigment epithelial cells using ARPE-19 cells indicated that lutein/zeaxanthin could modulate inflammatory responses due to photooxidation. This may be due to the protection of proteasome from oxidative inactivation [189]. Tuzcu *et al.*, (2017) showed that lutein/zeaxanthin supplementation to rats fed with a high-fat diet was able to modulate genes involved in oxidative stress and inflammation in retina like NF-κB and Nrf2 signaling pathways which can prevent damage to the retina [190]. Thus, based on several clinical studies, supplementation of lutein/zeaxanthin may be considered as an alternative for the prevention of progression of AMD. Lutein may enhance glial cell survival after hypoxic injury, an *in vitro* study done on Muller cells, through regulating both apoptosis and autophagy which suggested it to be beneficial in many ocular disorders like glaucoma and DR [191]. An early hypothesis states that higher concentrations of these carotenoids in retina correlate with higher levels in the lens affecting the progression of cataract [192]. This hypothesis was supported by epidemiological studies where it was found that higher intake of lutein and zeaxanthin was associated with a 20% reduced risk of development of cataract [193, 194]. Another study reported a decreased risk of nuclear opacity by 50% in younger subjects who were having a high dietary intake of lutein [195] while other studies showed a 50% reduced rate of posterior subcapsular cataract [196]. A study performed on 3271 patients in Australia also reported a reduction in the incidence of nuclear cataract by 36%. However, posterior subcapsular and cortical cataract remains unaffected [197]. A large 10-year prospective study done in 35,551 patients indicated an 18% lower risk of cataract with a higher intake of carotenoids [198]. However, the study of 3115 patients revealed no statistical significance between the dietary intake of lutein and the development of cataracts [199]. Thus, further studies are warranted to confirm the beneficial role in the progress of cataractogenesis. Animal studies have suggested improvement in the retinal function mainly by inhibiting the pathways of oxidative stress [200, 201]. Lutein has also shown neuroprotective effects in the diabetic retina in some animal studies [200, 202]. Brazionis *et al.* (2009) reported a 66% reduced risk of DR in patients with higher concentrations of lutein/zeaxanthin and lycopene [203]. Another study was done with supplementation of these carotenoids also showed improved MPOD and visual acuity in non-proliferative DR patients [204]. Neelam *et al.* (2017) have reviewed several animal and human studies for the effect on DR and found the discrepancy between animal and human studies [205]. The discrepancy may be due to inappropriate models of DR in animals since the disease in humans is usually full-blown with detectable changes in the retina. Thus, a quality prospective study in patients of type II diabetes with DR is warranted to have confirmed results for the use of lutein/zeaxanthin.

Other Phytochemicals

Omega-3-fatty Acids

Omega-3-fatty acids are long-chain polyunsaturated fatty acids including eicosapentaenoic acid (EPA) and docosahexaenoic acid (DHA) which are majorly our dietary fatty acids with health benefits. Both fatty acids are mainly fish-derived omega-3 fatty acids which have been well associated with fetal development, neuronal, retinal, immune and cardiovascular functions, and Alzheimer's disease. Omega-3 fatty acids have been shown since long to have some clinical evidence in protecting the progression of AMD [206]. Hodge *et al.* (2007) reviewed a randomized clinical trial and prospective cohort study which reported effectiveness in slowing the progression of AMD [207]. Souied *et al.* (2015) conducted a systematic review of various studies done on omega-3 supplementation and showed an association of fish consumption or omega-3 fatty acids intakes from food with a lower risk of AMD progression [208]. However, a review conducted for the evidence of the preventive effect of omega-3 fatty acids in AMD showed no risk reduction or reduction in the progression of AMD in people taking omega-3 supplementation for five years [209]. Wu *et al.* (2017) conducted a prospective cohort study and found that higher intakes of EPA and DHA may have a potential to delay the development of intermediate AMD but no co-relation with advanced AMD [210].

The effect of dietary omega-3-fatty acids has also been evaluated on IOP in an animal model which has suggested it to be a modifiable factor for IOP control [211]. However, more studies are required to consider their role in the prevention or treatment of glaucoma. Cross-sectional studies have reported no beneficial effect of dietary omega-3- fatty acids on the slowing of progression of nuclear cataracts while one study reported it to be effective for cortical cataracts [212]. Lu *et al.* (2005) also reported a reduction in the risk of cataract development by omega-3-fatty acids [213]. A recent randomized clinical trial has shown that omega-3 dietary supplementation after cataract surgery has an additive effect on tear film indices of dry eye syndrome patients [214]. Hobbs and Bernstein (2014) have reported that supplementation of omega-3 fatty acids did not show any added benefit in AMD or cataract from their review [215]. Thus, the results of omega-3 supplementation are still under conflict for the prevention of cataract progression.

α-Lipoic Acid

α-Lipoic acid (ALA) is a potent antioxidant found in plants that scavenge free radicals, reduces inflammation and also known to slow the aging process. Humans are also capable of synthesizing ALA on their own in small amounts. It is also known as mitochondrial targeted anti-oxidant or mitochondrial nutrient [216]. A study done on APRE-19 cells suggests that ALA can protect the retinal cells against toxicity by acrolein exposure through its anti-oxidant mechanism [217]. This may help reduce the chronic oxidative induced retinal cell degeneration as in AMD. ALA supplementation has also been predicted to have possible preventive action in AMD as seen by an apparent increase in serum SOD activity in AMD patients [218]. Tao *et al.* (2016) studied the vision-related quality of life in patients with AMD supplemented with ALA. Their results supported the benefit of ALA treatment in patients with dry AMD [219]. However, high dose ALA may not be tolerable by elderly patients while 600 mg dose daily was well tolerated [220]. ALA supplementation, both prophylactic and therapeutic, in the DBA/2J mouse model of glaucoma showed significant increased antioxidant gene and protein expression and increased protection of retinal ganglionic cells thus demonstrating the use of dietary therapy for such chronic disorders [221]. Furthermore, ALA application to rabbit eyes after trabeculectomy was effective in preventing or reducing fibrosis and thus can also be implicated for delaying tissue regeneration after trabeculectomy [222]. The anti-oxidative property of ALA has been attributed to Nrf2 activation, NF-κB inhibition, and activation of 5' adenosine monophosphate-activated protein kinase (AMPK) [223].

The potential of ALA to be used in the prevention of cataract has been long back proposed from the study done using buthionine sulfoximine-induced cataract formation in newborn rats where it showed significant antioxidant activity [224]. This was additionally supported by Kilic *et al.* (1998) showing *in vitro* effect of ALA on glutathione concentrations in lens suggesting a role in the diabetic cataract [225]. Another study done in diabetic rats also showed inhibited cataract development by ALA injection through reduced aldose reductase activity and increased glutathione levels in the lens [226]. ALA oral ingestion has shown it to be effective in inhibiting diabetic cataractogenesis [227, 228]. Chen *et al.* (2010) showed for the first time that ALA was able to inhibit the post-translational modifications induced by naphthalene induced lens opacity [229]. ALA was also proposed to protect the lens from H2O2 induced cataract by inhibiting epithelial cell apoptosis and anti-oxidative activity [230]. However, it was not found to be very effective against diabetic cataract induced by streptozotocin in Balb/c mice [231]. A randomized double-blind placebo-controlled trial was done to evaluate the efficacy of the ALA in the prevention of diabetic macular edema but was not found to be effective [232].

ALA is also been evaluated in DR in animals. ALA supplementation in streptozotocin-induced diabetic rats revealed beneficial effects on the development of DR by inhibition of accumulation of oxidized DNA and nitrotyrosine in retinal cells [233]. ALA supplementation has also been investigated on late-phase supernormal retinal oxygenation response in experimental DR where it was found beneficial due to its anti-oxidative capacity [234]. Different formulations of ALA were also tried for non-oral administration in streptozotocin-induced diabetic rats and found that even intra-vitreal or intraperitoneal administration was effective in reducing microvascular complications like retinopathy [235].

Coenzyme Q10

Coenzyme Q10 (CoQ10), a well-known ubiquitous enzyme observed in the biological system, is also referred to as ubidecarenone, ubiquinone and vitamin Q10. It is obtained by the conjugation of the benzoquinone ring with the isoprenoid chain variable in lengths. CoQ10 has a property of scavenging free radicals and protects against lipid peroxidation of phospholipids and membrane protein by regeneration of α-tocopherol. Thus, it has anti-oxidant properties. It is located in the inner membrane of the mitochondria, involved in the transmission of the electron from dehydrogenases bounded to the membrane to complex III of the electron transport chain [236].

Blasi *et al.* (2001) studied the concept of opposing oxidative stress in patients with AMD and found the pathogenetic role of free radicals in AMD using coenzyme Q10 [237]. As age advances, the retinal levels of CoQ10 also reduce by about 40%. This reduction may lead to a decrease in the anti-oxidative ability of retina and a decrease in the rate of ATP synthesis in the retina which gradually associated with macular degeneration [238]. CoQ10 is believed to be beneficial in several retinal disorders by inhibiting the production of reactive oxygen species and thus protection against oxidative stress. CoQ10 can improve the visual function in AMD patients, enhancement of visual cortical response in glaucoma patients, preventing oxidative stress in DR as well as retinitis pigmentosa [239].

Kernt *et al.* (2010) investigated the role of CoQ10 in human lens epithelial cells which were exposed to white light leading to increased apoptosis, intracellular ROS and BAX expression and reduced BCL-2 expression [240]. These changes were significantly reduced when the cells were pre-incubated with CoQ10 which suggests that it may help prevent cataract formation *in vivo* [240]. More recently, CoQ10 encapsulated into liposomes were studied for its preventive effect on selenite induced cataract in rat pups. It was concluded that CoQ10 alone, as well as liposomal CoQ10, were effective in reducing the progression of cataract by improving the soluble protein levels as well as antioxidant status [241]. Furthermore, it was also found in a recent prospective, randomized clinical study that pseudo-exfoliative glaucoma patients pre-treated with CoQ10 and vitamin E eye drop 1 month before cataract surgery were having significantly lower SOD levels as compared to the patients not receiving drops [242].

A study was carried out in diabetic patients to understand the relation between proliferative DR and plasma CoQ10 levels. It suggested that high levels of plasma ubiquinol-10/ubiquinone-10 ratio indicating a protective effect on DR [243]. Domanico *et al.* (2015) showed a reduction in ROS in non-proliferative DR due to the antioxidant formulation containing pycnogenol, vitamin E and coenzyme Q10 [244]. Another, randomized, double-blind, phase IIa, placebo-controlled, clinical trial in patients with non-proliferative DR wherein coenzyme Q10 and combined antioxidant therapy was given for 6 months, also showed improvement in the oxidative stress in DR patients [245].

Citicoline

Citicoline is also referred to as cytidine 5′-diphosphocholine (CDP-choline) is found endogenously for the synthesis of important phospholipid for the cell membrane. Citicoline tends to stabilize cell membranes and decreases the level of free radicals thus it has been proposed to use it in various brain diseases like vascular dementia, stroke, Parkinson and brain aging [246].

The beneficial effect of citicoline on retinal function and cortical responses in patients with glaucoma was studied in a randomized clinical trial consisting of forty patients with open-angle glaucoma. It was found that citicoline may induce improvement in the retinal and visual pathway functions in glaucoma patients [247]. Similar responses were also observed when citicoline was given orally to glaucoma patients [248]. Another study was carried to confirm the neuroprotective effect of citicoline in glaucoma patients wherein the treatment period was extended up to 8 years. This study reflected the stabilization in the improvement of the visual function in glaucomatous eyes [249]. Frolov *et al.* (2011) also studied the effect of parenteral citicoline on the visual functions and life quality of primary open-angle glaucoma patients. The study was conducted on 40 patients with normalized intraocular pressure and divided equally into the experimental and control group [250]. All the patients were given intravenous citicoline for 10 days wherein it was found that it had a significant neuroprotective effect by preventing apoptosis [250]. Another study carried out for 2 years in patients supplemented with oral citicoline also showed a similar beneficial effect in slowing the progression of glaucoma in patients [251]. Parisi *et al.* (2015) studied topical citicoline in open-angle glaucoma patients and found improvement in the bioelectrical activity of the visual cortex [252]. All these studied indicated a beneficial effect of citicoline in glaucoma patients and thus could be considered as a molecule to be developed for the treatment of glaucoma patients.

Pycnogenol

Pycnogenol extracted from French maritime pine (*Pinus pinaster Ait*), is a standardized flavonoid [253]. It is being used as a nutritional supplement as well as a phytochemical constituent for the treatment of various diseases stretching from circulatory disorders to chronic inflammation. Pycnogenol, also has other beneficial applications as anti-oxidant, modulation of gene expression, reducing enzyme activity as well as free radical scavenging activity [254].

The effect of pycnogenol was investigated in a total of 40 patients with diabetes, atherosclerosis and other vascular diseases involving the retina. The study demonstrated the beneficial effect of pycnogenol on the progression of retinopathy. Significant recovery of visual acuity and improvement of retinal vascularization were observed in treated patients suggesting that it may be beneficial in reducing the progression of DR. The proposed mechanism was suggested to be free radical scavenging, anti-inflammatory and capillary protective activities [255]. Schönlau and Rohdewal (2001) reviewed five clinical trials of pycnogenol used for the treatment and prevention of retinopathy [256]. It was found that pycnogenol was able to improve capillary resistance and reduce leakages into the retina indicating beneficial effect in DR [256]. A study done in streptozotocin-induced diabetic rats with a low carbohydrate diet found that pycnogenol could be an effective antioxidative therapy that can reduce the risk of cataract and DR [257]. It was also observed that supplementation of pycnogenol in the early stages of retinopathy could increase retinal blood circulation leading to a reduction in edema and thus an improvement in the vision of the patients [258]. Trevithick *et al.* (2013) studied pycnogenol both *in vitro* incubated lenses and in streptozotocin-induced diabetic rats *in vivo* [259]. They concluded that pycnogenol was having a cataractogenic effect *in vitro* however; it was showing a marginally protective effect *in vivo* and was able to reduce glycation of proteins [259].

Trans-anethole

Foeniculum vulgare is a medicinal plant and has diuretic, antipyretic and antioxidant properties [260]. Trans-anethole, estragole, limonene, and fenchone are the major component of the essential oil of *Foeniculum vulgare* [261]. Trans-anethole is non-toxic in nature and used as a flavoring agent in food. It also has great potential to control the secondary complications in diabetes mellitus. Improvement in blood glucose, lipid profile, glycated hemoglobin and other parameters observed by prolonged treatment with *F. vulgare* distillate in streptozotocin-induced diabetic rats [262]. Trans-anethole can prevent cataract formation by increasing soluble lens protein, reducing glutathione, catalase, and

SOD [263].

Caffeine

Caffeine is an alkaloid and abundantly present in coffee [263]. Caffeine solution is very stable and resistant to photodynamic degradation. Therefore, it has been tested for the prevention of cataract formation induced by UV radiation protection. Kronschläger *et al.* (2014) demonstrated that caffeine eye drops with 0.9% hydroxypropylmethylcellulose showed a protective effect against cataracts induced by exposure of UV-B-type radiation in rats (263). Similarly, Varma *et al.* (2016) showed that caffeine has a protective effect against cataract formation induced by UV exposure both *in vitro* and *in vivo* [264]. Zhang *et al.* (2017) demonstrated that caffeine protects against oxygen-induced retinopathy (OIR) in mice without interfering with normal retinal vascularization development [265]. Varma SD (2016) demonstrated that cataract blindness incidence was significantly lowered in higher coffee intake groups as compared to lower coffee intake groups [264].

Squalamine

Squalamine is an aminosterol and generally extracted from the cartilage of the dogfish shark. It has anti-angiogenic properties and lower systemic toxicity [266]. Higgins *et al.* (2000) showed the antiangiogenic effect of squalamine in the mouse model of retinopathy of prematurity [266]. They significantly inhibited retinal neovascularization in this model through intra-peritoneal injection at a daily dose of 40 mg/kg squalamine. Besides, Ciulla *et al.* (2003) demonstrate that systemic administration of squalamine lactate partially reduced choroidal neovascular membrane development in the rat model, which was induced by laser trauma [267]. Similarly, systemically injected squalamine inhibited iris neovasculari-zation and partially regressed new vessels in the primate model, but intravitreally injected squalamine did not affect neovascularization [268]. Wroblewski *et al.* (2016) done a study in patients with retinal vein occlusion related macular edema (ME), topical squalamine in combination with ranibizumab enhanced visual recovery as compared to ranibizumab alone [269]. Combination therapy of ranibizumab and squalamine appeared safe and well-tolerated.

Chitosan

The ocular mucosal surface is negatively charged due to the existence of sialic acid in the mucin layer, which led to the consideration of positively charged adhering polymers to the cornea's surface [270]. Thus, a cationic polymer can deliver drugs to the cornea through adhering to it. Chitosan is a suitable candidate for this use due to its bioavailability and mucoadhesive character [271]. It is obtained by the deacetylation of chitin, which is generally present in the exoskeleton of crustaceans [272]. The protonated amine group of chitosan allows it to interact with negative charges of cornea and conjunctiva surface. Thus, chitosan plays an excellent role in ocular drug delivery [271]. In a recent study, a novel insulin delivery system was developed for DR *via* loading insulin onto chitosan nanoparticles /poly (lactic-co-glycolic acid)-poly (ethylene glycol)-poly (lactic-co-glycolic acid) hydrogel (ICNPH) [273]. This study suggests that ICNPH facilitates controlled insulin delivery and has a neuroprotective effect on the retina by sub-conjunctival injection in diabetic retinopathic rats. It might be useful therapeutic strategies for the treatment of DR shortly.

Saffron

Saffron is one type of spice and normally used in traditional medicine. Dietary supplementation of saffron may show a protective effect against cell death through the maintenance of the GSH levels [274]. In rats, the supplementation of saffron showed the effects of continuous bright light exposure were significantly diminished [275]. Whereas, in human clinical trials of early AMD patients, saffron supplementation (20mg/day for 90 days) showed a significant enhancement of some macular photopic flash electroretinogram (fERG) parameters, such as amplitude and modulation threshold [276]. Some preclinical studies showed that saffron displays neuroprotective properties, and previous studies on rats provide evidence for the inhibition of cell death when they exposed to intense light [275]. The results of clinical trials specified that saffron supplementation may induce a short-term improvement in retinal function in early AMD patients. Also, saffron has been shown to prevent the development of selenite-induced cataract in Wistar rats by proteolytic inhibition of the lens's water-soluble protein fractions [277]. Although the studies do not conclusively demonstrate the neuroprotective effect of saffron in AMD and prevention of cataracts, this data seems promising for therapeutic uses of dietary supplements against the ocular diseases.

Atropine

Atropine is naturally occurring alkaloid and commonly found in *Atropa belladonna*. Atropine is used in the eye drops and can induce mydriasis through blocking the contraction of the circular pupillary sphincter muscle and by permitting the radial pupillary dilator muscle to contract ultimately leading to dilation of the pupil. Atropine also induces cycloplegia through paralyzing the ciliary muscles, which is responsible for the accommodation to allow accurate refraction in children, helps to treat ciliary block (malignant) glaucoma and relaxation in iridocyclitis pain associated with iridocyclitis [278].

NATURAL COMPOUNDS AS A VISCOELASTIC SUBSTANCE

Viscoelastic substances provide numerous advantages to the ophthalmic surgeon such as maintenance of tissue planes, gentle creation of surgical spaces and protection of tissues against intracellular trauma. There are several criteria of viscoelastic substance for their use in ophthalmology. They must be sterile, nontoxic and non-immunogenic in nature, should not affect the normal metabolism of cells [279]. Currently, three viscoelastic substances are in clinical use: Hyaluronic acid or sodium hyaluronate (SH), hydroxypropyl methyl-cellulose (HPMC) and chondroitin sulfate (CS) [280 - 282].

Hyaluronic Acid

Hyaluronic acid is a natural unbranched glycosaminoglycan containing repeated units of N-acetyl-D-glucosamine and D-glucuronic acid with distinct physicochemical properties, which is important for their applicability as a lubricating or viscoelastic and shock absorbing fluid tool in ophthalmological surgery constitutes the main ingredient in artificial tear formulation for the relief of dry eye [283, 284]. It is commonly used in several ophthalmological surgeries such as trabeculectomy, cataract removal, refractive surgery, and corneal plastic surgery [283]. The elasticity of hyaluronic acid can be strengthened by increasing its molecular weight and it is responsible for the protection of ocular cells from damage, which is caused by contact with surgical instruments and implants. For clinical use, exogenous hyaluronic acid formulations are derived from rooster combs or by fermentation of streptococcal cultures [284]. High molecular mass containing hyaluronic acid acts as a good barrier to the inflammatory process, defends against the effects of free radicals and reduces chemotaxis of inflammatory cells [285, 286]. Van Beek *et al.* (2008) discovered that hyaluronic acid may be used in silicone hydrogel contact lenses without affecting its optical properties and its gradual release from the lens prevents protein layer formation on the contact lens [287].

Hydroxypropyl Methylcellulose

Since 1976, methylcellulose is used to avoid damage to corneal endothelium during implantation of intraocular lenses. Once, a drop of 1% methylcellulose solution placed on the artificial lens than the anterior chamber filled with 2% methylcellulose solution before implantation [288]. In this manner, it is possible to keep a space between the cornea and iris, even if vitreous pressure is present and to operate without any kind of risk to the corneal endothelium [288]. It is also widely used as a food additive. It contains long chains of glucose molecules through replacement of hydrogen of the hydroxyl group by methoxy (up to 29%) and hydroxypropyl (up to 8.5%) side chains, which is responsible for its high hydrophilicity over the methylcellulose. Methylcellulose is widely distributed in nature (in wood and cotton), whereas hydroxypropyl methylcellulose synthesized from methylcellulose by various chemical industries. It has been reported to be a safe and effective viscoelastic compound in human cataract surgery by several investigators [279, 281, 288].

Chondroitin Sulfate

Chondroitin sulfate is commonly present in the extracellular matrix of animals. It is the main constituent of connective tissue such as cartilage. Within the ocular tissue, it is present widely in the cornea at high concentration. It is a sulfated glycosaminoglycan (GAG), which is generally present in the form of proteoglycans and at least one side chain covalently attached to the core protein [289]. For medicinal use, chondroitin sulfate is isolated from shark fin cartilage. Viscoat® is a combination of 3% sodium hyaluronate and 4% chondroitin sulfate and contains typical dispersive properties [290].

Clinical and Preclinical Trials of Natural Compounds

Although several natural compounds in a crude form are in use today for the prevention and treatment of various ocular diseases, few isolated natural compounds have reached the preclinical stage and clinical stages of evaluation. Natural compounds such as curcumin, resveratrol, caffeine, saffron, folic acid, α-tocopherol, carnitine, lutein, zeaxanthin, coenzyme Q10, citicoline, and squalamine have been tested in clinical trials. Table **2** provides a list of natural compounds that are in various preclinical and clinical stages.

Table 2. Natural compounds in clinical and preclinical trials against ocular diseases.

Natural compounds	Preclinical	Clinical
Curcumin	Cataract [21, 22]; DR [23]; Conjunctivitis [24]; Glaucoma [25]; Chronic anterior uveitis [26]	Chronic anterior uveitis [26]
Quercetin	Dry eye [291]	-
Catechin	Dry eye [28]; cataract [29]	-
Resveratrol	DR [32]	AMD [292]
Acetyl-11-keto-b-boswellic acid	DR [36]	-
Pycnogenol	Conjunctivitis [293]	-
Caffeine	Diabetic cataract [39]	Cataract blindness [264]
Saffron	Cataract [277]	AMD [294]

(Table 2) cont.....

Natural compounds	Preclinical	Clinical
Folic acid	Cataract [14]	Cataract [295]
α-tocopherol	Glaucoma [116]	AMD [110], cataract [122]
Methylcobalamin	-	Cataract [295] Glaucoma [130]
L-glutathione	-	Glaucoma [138, 139]
Carnitine	Cataract [157]	AMD [151]
Lutein and zeaxanthin	IOP [211]	Cataract [197], DR [203]
α-lipoic acid	Glaucoma [221]; DR [233]	-
Coenzyme Q10	Cataract [240]	AMD [239]; Glaucoma [239] DR [245]
Citicoline	Glaucoma [296]	Glaucoma [247, 252]
Squalamine	Retinopathy [266]	ME [269]

Ocular Barriers

The eye is provided with three barriers. These are corneal epithelial barrier (CEB), blood-aqueous barrier (BAB) and blood-retinal barriers (BRB) (Fig. **3**). These ocular drug barriers pose a major challenge to the delivery of therapeutics agents inside the eye and have limited use of many proposed drugs including phytochemicals for the treatment of ocular diseases. The cornea is an avascular transparent structure with multilayered epithelium towards its external surface [297]. This corneal epithelial layer provides the main barrier against the topically administered drugs to the eye such as eye drops, gels, and emulsions used for the treatment of anterior segment-related diseases [297, 298]. Tight junctions between the cells of corneal epithelium prevent the permeation of hydrophilic drugs, whereas hydrophobic drugs are comparatively highly permeable [298]. The BAB is composed of endothelial cells of blood vessels in the iris and the non-pigmented cell layer of the ciliary epithelium, posterior iridial epithelium, and endothelium of the iridial blood vessels [299]. Inflammation conditions in the anterior chamber of the eye can disrupt the function of this barrier [300]. BRB is located at the posterior portion of the eye and is composed of retinal pigment epithelial (RPE) cells and it regulates the movement of solutes and nutrients from the choroid to the sub-retinal space. The diffusion of drugs across BRB is based on their lipid solubility. The entry of drugs from the paracellular route is restricted by BRB and BAB because both contain epithelium and endothelium with tight junctions [298].

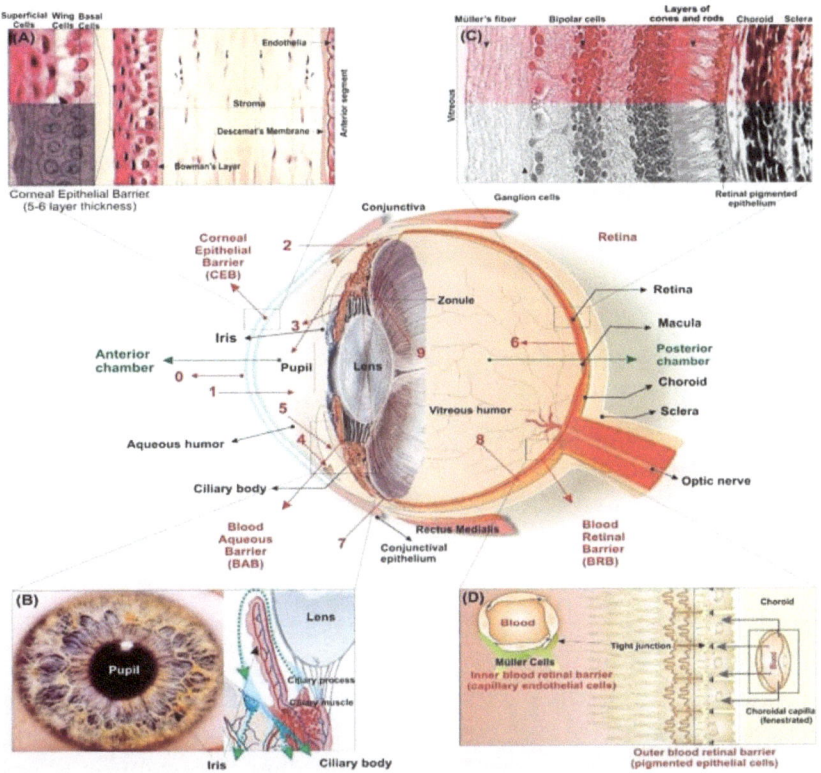

Fig. (3). Ocular barriers. The eye has a corneal epithelial barrier (CEB, A), the blood-aqueous barrier (BAB, B), the biostructures of the retina (C), and the blood-retinal barriers (BRB, D). Several static and dynamic barriers in the eye affect the movement of the drug and its metabolites in the eye. Tear film can modulate topically administered drugs (0). The cornea does not allow any topically administered drugs to directly reach the interior of the eye (1). The conjunctiva and sclera provide excess to hydrophilic drugs (2). Systemically administered drugs reach the eye through iris blood vessels into the anterior chamber (3). Aqueous blood flow can regulate the concentration of drug into the aqueous humor (4). The drug which has reached eye can be removed from the eye by BAB (5). Most of the systemically administered drugs enter the eye through the BRBs which is composed of retinal pigment epithelial (RPE) and the retinal capillary endothelium (RCE) (6). Drugs can be directly injected into the vitreous chamber (7) and can be removed from here by BRB (8). Drugs reaching vitreous humor can be diffused to the anterior chamber (9). Reproduced with permission from Brar *et al.*, 2016 [297].

FUTURE PROSPECTS

Nature has provided us with thousands of molecules with different biological properties and hence can be utilized as a medicine for the treatment of various ailments including ocular diseases. Several herbal and other nature-based medicines are used worldwide for the treatment of ocular diseases, however, the only fraction of them is studied utilizing scientific methods. Several researchers have focused their studies on identifying the natural compounds for the prevention and treatment of ocular diseases. These have led to an exponential increase in the number of natural compounds that can be implemented for the treatment of ocular diseases. However, exact molecular/cellular targets and underlying mechanisms of action remain to be studied. For those natural compounds, even if the targets are identified, studies at the level of preclinical and clinical trials are lacking and hence the thorough scientific support is negligible. Several herbal or nature-based medicines have several active compounds and they can interact with multiple targets and can elicit varied molecular, cellular and physiological effects. To identify the exact molecular targets, modern approaches including the use of bioinformatics tools and omics-based studies should be utilized. Consideration of different responsive studies such as expressional change of genes, proteins, microRNA and other metabolites may effectively generate strong hypothesis or predict specific pharmacological activity for the utilization of natural compounds for the prevention of ocular disease. Recent discoveries in the improvement of drug delivery may also be implicated to optimize the pharmacokinetics of natural compounds to achieve greater efficacy with fewer side effects.

CONCLUSION

Various natural compounds are used for the treatment of various ocular disorders from ancient times. Major ocular disorders, such as AMD, glaucoma, cataract and DR are associated with oxidative stress, inflammation, abnormal protein folding and response, secretion of various cytokines, abnormal proliferation, migration and differentiation of cells, abnormal level of nutrients or pro-nutrients, and cell death. Amongst them, oxidative stress and resultant abnormal behavior of cells can be targeted by several natural compounds. The certain specific characteristic of natural compounds to modulate particular cellular processes and cell signaling events have found its use in the treatment of various ocular disorders. However, poor solubility, stability in the alimentary canal and body fluids and bioavailability is a major concern. The invention of new technologies in drug delivery particularly the targeted drug therapy, nano-formulations, and liposomes. can be utilized to take care of the above-listed concerns. Natural compounds are also required for the formation and maintenance of the visual pigments. Certain natural compounds have a very specific use in ophthalmology such as atropine as iris diluent. Highly viscous natural compounds or derivatives of natural compounds such as sodium hyaluronate, chondroitin sulfate, methylcellulose is used as a visco-elastic device during ophthalmic surgery. The known use of the natural compounds is only for the fractions ocular disorders and there is an immense possibility to utilize the natural compounds for the treatment of several other ocular disorders and abnormalities. Several new natural compounds are identified from newly discovered species and their application in the field of ophthalmology remains to be evaluated.

CONSENT FOR PUBLICATION

Not applicable.

CONFLICT OF INTEREST

The author confirms that this chapter contents have no conflict of interest.

ACKNOWLEDGEMENT

Declared none.

REFERENCES

[1]   Farnsworth NR, Akerele O, Bingel AS, Soejarto DD, Guo Z. Medicinal plants in therapy. Bull World Health Organ 1985; 63(6): 965-81.
[PMID: 3879679]

[2]   Khoo HE, Ng HS, Yap W-S, Goh HJH, Yim HS. Nutrients for prevention of macular degeneration and eye-related diseases. Antioxidants 2019; 8(4): 85.
[http://dx.doi.org/10.3390/antiox8040085] [PMID: 30986936]

[3]   Huynh T-P, Mann SN, Mandal NA. Botanical compounds: effects on major eye diseases. Evid Based Complement Alternat Med 2013; 2013549174
[http://dx.doi.org/10.1155/2013/549174] [PMID: 23843879]

[4]   Elshout M, Webers CA, van der Reis MI, de Jong-Hesse Y, Schouten JS. Tracing the natural course of visual acuity and quality of life in neovascular age-related macular degeneration: a systematic review and quality of life study. BMC Ophthalmol 2017; 17(1): 120.
[http://dx.doi.org/10.1186/s12886-017-0514-3] [PMID: 28693519]

[5]   Zhao B, Wang M, Xu J, Li M, Yu Y. Identification of pathogenic genes and upstream regulators in age-related macular degeneration. BMC Ophthalmol 2017; 17(1): 102.
[http://dx.doi.org/10.1186/s12886-017-0498-z] [PMID: 28651595]

[6]   Lim LS, Mitchell P, Seddon JM, Holz FG, Wong TY. Age-related macular degeneration. Lancet 2012; 379(9827): 1728-38.
[http://dx.doi.org/10.1016/S0140-6736(12)60282-7] [PMID: 22559899]

[7]   Moore NA, Bracha P, Hussain RM, Morral N, Ciulla TA. Gene therapy for age-related macular degeneration. Expert Opin Biol Ther 2017; 17(10): 1235-44.
[http://dx.doi.org/10.1080/14712598.2017.1356817] [PMID: 28726562]

[8]   Carneiro Â, Andrade JP. Nutritional and Lifestyle interventions for age-related macular degeneration: A Review. Oxid Med Cell Longev 2017; 2017: 1-13.

[9]   Chiu C-J, Chang M-L, Li T, Gensler G, Taylor A. Visualization of dietary patterns and their associations with age-related macular degeneration. Invest Ophthalmol Vis Sci 2017; 58(3): 1404-10.
[http://dx.doi.org/10.1167/iovs.16-20454] [PMID: 28253403]

[10]   Pinazo-Duran MD, Shoaie-Nia K, Zanon-Moreno V, Sanz-Gonzalez SM, Del Castillo JB, Garcia-Medina JJ. Strategies to reduce oxidative stress in glaucoma patients. curr neuropharmacol 2018; 16: 903-18.

[11]   Bussel II, Aref AA. Dietary factors and the risk of glaucoma: a review. Ther Adv Chronic Dis 2014; 5(4): 188-94.
[http://dx.doi.org/10.1177/2040622314530181] [PMID: 24982753]

[12]   Almasieh M, Levin LA. Neuroprotection in glaucoma: animal models and clinical trials. Annu Rev

Vis Sci 2017; 3: 91-120.
[http://dx.doi.org/10.1146/annurev-vision-102016-061422] [PMID: 28731838]

[13] Zhu X, Zhang S, Chang R, Lu Y. New cataract markers: Mechanisms of disease. Clin Chim Acta 2017; 472: 41-5.
[http://dx.doi.org/10.1016/j.cca.2017.07.010] [PMID: 28705775]

[14] Gupta VB, Rajagopala M, Ravishankar B. Etiopathogenesis of cataract: an appraisal. Indian J Ophthalmol 2014; 62(2): 103-10.
[http://dx.doi.org/10.4103/0301-4738.121141] [PMID: 24618482]

[15] Kupfer C. Bowman lecture. The conquest of cataract: a global challenge. Trans Ophthalmol Soc U K 1985; 104(Pt 1): 1-10.
[PMID: 3855332]

[16] Yonova-Doing E, Forkin ZA, Hysi PG, *et al.* Genetic and dietary factors influencing the progression of nuclear cataract. Ophthalmology 2016; 123(6): 1237-44.
[http://dx.doi.org/10.1016/j.ophtha.2016.01.036] [PMID: 27016950]

[17] Zhao L-Q, Li L-M, Zhu H, The Epidemiological Evidence-Based Eye Disease Study Research Group EY. The effect of multivitamin/mineral supplements on age-related cataracts: a systematic review and meta-analysis. Nutrients 2014; 6(3): 931-49.
[http://dx.doi.org/10.3390/nu6030931] [PMID: 24590236]

[18] Eshaq RS, Aldalati AMZ, Alexander JS, Harris NR. Diabetic retinopathy: Breaking the barrier. Pathophysiology 2017; 24(4): 229-41.
[http://dx.doi.org/10.1016/j.pathophys.2017.07.001] [PMID: 28732591]

[19] Duh EJ, Sun JK, Stitt AW. Diabetic retinopathy: current understanding, mechanisms, and treatment strategies. JCI Insight 2017; 2(14): 93751.
[http://dx.doi.org/10.1172/jci.insight.93751] [PMID: 28724805]

[20] Radomska-Leśniewska DM, Osiecka-Iwan A, Hyc A, Góźdź A, Dąbrowska AM, Skopiński P. Therapeutic potential of curcumin in eye diseases. Cent Eur J Immunol 2019; 44(2): 181-9.
[http://dx.doi.org/10.5114/ceji.2019.87070] [PMID: 31530988]

[21] Manikandan R, Thiagarajan R, Beulaja S, Sudhandiran G, Arumugam M. Effect of curcumin on selenite-induced cataractogenesis in Wistar rat pups. Curr Eye Res 2010; 35(2): 122-9.
[http://dx.doi.org/10.3109/02713680903447884] [PMID: 20136422]

[22] Raju TN, Kumar CS, Kanth VR, *et al.* Cumulative antioxidant defense against oxidative challenge in galactose-induced cataractogenesis in Wistar rats. Indian J Exp Biol 2006; 44(9): 733-9.
[PMID: 16999028]

[23] Gupta SK, Kumar B, Nag TC, *et al.* Curcumin prevents experimental diabetic retinopathy in rats through its hypoglycemic, antioxidant, and anti-inflammatory mechanisms. J Ocul Pharmacol Ther 2011; 27(2): 123-30.
[http://dx.doi.org/10.1089/jop.2010.0123] [PMID: 21314438]

[24] Chung S-H, Choi SH, Choi JA, Chuck RS, Joo C-K. Curcumin suppresses ovalbumin-induced allergic conjunctivitis. Mol Vis 2012; 18: 1966-72.
[PMID: 22876123]

[25] Davis BM, Pahlitzsch M, Guo L, *et al.* Topical curcumin nanocarriers are neuroprotective in eye disease. Sci Rep 2018; 8(1): 11066.
[http://dx.doi.org/10.1038/s41598-018-29393-8] [PMID: 30038334]

[26] Allegri P, Mastromarino A, Neri P. Management of chronic anterior uveitis relapses: efficacy of oral phospholipidic curcumin treatment. Long-term follow-up. Clin Ophthalmol 2010; 4: 1201-6.
[PMID: 21060672]

[27] Sutherland BA, Rahman RM, Appleton I. Mechanisms of action of green tea catechins, with a focus on ischemia-induced neurodegeneration. J Nutr Biochem 2006; 17(5): 291-306.

[http://dx.doi.org/10.1016/j.jnutbio.2005.10.005] [PMID: 16443357]

[28]　Lee H, Shim W, Kim CE, Choi SY, Lee H, Yang J. Therapeutic efficacy of nanocomplex of poly(ethylene glycol) and catechin for dry eye disease in a mouse model. Invest Ophthalmol Vis Sci 2017; 58(3): 1682-91.
[http://dx.doi.org/10.1167/iovs.16-20843] [PMID: 28319642]

[29]　Ergen I, Turgut B, Ilhan N. Comparison of the impact of epigallocatechin gallate and ellagic acid in an experimental cataract model induced by sodium selenite. Int J Ophthalmol 2017; 10(4): 499-506.
[PMID: 28503419]

[30]　Chen X, Han R, Hao P, *et al.* Nepetin inhibits IL-1β induced inflammation *via* NF-κB and MAPKs signaling pathways in ARPE-19 cells. Biomed Pharmacother 2018; 101: 87-93.
[http://dx.doi.org/10.1016/j.biopha.2018.02.054] [PMID: 29477475]

[31]　Li D, Liu N, Zhao HH, *et al.* Interactions between Sirt1 and MAPKs regulate astrocyte activation induced by brain injury *in vitro* and *in vivo*. J Neuroinflammation 2017; 14(1): 67.
[http://dx.doi.org/10.1186/s12974-017-0841-6] [PMID: 28356158]

[32]　Soufi FG, Mohammad-Nejad D, Ahmadieh H. Resveratrol improves diabetic retinopathy possibly through oxidative stress - nuclear factor κB - apoptosis pathway. Pharmacol Rep 2012; 64(6): 1505-14.
[http://dx.doi.org/10.1016/S1734-1140(12)70948-9] [PMID: 23406761]

[33]　Richer S, Stiles W, Ulanski L, Carroll D, Podella C. Observation of human retinal remodeling in octogenarians with a resveratrol based nutritional supplement. Nutrients 2013; 5(6): 1989-2005.
[http://dx.doi.org/10.3390/nu5061989] [PMID: 23736827]

[34]　Popescu M, Bogdan C, Pintea A, Rugină D, Ionescu C. Antiangiogenic cytokines as potential new therapeutic targets for resveratrol in diabetic retinopathy. Drug Des Devel Ther 2018; 12: 1985-96.
[http://dx.doi.org/10.2147/DDDT.S156941] [PMID: 30013318]

[35]　Chang CC, Duann YF, Yen TL, *et al.* Andrographolide, a Novel NF-κB Inhibitor, Inhibits Vascular Smooth Muscle Cell Proliferation and Cerebral Endothelial Cell Inflammation. Acta Cardiol Sin 2014; 30(4): 308-15.
[PMID: 27122804]

[36]　Kumar M, Dhatwalia SK, Dhawan DK. Role of angiogenic factors of herbal origin in regulation of molecular pathways that control tumor angiogenesis. Tumour Biol 2016; 37(11): 14341-54.
[http://dx.doi.org/10.1007/s13277-016-5330-5] [PMID: 27614685]

[37]　Rossino MG, Casini G. Nutraceuticals for the treatment of diabetic retinopathy. Nutrients 2019; 11(4): 771.
[http://dx.doi.org/10.3390/nu11040771] [PMID: 30987058]

[38]　Dongare V, Kulkarni C, Kondawar M, Magdum C, Haldavnekar V, Arvindekar A. Inhibition of aldose reductase and anti-cataract action of trans-anethole isolated from *Foeniculum vulgare* Mill. fruits. Food Chem 2012; 132(1): 385-90.
[http://dx.doi.org/10.1016/j.foodchem.2011.11.005] [PMID: 26434305]

[39]　Varma SD, Kovtun S, Hegde K. Effectiveness of topical caffeine in cataract prevention: studies with galactose cataract. Mol Vis 2010; 16: 2626-33.
[PMID: 21179241]

[40]　Hewlings SJ, Kalman DS. Curcumin: A review of its' effects on human health. Foods 2017; 6(10)E92
[http://dx.doi.org/10.3390/foods6100092] [PMID: 29065496]

[41]　Fadus MC, Lau C, Bikhchandani J, Lynch HT. Curcumin: An age-old anti-inflammatory and anti-neoplastic agent. J Tradit Complement Med 2016; 7(3): 339-46.
[http://dx.doi.org/10.1016/j.jtcme.2016.08.002] [PMID: 28725630]

[42]　Din FU, Aman W, Ullah I, *et al.* Effective use of nanocarriers as drug delivery systems for the treatment of selected tumors. Int J Nanomedicine 2017; 12: 7291-309.
[http://dx.doi.org/10.2147/IJN.S146315] [PMID: 29042776]

[43] Menon VP, Sudheer AR. Antioxidant and anti-inflammatory properties of curcumin. Adv Exp Med Biol 2007; 595: 105-25.
[http://dx.doi.org/10.1007/978-0-387-46401-5_3] [PMID: 17569207]

[44] Momtazi AA, Derosa G, Maffioli P, Banach M, Sahebkar A. Role of microRNAs in the therapeutic effects of curcumin in non-cancer diseases. Mol Diagn Ther 2016; 20(4): 335-45.
[http://dx.doi.org/10.1007/s40291-016-0202-7] [PMID: 27241179]

[45] Goel A, Kunnumakkara AB, Aggarwal BB. Curcumin as "Curecumin": from kitchen to clinic. Biochem Pharmacol 2008; 75(4): 787-809.
[http://dx.doi.org/10.1016/j.bcp.2007.08.016] [PMID: 17900536]

[46] Abe Y, Hashimoto S, Horie T. Curcumin inhibition of inflammatory cytokine production by human peripheral blood monocytes and alveolar macrophages. Pharmacol Res 1999; 39(1): 41-7.
[http://dx.doi.org/10.1006/phrs.1998.0404] [PMID: 10051376]

[47] Liu X-F, Hao J-L, Xie T, et al. Curcumin, a potential therapeutic candidate for anterior segment eye diseases: a review. Front Pharmacol 2017; 8: 66.
[http://dx.doi.org/10.3389/fphar.2017.00066] [PMID: 28261099]

[48] Lal B, Kapoor AK, Asthana OP, et al. Efficacy of curcumin in the management of chronic anterior uveitis. Phytother Res 1999; 13(4): 318-22.
[http://dx.doi.org/10.1002/(SICI)1099-1573(199906)13:4<318::AID-PTR445>3.0.CO;2-7]   [PMID: 10404539]

[49] Mandal MNA, Patlolla JMR, Zheng L, et al. Curcumin protects retinal cells from light-and oxidant stress-induced cell death. Free Radic Biol Med 2009; 46(5): 672-9.
[http://dx.doi.org/10.1016/j.freeradbiomed.2008.12.006] [PMID: 19121385]

[50] Xie P, Zhang W, Yuan S, et al. Suppression of experimental choroidal neovascularization by curcumin in mice. PLoS One 2012; 7(12)e53329
[http://dx.doi.org/10.1371/journal.pone.0053329] [PMID: 23285282]

[51] Zhu W, Wu Y, Meng YF, et al. Effect of curcumin on aging retinal pigment epithelial cells. Drug Des Devel Ther 2015; 9: 5337-44.
[PMID: 26445530]

[52] Aldebasi YH, Aly SM, Rahmani AH. Therapeutic implications of curcumin in the prevention of diabetic retinopathy via modulation of anti-oxidant activity and genetic pathways. Int J Physiol Pathophysiol Pharmacol 2013; 5(4): 194-202.
[PMID: 24379904]

[53] Li J, Wang P, Ying J, Chen Z, Yu S. Curcumin attenuates retinal vascular leakage by inhibiting calcium/calmodulin-dependent protein kinase II activity in streptozotocin-induced diabetes. Cell Physiol Biochem 2016; 39(3): 1196-208.
[http://dx.doi.org/10.1159/000447826] [PMID: 27595397]

[54] Wang L, Li C, Guo H, Kern TS, Huang K, Zheng L. Curcumin inhibits neuronal and vascular degeneration in retina after ischemia and reperfusion injury. PLoS One 2011; 6(8)e23194
[http://dx.doi.org/10.1371/journal.pone.0023194] [PMID: 21858029]

[55] Matteucci A, Frank C, Domenici MR, et al. Curcumin treatment protects rat retinal neurons against excitotoxicity: effect on N-methyl-D: -aspartate-induced intracellular Ca^{2+} increase. Exp Brain Res 2005; 167(4): 641-8.
[http://dx.doi.org/10.1007/s00221-005-0068-0] [PMID: 16078027]

[56] Yue Y-K, Mo B, Zhao J, et al. Neuroprotective effect of curcumin against oxidative damage in BV-2 microglia and high intraocular pressure animal model. J Ocul Pharmacol Ther 2014; 30(8): 657-64.
[http://dx.doi.org/10.1089/jop.2014.0022] [PMID: 24963995]

[57] Gupta SK, Selvan VK, Agrawal SS, Saxena R. Advances in pharmacological strategies for the prevention of cataract development. Indian J Ophthalmol 2009; 57(3): 175-83.

[http://dx.doi.org/10.4103/0301-4738.49390] [PMID: 19384010]

[58]   Pari L, Tewas D, Eckel J. Role of curcumin in health and disease. Arch Physiol Biochem 2008; 114(2): 127-49.
[http://dx.doi.org/10.1080/13813450802033958] [PMID: 18484280]

[59]   Suryanarayana P, Saraswat M, Mrudula T, Krishna TP, Krishnaswamy K, Reddy GB. Curcumin and turmeric delay streptozotocin-induced diabetic cataract in rats. Invest Ophthalmol Vis Sci 2005; 46(6): 2092-9.
[http://dx.doi.org/10.1167/iovs.04-1304] [PMID: 15914628]

[60]   Murugan P, Pari L. Antioxidant effect of tetrahydrocurcumin in streptozotocin-nicotinamide induced diabetic rats. Life Sci 2006; 79(18): 1720-8.
[http://dx.doi.org/10.1016/j.lfs.2006.06.001] [PMID: 16806281]

[61]   Grama CN, Suryanarayana P, Patil MA, *et al*. Efficacy of biodegradable curcumin nanoparticles in delaying cataract in diabetic rat model. PLoS One 2013; 8(10)e78217
[http://dx.doi.org/10.1371/journal.pone.0078217] [PMID: 24155984]

[62]   Berthoud VM, Minogue PJ, Yu H, Snabb JI, Beyer EC. Connexin46fs380 causes progressive cataracts. Invest Ophthalmol Vis Sci 2014; 55(10): 6639-48.
[http://dx.doi.org/10.1167/iovs.14-15012] [PMID: 25103261]

[63]   Moreau KL, King JA. Protein misfolding and aggregation in cataract disease and prospects for prevention. Trends Mol Med 2012; 18(5): 273-82.
[http://dx.doi.org/10.1016/j.molmed.2012.03.005] [PMID: 22520268]

[64]   Kumar PA, Haseeb A, Suryanarayana P, Ehtesham NZ, Reddy GB. Elevated expression of alphaA- and alphaB-crystallins in streptozotocin-induced diabetic rat. Arch Biochem Biophys 2005; 444(2): 77-83.
[http://dx.doi.org/10.1016/j.abb.2005.09.021] [PMID: 16309625]

[65]   Manikandan R, Beulaja M, Thiagarajan R, Arumugam M. Effect of curcumin on the modulation of αA- and αB-crystallin and heat shock protein 70 in selenium-induced cataractogenesis in Wistar rat pups. Mol Vis 2011; 17: 388-94.
[PMID: 21311744]

[66]   Manikandan R, Thiagarajan R, Beulaja S, Sudhandiran G, Arumugam M. Curcumin prevents free radical-mediated cataractogenesis through modulations in lens calcium. Free Radic Biol Med 2010; 48(4): 483-92.
[http://dx.doi.org/10.1016/j.freeradbiomed.2009.11.011] [PMID: 19932168]

[67]   Hu YH, Huang XR, Qi MX, Hou BY. Curcumin inhibits proliferation of human lens epithelial cells: a proteomic analysis. J Zhejiang Univ Sci B 2012; 13(5): 402-7.
[http://dx.doi.org/10.1631/jzus.B1100278] [PMID: 22556179]

[68]   Huang XR, Qi MX, Kang KR. [Apoptosis of lens epithelial cell induced by curcumin and its mechanism]. Zhonghua Yan Ke Za Zhi 2006; 42(7): 649-53.
[PMID: 17081427]

[69]   Anand David AV, Arulmoli R, Parasuraman S. Overviews of biological importance of quercetin: a bioactive flavonoid. Pharmacogn Rev 2016; 10(20): 84-9.
[http://dx.doi.org/10.4103/0973-7847.194044] [PMID: 28082789]

[70]   Kennedy DOB. Vitamins and the brain: mechanisms, dose and efficacy - a review. Nutrients 2016; 8(2): 68.
[http://dx.doi.org/10.3390/nu8020068] [PMID: 26828517]

[71]   Cao X, Liu M, Tuo J, Shen D, Chan C-C. The effects of quercetin in cultured human RPE cells under oxidative stress and in Ccl2/Cx3cr1 double deficient mice. Exp Eye Res 2010; 91(1): 15-25.
[http://dx.doi.org/10.1016/j.exer.2010.03.016] [PMID: 20361964]

[72]   Manjeet K R, Ghosh B. Quercetin inhibits LPS-induced nitric oxide and tumor necrosis factor-alpha

production in murine macrophages. Int J Immunopharmacol 1999; 21(7): 435-43.
[http://dx.doi.org/10.1016/S0192-0561(99)00024-7] [PMID: 10454017]

[73]   van Jaarsveld H, Kuyl JM, Schulenburg DH, Wiid NM. Effect of flavonoids on the outcome of myocardial mitochondrial ischemia/reperfusion injury. Res Commun Mol Pathol Pharmacol 1996; 91(1): 65-75.
[PMID: 8824932]

[74]   Arts IC, van de Putte B, Hollman PC. Catechin contents of foods commonly consumed in The Netherlands. 1. Fruits, vegetables, staple foods, and processed foods. J Agric Food Chem 2000; 48(5): 1746-51.
[http://dx.doi.org/10.1021/jf000025h] [PMID: 10820089]

[75]   Zhang B, Osborne NN. Oxidative-induced retinal degeneration is attenuated by epigallocatechin gallate. Brain Res 2006; 1124(1): 176-87.
[http://dx.doi.org/10.1016/j.brainres.2006.09.067] [PMID: 17084820]

[76]   Zhang B, Rusciano D, Osborne NN. Orally administered epigallocatechin gallate attenuates retinal neuronal death *in vivo* and light-induced apoptosis *in vitro*. Brain Res 2008; 1198: 141-52.
[http://dx.doi.org/10.1016/j.brainres.2007.12.015] [PMID: 18255049]

[77]   Costa BL, Fawcett R, Li GY, Safa R, Osborne NN. Orally administered epigallocatechin gallate attenuates light-induced photoreceptor damage. Brain Res Bull 2008; 76(4): 412-23.
[http://dx.doi.org/10.1016/j.brainresbull.2008.01.022] [PMID: 18502318]

[78]   Lee SM, Ko I-G, Kim S-E, Kim DH, Kang BN. Protective effect of catechin on apoptosis of the lens epithelium in rats with N-methyl-N-nitrosourea-induced cataracts. Korean J Ophthalmol 2010; 24(2): 101-7.
[http://dx.doi.org/10.3341/kjo.2010.24.2.101] [PMID: 20379460]

[79]   Chan C-M, Huang J-H, Chiang H-S, *et al.* Effects of (-)-epigallocatechin gallate on RPE cell migration and adhesion. Mol Vis 2010; 16: 586-95.
[PMID: 20376327]

[80]   Militão GCG, Albuquerque MRJR, Pessoa ODL, *et al.* Cytotoxic activity of nepetin, a flavonoid from Eupatorium ballotaefolium HBK. Pharmazie 2004; 59(12): 965-6.
[PMID: 15638088]

[81]   Patel K, Patel DK. Medicinal importance, pharmacological activities, and analytical aspects of hispidulin: A concise report. J Tradit Complement Med 2016; 7(3): 360-6.
[http://dx.doi.org/10.1016/j.jtcme.2016.11.003] [PMID: 28725632]

[82]   Brimson JM, Onlamoon N, Tencomnao T, Thitilertdecha P. Clerodendrum petasites S. Moore: The therapeutic potential of phytochemicals, hispidulin, vanillic acid, verbascoside, and apigenin. Biomed Pharmacother 2019; 118109319
[http://dx.doi.org/10.1016/j.biopha.2019.109319] [PMID: 31404773]

[83]   Sudha A, Srinivasan P. Physicochemical and phytochemical profiles of aerial parts of *Lippia nodiflora* L. Int J Pharm Sci Res 2013; 4: 4263-71.

[84]   Gao Y, Zhang Y, Fan Y. Eupafolin ameliorates lipopolysaccharide-induced cardiomyocyte autophagy *via* PI3K/AKT/mTOR signaling pathway. Iran J Basic Med Sci 2019; 22(11): 1340-6.
[PMID: 32128100]

[85]   Langcake P, Pryce RJ. A new class of phytoalexins from grapevines. Experientia 1977; 33(2): 151-2.
[http://dx.doi.org/10.1007/BF02124034] [PMID: 844529]

[86]   Abu-Amero KK, Kondkar AA, Chalam KV. Resveratrol and ophthalmic diseases. Nutrients 2016; 8(4): 200.
[http://dx.doi.org/10.3390/nu8040200] [PMID: 27058553]

[87]   Lippi G, Franchini M, Favaloro EJ, Targher G. Moderate red wine consumption and cardiovascular disease risk: beyond the "French paradox". Semin Thromb Hemost 2010; 36(1): 59-70.

[http://dx.doi.org/10.1055/s-0030-1248725] [PMID: 20391297]

[88] Wu JM, Hsieh TC. Resveratrol: a cardioprotective substance. Ann N Y Acad Sci 2011; 1215: 16-21.
[http://dx.doi.org/10.1111/j.1749-6632.2010.05854.x] [PMID: 21261637]

[89] Richard T, Pawlus AD, Iglésias M-L, *et al.* Neuroprotective properties of resveratrol and derivatives. Ann N Y Acad Sci 2011; 1215: 103-8.
[http://dx.doi.org/10.1111/j.1749-6632.2010.05865.x] [PMID: 21261647]

[90] Gusman J, Malonne H, Atassi G. A reappraisal of the potential chemopreventive and chemotherapeutic properties of resveratrol. Carcinogenesis 2001; 22(8): 1111-7.
[http://dx.doi.org/10.1093/carcin/22.8.1111] [PMID: 11470738]

[91] de la Lastra CA, Villegas I. Resveratrol as an anti-inflammatory and anti-aging agent: mechanisms and clinical implications. Mol Nutr Food Res 2005; 49(5): 405-30.
[http://dx.doi.org/10.1002/mnfr.200500022] [PMID: 15832402]

[92] King RE, Kent KD, Bomser JA. Resveratrol reduces oxidation and proliferation of human retinal pigment epithelial cells *via* extracellular signal-regulated kinase inhibition. Chem Biol Interact 2005; 151(2): 143-9.
[http://dx.doi.org/10.1016/j.cbi.2004.11.003] [PMID: 15698585]

[93] Luna C, Li G, Liton PB, *et al.* Resveratrol prevents the expression of glaucoma markers induced by chronic oxidative stress in trabecular meshwork cells. Food Chem Toxicol 2009; 47(1): 198-204.
[http://dx.doi.org/10.1016/j.fct.2008.10.029] [PMID: 19027816]

[94] Kaarniranta K, Salminen A, Haapasalo A, Soininen H, Hiltunen M. Age-related macular degeneration (AMD): Alzheimer's disease in the eye? J Alzheimers Dis 2011; 24(4): 615-31.
[http://dx.doi.org/10.3233/JAD-2011-101908] [PMID: 21297256]

[95] Koskela A, Reinisalo M, Hyttinen JMT, Kaarniranta K, Karjalainen RO. Pinosylvin-mediated protection against oxidative stress in human retinal pigment epithelial cells. Mol Vis 2014; 20: 760-9.
[PMID: 24940030]

[96] Nathu Z, Dwivedi DJ, Reddan JR, Sheardown H, Margetts PJ, West-Mays JA. Temporal changes in MMP mRNA expression in the lens epithelium during anterior subcapsular cataract formation. Exp Eye Res 2009; 88(2): 323-30.
[http://dx.doi.org/10.1016/j.exer.2008.08.014] [PMID: 18809398]

[97] Kayastha F, Johar K, Gajjar D, *et al.* Andrographolide suppresses epithelial mesenchymal transition by inhibition of MAPK signalling pathway in lens epithelial cells. J Biosci 2015; 40(2): 313-24.
[http://dx.doi.org/10.1007/s12038-015-9513-9] [PMID: 25963259]

[98] Kayastha F, Madhu H, Vasavada A, Johar K. Andrographolide reduces proliferation and migration of lens epithelial cells by modulating PI3K/Akt pathway. Exp Eye Res 2014; 128: 23-6.
[http://dx.doi.org/10.1016/j.exer.2014.09.002] [PMID: 25220506]

[99] Li W, Liu J, Fu W, *et al.* 3-O-acetyl-11-keto-β-boswellic acid exerts anti-tumor effects in glioblastoma by arresting cell cycle at G2/M phase. J Exp Clin Cancer Res 2018; 37(1): 132.
[http://dx.doi.org/10.1186/s13046-018-0805-4] [PMID: 29970196]

[100] Raja AF, Ali F, Khan IA, Shawl AS, Arora DS. Acetyl-11-keto-β-boswellic acid (AKBA); targeting oral cavity pathogens. BMC Res Notes 2011; 4: 406.
[http://dx.doi.org/10.1186/1756-0500-4-406] [PMID: 21992439]

[101] Lulli M, Cammalleri M, Fornaciari I, Casini G, Dal Monte M. Acetyl-11-keto-β-boswellic acid reduces retinal angiogenesis in a mouse model of oxygen-induced retinopathy. Exp Eye Res 2015; 135: 67-80.
[http://dx.doi.org/10.1016/j.exer.2015.04.011] [PMID: 25913458]

[102] Kunnumakkara AB, Nair AS, Sung B, Pandey MK, Aggarwal BB. Boswellic acid blocks signal transducers and activators of transcription 3 signaling, proliferation, and survival of multiple myeloma *via* the protein tyrosine phosphatase SHP-1. Mol Cancer Res 2009; 7(1): 118-28.

[http://dx.doi.org/10.1158/1541-7786.MCR-08-0154] [PMID: 19147543]

[103] Škovierová H, Vidomanová E, Mahmood S, *et al.* The molecular and cellular effect of homocysteine metabolism imbalance on human health. Int J Mol Sci 2016; 17(10): 1733.
[http://dx.doi.org/10.3390/ijms17101733] [PMID: 27775595]

[104] Ritch R, Prata TS, de Moraes CGV, *et al.* Association of exfoliation syndrome and central retinal vein occlusion: an ultrastructural analysis. Acta Ophthalmol 2010; 88(1): 91-5.
[http://dx.doi.org/10.1111/j.1755-3768.2009.01578.x] [PMID: 19725816]

[105] Bleich S, Jünemann A, von Ahsen N, *et al.* Homocysteine and risk of open-angle glaucoma. J Neural Transm (Vienna) 2002; 109(12): 1499-504.
[http://dx.doi.org/10.1007/s007020200097] [PMID: 12486490]

[106] Zappacosta B, Mastroiacovo P, Persichilli S, *et al.* Homocysteine lowering by folate-rich diet or pharmacological supplementations in subjects with moderate hyperhomocysteinemia. Nutrients 2013; 5(5): 1531-43.
[http://dx.doi.org/10.3390/nu5051531] [PMID: 23698160]

[107] Vessani RM, Ritch R, Liebmann JM, Jofe M. Plasma homocysteine is elevated in patients with exfoliation syndrome. Am J Ophthalmol 2003; 136(1): 41-6.
[http://dx.doi.org/10.1016/S0002-9394(03)00077-1] [PMID: 12834668]

[108] Clement CI, Goldberg I, Healey PR, Graham SL. Plasma homocysteine, MTHFR gene mutation, and open-angle glaucoma. J Glaucoma 2009; 18(1): 73-8.
[http://dx.doi.org/10.1097/IJG.0b013e31816f7631] [PMID: 19142139]

[109] Lobo V, Patil A, Phatak A, Chandra N. Free radicals, antioxidants and functional foods: Impact on human health. Pharmacogn Rev 2010; 4(8): 118-26.
[http://dx.doi.org/10.4103/0973-7847.70902] [PMID: 22228951]

[110] West S, Vitale S, Hallfrisch J, *et al.* Are antioxidants or supplements protective for age-related macular degeneration? Arch Ophthalmol 1994; 112(2): 222-7.
[http://dx.doi.org/10.1001/archopht.1994.01090140098031] [PMID: 8311777]

[111] Smith W, Mitchell P, Rochester C. Serum beta carotene, alpha tocopherol, and age-related maculopathy: the Blue Mountains Eye Study. Am J Ophthalmol 1997; 124(6): 838-40.
[http://dx.doi.org/10.1016/S0002-9394(14)71702-7] [PMID: 9402831]

[112] Christen WG, Glynn RJ, Chew EY, Buring JE. Vitamin E and age-related macular degeneration in a randomized trial of women. Ophthalmology 2010; 117(6): 1163-8.
[http://dx.doi.org/10.1016/j.ophtha.2009.10.043] [PMID: 20153900]

[113] Tanito M, Yoshida Y, Kaidzu S, *et al.* Acceleration of age-related changes in the retina in alpha-tocopherol transfer protein null mice fed a Vitamin E-deficient diet. Invest Ophthalmol Vis Sci 2007; 48(1): 396-404.
[http://dx.doi.org/10.1167/iovs.06-0872] [PMID: 17197560]

[114] Aoki A, Inoue M, Nguyen E, *et al.* Dietary n-3 Fatty Acid, α-Tocopherol, Zinc, vitamin D, vitamin C, and β-carotene are associated with age-related macular degeneration in Japan. Sci Rep 2016; 6: 20723.
[http://dx.doi.org/10.1038/srep20723] [PMID: 26846575]

[115] Vizzarri F, Palazzo M, Bartollino S, *et al.* Effects of an antioxidant protective topical formulation on eye exposed to ultraviolet-irradiation: a study in rabbit animal model. Physiol Res 2018; 67(3): 457-64.
[http://dx.doi.org/10.33549/physiolres.933759] [PMID: 29527920]

[116] Larrosa JM, Polo V, Ramirez T, Pinilla I, Pablo LE, Honrubia FM. Alpha-tocopherol derivatives and wound healing in an experimental model of filtering surgery. Ophthalmic Surg Lasers 2000; 31(2): 131-5.
[PMID: 10743924]

[117] Engin KN, Engin G, Kucuksahin H, Oncu M, Engin G, Guvener B. Clinical evaluation of the

neuroprotective effect of alpha-tocopherol against glaucomatous damage. Eur J Ophthalmol 2007; 17(4): 528-33.
[http://dx.doi.org/10.1177/112067210701700408] [PMID: 17671926]

[118] Goldblum D, Meyenberg A, Mojon D, Tappeiner C, Frueh BE. Dietary tocopherol supplementation after trabeculectomy and phacotrabeculectomy: double-blind randomized placebo-controlled trial. Ophthalmologica 2009; 223(4): 228-32.
[http://dx.doi.org/10.1159/000203367] [PMID: 19246952]

[119] Wang SY, Singh K, Lin SC. Glaucoma and vitamins A, C, and E supplement intake and serum levels in a population-based sample of the United States. Eye (Lond) 2013; 27(4): 487-94.
[http://dx.doi.org/10.1038/eye.2013.10] [PMID: 23429409]

[120] Ramdas WD, Schouten JSAG, Webers CAB. The effect of vitamins on glaucoma: a systematic review and meta-analysis. Nutrients 2018; 10(3): 359.
[http://dx.doi.org/10.3390/nu10030359] [PMID: 29547516]

[121] Teikari JM, Virtamo J, Rautalahti M, Palmgren J, Liesto K, Heinonen OP. Long-term supplementation with alpha-tocopherol and beta-carotene and age-related cataract. Acta Ophthalmol Scand 1997; 75(6): 634-40.
[http://dx.doi.org/10.1111/j.1600-0420.1997.tb00620.x] [PMID: 9527321]

[122] Olmedilla B, Granado F, Blanco I, Vaquero M. Lutein, but not alpha-tocopherol, supplementation improves visual function in patients with age-related cataracts: a 2-y double-blind, placebo-controlled pilot study. Nutrition 2003; 19(1): 21-4.
[http://dx.doi.org/10.1016/S0899-9007(02)00861-4] [PMID: 12507634]

[123] Pham DQ, Plakogiannis R. Vitamin E supplementation in Alzheimer's disease, Parkinson's disease, tardive dyskinesia, and cataract: Part 2. Ann Pharmacother 2005; 39(12): 2065-72.
[http://dx.doi.org/10.1345/aph.1G271] [PMID: 16288072]

[124] Nourmohammadi I, Modarress M, Khanaki K, Shaabani M. Association of serum alpha-tocopherol, retinol and ascorbic acid with the risk of cataract development. Ann Nutr Metab 2008; 52(4): 296-8.
[http://dx.doi.org/10.1159/000148189] [PMID: 18663288]

[125] Wang J, Löfgren S, Dong X, Galichanin K, Söderberg PG. Dose-response relationship for α-tocopherol prevention of ultraviolet radiation induced cataract in rat. Exp Eye Res 2011; 93(1): 91-7.
[http://dx.doi.org/10.1016/j.exer.2011.05.002] [PMID: 21620831]

[126] Pastor-Valero M. Fruit and vegetable intake and vitamins C and E are associated with a reduced prevalence of cataract in a Spanish Mediterranean population. BMC Ophthalmol 2013; 13: 52.
[http://dx.doi.org/10.1186/1471-2415-13-52] [PMID: 24106773]

[127] Millen AE, Gruber M, Klein R, Klein BEK, Palta M, Mares JA. Relations of serum ascorbic acid and alpha-tocopherol to diabetic retinopathy in the Third National Health and Nutrition Examination Survey. Am J Epidemiol 2003; 158(3): 225-33.
[http://dx.doi.org/10.1093/aje/kwg116] [PMID: 12882944]

[128] Kunisaki M, Bursell SE, Umeda F, Nawata H, King GL. Prevention of diabetes-induced abnormal retinal blood flow by treatment with d-alpha-tocopherol. Biofactors 1998; 7(1-2): 55-67.
[http://dx.doi.org/10.1002/biof.5520070109] [PMID: 9523029]

[129] Gan L, Qian M, Shi K, *et al.* Restorative effect and mechanism of mecobalamin on sciatic nerve crush injury in mice. Neural Regen Res 2014; 9(22): 1979-84.
[http://dx.doi.org/10.4103/1673-5374.145379] [PMID: 25598780]

[130] Ritch R. Natural compounds: evidence for a protective role in eye disease. Can J Ophthalmol 2007; 42(3): 425-38.
[http://dx.doi.org/10.3129/i07-044] [PMID: 17508040]

[131] Kikuchi M, Kashii S, Honda Y, Tamura Y, Kaneda K, Akaike A. Protective effects of methylcobalamin, a vitamin B12 analog, against glutamate-induced neurotoxicity in retinal cell

culture. Invest Ophthalmol Vis Sci 1997; 38(5): 848-54.
[PMID: 9112980]

[132]   Ripps H, Shen W. Review: taurine: a "very essential" amino acid. Mol Vis 2012; 18: 2673-86.
[PMID: 23170060]

[133]   Militante JD, Lombardini JB. Taurine: evidence of physiological function in the retina. Nutr Neurosci 2002; 5(2): 75-90.
[http://dx.doi.org/10.1080/10284150290018991] [PMID: 12000086]

[134]   Di Leo MAS, Santini SA, Cercone S, *et al.* Chronic taurine supplementation ameliorates oxidative stress and Na+ K+ ATPase impairment in the retina of diabetic rats. Amino Acids 2002; 23(4): 401-6.
[http://dx.doi.org/10.1007/s00726-002-0202-2] [PMID: 12436207]

[135]   Cubillos S, Fazzino F, Lima L. Medium requirements for neuritic outgrowth from goldfish retinal explants and the trophic effect of taurine. Int J Dev Neurosci 2002; 20(8): 607-17.
[http://dx.doi.org/10.1016/S0736-5748(02)00105-3] [PMID: 12526891]

[136]   Pasantes-Morales H, Quiroz H, Quesada O. Treatment with taurine, diltiazem, and vitamin E retards the progressive visual field reduction in retinitis pigmentosa: a 3-year follow-up study. Metab Brain Dis 2002; 17(3): 183-97.
[http://dx.doi.org/10.1023/A:1019926122125] [PMID: 12322788]

[137]   Bains VK, Bains R. The antioxidant master glutathione and periodontal health. Dent Res J (Isfahan) 2015; 12(5): 389-405.
[http://dx.doi.org/10.4103/1735-3327.166169] [PMID: 26604952]

[138]   Unal M, Güven M, Devranoğlu K, *et al.* Glutathione S transferase M1 and T1 genetic polymorphisms are related to the risk of primary open-angle glaucoma: a study in a Turkish population. Br J Ophthalmol 2007; 91(4): 527-30.
[http://dx.doi.org/10.1136/bjo.2006.102418] [PMID: 16973661]

[139]   Yang J, Tezel G, Patil RV, Romano C, Wax MB. Serum autoantibody against glutathione S-transferase in patients with glaucoma. Invest Ophthalmol Vis Sci 2001; 42(6): 1273-6.
[PMID: 11328739]

[140]   Wei Z, Caty J, Whitson J, *et al.* Reduced glutathione level promotes epithelial-mesenchymal transition in lens epithelial cells *via* a Wnt/β-catenin–Mediated Pathway. Am J Pathol 2017; 187(11): 2399-412.
[http://dx.doi.org/10.1016/j.ajpath.2017.07.018] [PMID: 28827139]

[141]   Mokhtari V, Afsharian P, Shahhoseini M, Kalantar SM, Moini A. A review on various uses of n-acetyl cysteine. Cell J 2017; 19(1): 11-7.
[PMID: 28367412]

[142]   Denis U, Lecomte M, Paget C, Ruggiero D, Wiernsperger N, Lagarde M. Advanced glycation end-products induce apoptosis of bovine retinal pericytes in culture: involvement of diacylglycerol/ceramide production and oxidative stress induction. Free Radic Biol Med 2002; 33(2): 236-47.
[http://dx.doi.org/10.1016/S0891-5849(02)00879-1] [PMID: 12106819]

[143]   England K, O'Driscoll C, Cotter TG. Carbonylation of glycolytic proteins is a key response to drug-induced oxidative stress and apoptosis. Cell Death Differ 2004; 11(3): 252-60.
[http://dx.doi.org/10.1038/sj.cdd.4401338] [PMID: 14631408]

[144]   Hori K, Katayama M, Sato N, Ishii K, Waga S, Yodoi J. Neuroprotection by glial cells through adult T cell leukemia-derived factor/human thioredoxin (ADF/TRX). Brain Res 1994; 652(2): 304-10.
[http://dx.doi.org/10.1016/0006-8993(94)90241-0] [PMID: 7953744]

[145]   Chotikavanich S, de Paiva CS, Li Q, *et al.* Production and activity of matrix metalloproteinase-9 on the ocular surface increase in dysfunctional tear syndrome. Invest Ophthalmol Vis Sci 2009; 50(7): 3203-9.
[http://dx.doi.org/10.1167/iovs.08-2476] [PMID: 19255163]

[146] Ramaesh T, Ramaesh K, Riley SC, West JD, Dhillon B. Effects of N-acetylcysteine on matrix metalloproteinase-9 secretion and cell migration of human corneal epithelial cells. Eye (Lond) 2012; 26(8): 1138-44.
[http://dx.doi.org/10.1038/eye.2012.135] [PMID: 22766540]

[147] Vidal-Casariego A, Burgos-Peláez R, Martínez-Faedo C, *et al.* Metabolic effects of L-carnitine on type 2 diabetes mellitus: systematic review and meta-analysis. Exp Clin Endocrinol Diabetes 2013; 121(4): 234-8.
[http://dx.doi.org/10.1055/s-0033-1333688] [PMID: 23430574]

[148] Ferreira GC, McKenna MC. L-carnitine and acetyl-L-carnitine roles and neuroprotection in developing brain. Neurochem Res 2017; 42(6): 1661-75.
[http://dx.doi.org/10.1007/s11064-017-2288-7] [PMID: 28508995]

[149] Vogt C, Georgi A, Werner G. Enantiomeric separation of D/L-carnitine using HPLC and CZE after derivatization. Chromatographia 1995; 40: 287-95.
[http://dx.doi.org/10.1007/BF02290359]

[150] Vaz FM, Wanders RJ. Carnitine biosynthesis in mammals. Biochem J 2002; 361(Pt 3): 417-29.
[http://dx.doi.org/10.1042/bj3610417] [PMID: 11802770]

[151] Ates O, Alp HH, Mumcu U, *et al.* The effect of L-carnitine treatment on levels of malondialdehyde and glutathione in patients with age related macular degeneration. Eurasian J Med 2008; 40(1): 1-5.
[PMID: 25610013]

[152] Feher J, Kovacs B, Kovacs I, Schveoller M, Papale A, Balacco Gabrieli C. Improvement of visual functions and fundus alterations in early age-related macular degeneration treated with a combination of acetyl-L-carnitine, n-3 fatty acids, and coenzyme Q10. Ophthalmologica 2005; 219(3): 154-66.
[http://dx.doi.org/10.1159/000085248] [PMID: 15947501]

[153] Pescosolido N, Imperatrice B, Karavitis P. The aging eye and the role of L-carnitine and its derivatives. Drugs R D 2008; 9 (Suppl. 1): 3-14.
[http://dx.doi.org/10.2165/0126839-200809001-00002] [PMID: 19105587]

[154] Calandrella N, De Seta C, Scarsella G, Risuleo G. Carnitine reduces the lipoperoxidative damage of the membrane and apoptosis after induction of cell stress in experimental glaucoma. Cell Death Dis 2010; 1e62
[http://dx.doi.org/10.1038/cddis.2010.40] [PMID: 21364667]

[155] Pessotto P, Valeri P, Arrigoni-Martelli E. The presence of L-carnitine in ocular tissues of the rabbit. J Ocul Pharmacol 1994; 10(4): 643-51.
[http://dx.doi.org/10.1089/jop.1994.10.643] [PMID: 7714408]

[156] Gawecki M, Raczyńska K, Homziuk M, Iwaszkiewicz-Bilikiewicz B. Carnitine level in human lens and density of cataract. Klin Oczna 2004; 106(3) (Suppl.): 409-10.
[PMID: 15636217]

[157] Kocer I, Taysi S, Ertekin MV, *et al.* The effect of L-carnitine in the prevention of ionizing radiation-induced cataracts: a rat model. Graefes Arch Clin Exp Ophthalmol 2007; 245(4): 588-94.
[http://dx.doi.org/10.1007/s00417-005-0097-1] [PMID: 16915402]

[158] Geraldine P, Sneha BB, Elanchezhian R, *et al.* Prevention of selenite-induced cataractogenesis by acetyl-L-carnitine: an experimental study. Exp Eye Res 2006; 83(6): 1340-9.
[http://dx.doi.org/10.1016/j.exer.2006.07.009] [PMID: 16962580]

[159] Elanchezhian R, Ramesh E, Sakthivel M, *et al.* Acetyl-L-carnitine prevents selenite-induced cataractogenesis in an experimental animal model. Curr Eye Res 2007; 32(11): 961-71.
[http://dx.doi.org/10.1080/02713680701673470] [PMID: 18027172]

[160] Elanchezhian R, Sakthivel M, Geraldine P, Thomas PA. The effect of acetyl-L-carnitine on lenticular calpain activity in prevention of selenite-induced cataractogenesis. Exp Eye Res 2009; 88(5): 938-44.

[http://dx.doi.org/10.1016/j.exer.2008.12.009] [PMID: 19150348]

[161] Elanchezhian R, Sakthivel M, Geraldine P, Thomas PA. Regulatory effect of acetyl-l-carnitine on expression of lenticular antioxidant and apoptotic genes in selenite-induced cataract. Chem Biol Interact 2010; 184(3): 346-51.
[http://dx.doi.org/10.1016/j.cbi.2010.01.006] [PMID: 20067779]

[162] Farghaly LM, Ghobashy WA, Shoukry Y, El-Azab MF. Ameliorative effect of acetyl-L-carnitine and/or nifedipine against selenite-induced cataractogenesis in young albino rats. Eur J Pharmacol 2014; 729: 1-9.
[http://dx.doi.org/10.1016/j.ejphar.2014.02.005] [PMID: 24530554]

[163] Yang SP, Yang XZ, Cao GP. Acetyl-l-carnitine prevents homocysteine-induced suppression of Nrf2/Keap1 mediated antioxidation in human lens epithelial cells. Mol Med Rep 2015; 12(1): 1145-50.
[http://dx.doi.org/10.3892/mmr.2015.3490] [PMID: 25776802]

[164] Poorabbas A, Fallah F, Bagdadchi J, *et al.* Determination of free L-carnitine levels in type II diabetic women with and without complications. Eur J Clin Nutr 2007; 61(7): 892-5.
[http://dx.doi.org/10.1038/sj.ejcn.1602594] [PMID: 17311064]

[165] Liepinsh E, Skapare E, Vavers E, *et al.* High L-carnitine concentrations do not prevent late diabetic complications in type 1 and 2 diabetic patients. Nutr Res 2012; 32(5): 320-7.
[http://dx.doi.org/10.1016/j.nutres.2012.03.010] [PMID: 22652370]

[166] Cao Y, Li X, Shi P, Wang LX, Sui ZG. Effects of L-carnitine on high glucose-induced oxidative stress in retinal ganglion cells. Pharmacology 2014; 94(3-4): 123-30.
[http://dx.doi.org/10.1159/000363062] [PMID: 25247444]

[167] Cao Y, Li X, Wang C-J, *et al.* Role of NF-E2-related factor 2 in neuroprotective effect of l-carnitine against high glucose-induced oxidative stress in the retinal ganglion cells. Biomed Pharmacother 2015; 69: 345-8.
[http://dx.doi.org/10.1016/j.biopha.2014.12.030] [PMID: 25661380]

[168] Galasso C, Corinaldesi C, Sansone C. Carotenoids from marine organisms: biological functions and industrial applications. Antioxidants 2017; 6(4): 6.
[http://dx.doi.org/10.3390/antiox6040096] [PMID: 29168774]

[169] Yuan H, Zhang J, Nageswaran D, Li L. Carotenoid metabolism and regulation in horticultural crops. Hortic Res 2015; 2: 15036.
[http://dx.doi.org/10.1038/hortres.2015.36] [PMID: 26504578]

[170] Khoo H-E, Prasad KN, Kong K-W, Jiang Y, Ismail A. Carotenoids and their isomers: color pigments in fruits and vegetables. Molecules 2011; 16(2): 1710-38.
[http://dx.doi.org/10.3390/molecules16021710] [PMID: 21336241]

[171] Rodrigo-Baños M, Garbayo I, Vílchez C, Bonete MJ, Martínez-Espinosa RM. Carotenoids from haloarchaea and their potential in biotechnology. Mar Drugs 2015; 13(9): 5508-32.
[http://dx.doi.org/10.3390/md13095508] [PMID: 26308012]

[172] Liu RH. Health-promoting components of fruits and vegetables in the diet. Adv Nutr 2013; 4(3): 384S-92S.
[http://dx.doi.org/10.3945/an.112.003517] [PMID: 23674808]

[173] Mourvaki E, Gizzi S, Rossi R, Rufini S, Rufini S. Passionflower fruit-a "new" source of lycopene? J Med Food 2005; 8(1): 104-6.
[http://dx.doi.org/10.1089/jmf.2005.8.104] [PMID: 15857218]

[174] Toti E, Chen CO, Palmery M, Villaño Valencia D, Peluso I. Non-provitamin A and provitamin A carotenoids as immunomodulators: recommended dietary allowance, therapeutic index, or personalized nutrition? Oxid Med Cell Longev 2018; 20184637861
[http://dx.doi.org/10.1155/2018/4637861] [PMID: 29861829]

[175] Tapiero H, Townsend DM, Tew KD. The role of carotenoids in the prevention of human pathologies. Biomed Pharmacother 2004; 58(2): 100-10.
[http://dx.doi.org/10.1016/j.biopha.2003.12.006] [PMID: 14992791]

[176] Fiedor J, Burda K. Potential role of carotenoids as antioxidants in human health and disease. Nutrients 2014; 6(2): 466-88.
[http://dx.doi.org/10.3390/nu6020466] [PMID: 24473231]

[177] Jia YP, Sun L, Yu HS, *et al.* The pharmacological effects of lutein and zeaxanthin on visual disorders and cognition diseases. Molecules 2017; 22(4): 610.
[http://dx.doi.org/10.3390/molecules22040610] [PMID: 28425969]

[178] Ma L, Yan S-F, Huang Y-M, *et al.* Effect of lutein and zeaxanthin on macular pigment and visual function in patients with early age-related macular degeneration. Ophthalmology 2012; 119(11): 2290-7.
[http://dx.doi.org/10.1016/j.ophtha.2012.06.014] [PMID: 22858124]

[179] Chew EY, Clemons TE, Sangiovanni JP, *et al.* Secondary analyses of the effects of lutein/zeaxanthin on age-related macular degeneration progression: AREDS2 report No. 3. JAMA Ophthalmol 2014; 132(2): 142-9.
[http://dx.doi.org/10.1001/jamaophthalmol.2013.7376] [PMID: 24310343]

[180] Wang X, Jiang C, Zhang Y, Gong Y, Chen X, Zhang M. Role of lutein supplementation in the management of age-related macular degeneration: meta-analysis of randomized controlled trials. Ophthalmic Res 2014; 52(4): 198-205.
[http://dx.doi.org/10.1159/000363327] [PMID: 25358528]

[181] Murray IJ, Makridaki M, van der Veen RLP, Carden D, Parry NRA, Berendschot TTJM. Lutein supplementation over a one-year period in early AMD might have a mild beneficial effect on visual acuity: the CLEAR study. Invest Ophthalmol Vis Sci 2013; 54(3): 1781-8.
[http://dx.doi.org/10.1167/iovs.12-10715] [PMID: 23385792]

[182] Liu R, Wang T, Zhang B, *et al.* Lutein and zeaxanthin supplementation and association with visual function in age-related macular degeneration. Invest Ophthalmol Vis Sci 2014; 56(1): 252-8.
[http://dx.doi.org/10.1167/iovs.14-15553] [PMID: 25515572]

[183] Beatty S, Chakravarthy U, Nolan JM, *et al.* Secondary outcomes in a clinical trial of carotenoids with coantioxidants *versus* placebo in early age-related macular degeneration. Ophthalmology 2013; 120(3): 600-6.
[http://dx.doi.org/10.1016/j.ophtha.2012.08.040] [PMID: 23218821]

[184] Huang YM, Dou HL, Huang FF, *et al.* Changes following supplementation with lutein and zeaxanthin in retinal function in eyes with early age-related macular degeneration: a randomised, double-blind, placebo-controlled trial. Br J Ophthalmol 2015; 99(3): 371-5.
[http://dx.doi.org/10.1136/bjophthalmol-2014-305503] [PMID: 25228440]

[185] Wu J, Cho E, Willett WC, Sastry SM, Schaumberg DA. Intakes of lutein, zeaxanthin, and other carotenoids and age-related macular degeneration during 2 decades of prospective follow-up. JAMA Ophthalmol 2015; 133(12): 1415-24.
[http://dx.doi.org/10.1001/jamaophthalmol.2015.3590] [PMID: 26447482]

[186] Eggersdorfer M, Wyss A. Carotenoids in human nutrition and health. Arch Biochem Biophys 2018; 652: 18-26.
[http://dx.doi.org/10.1016/j.abb.2018.06.001] [PMID: 29885291]

[187] Krinsky NI, Landrum JT, Bone RA. Biologic mechanisms of the protective role of lutein and zeaxanthin in the eye. Annu Rev Nutr 2003; 23: 171-201.
[http://dx.doi.org/10.1146/annurev.nutr.23.011702.073307] [PMID: 12626691]

[188] Haegerstrom-Portnoy G. Short-wavelength-sensitive-cone sensitivity loss with aging: a protective role for macular pigment? J Opt Soc Am A 1988; 5(12): 2140-4.

[http://dx.doi.org/10.1364/JOSAA.5.002140] [PMID: 3230483]

[189] Bian Q, Gao S, Zhou J, *et al.* Lutein and zeaxanthin supplementation reduces photooxidative damage and modulates the expression of inflammation-related genes in retinal pigment epithelial cells. Free Radic Biol Med 2012; 53(6): 1298-307.
[http://dx.doi.org/10.1016/j.freeradbiomed.2012.06.024] [PMID: 22732187]

[190] Tuzcu M, Orhan C, Muz OE, Sahin N, Juturu V, Sahin K. Lutein and zeaxanthin isomers modulates lipid metabolism and the inflammatory state of retina in obesity-induced high-fat diet rodent model. BMC Ophthalmol 2017; 17(1): 129.
[http://dx.doi.org/10.1186/s12886-017-0524-1] [PMID: 28738845]

[191] Fung FKC, Law BYK, Lo ACY. Lutein attenuates both apoptosis and autophagy upon cobalt (ii) chloride-induced hypoxia in rat müller cells. PLoS One 2016; 11(12)e0167828
[http://dx.doi.org/10.1371/journal.pone.0167828] [PMID: 27936094]

[192] Hammond BR Jr, Wooten BR, Snodderly DM. Density of the human crystalline lens is related to the macular pigment carotenoids, lutein and zeaxanthin. Optom Vis Sci 1997; 74(7): 499-504.
[http://dx.doi.org/10.1097/00006324-199707000-00017] [PMID: 9293517]

[193] Chasan-Taber L, Willett WC, Seddon JM, *et al.* A prospective study of carotenoid and vitamin A intakes and risk of cataract extraction in US women. Am J Clin Nutr 1999; 70(4): 509-16.
[http://dx.doi.org/10.1093/ajcn/70.4.509] [PMID: 10500020]

[194] Brown L, Rimm EB, Seddon JM, *et al.* A prospective study of carotenoid intake and risk of cataract extraction in US men. Am J Clin Nutr 1999; 70(4): 517-24.
[http://dx.doi.org/10.1093/ajcn/70.4.517] [PMID: 10500021]

[195] Lyle BJ, Mares-Perlman JA, Klein BEK, Klein R, Greger JL. Antioxidant intake and risk of incident age-related nuclear cataracts in the Beaver Dam Eye Study. Am J Epidemiol 1999; 149(9): 801-9.
[http://dx.doi.org/10.1093/oxfordjournals.aje.a009895] [PMID: 10221316]

[196] Gale CR, Hall NF, Phillips DI, Martyn CN. Plasma antioxidant vitamins and carotenoids and age-related cataract. Ophthalmology 2001; 108(11): 1992-8.
[http://dx.doi.org/10.1016/S0161-6420(01)00833-8] [PMID: 11713067]

[197] Vu HTV, Robman L, Hodge A, McCarty CA, Taylor HR. Lutein and zeaxanthin and the risk of cataract: the Melbourne visual impairment project. Invest Ophthalmol Vis Sci 2006; 47(9): 3783-6.
[http://dx.doi.org/10.1167/iovs.05-0587] [PMID: 16936087]

[198] Christen WG, Liu S, Glynn RJ, Gaziano JM, Buring JE. Dietary carotenoids, vitamins C and E, and risk of cataract in women: a prospective study. Arch Ophthalmol (Chicago, Ill 1960) 2008; 126: 102-9.

[199] Glaser TS, Doss LE, Shih G, *et al.* The association of dietary lutein plus zeaxanthin and b vitamins with cataracts in the age-related eye disease study: AREDS Report No. 37. Ophthalmology 2015; 122(7): 1471-9.
[http://dx.doi.org/10.1016/j.ophtha.2015.04.007] [PMID: 25972257]

[200] Sasaki M, Ozawa Y, Kurihara T, *et al.* Neurodegenerative influence of oxidative stress in the retina of a murine model of diabetes. Diabetologia 2010; 53(5): 971-9.
[http://dx.doi.org/10.1007/s00125-009-1655-6] [PMID: 20162412]

[201] Arnal E, Miranda M, Johnsen-Soriano S, *et al.* Beneficial effect of docosahexanoic acid and lutein on retinal structural, metabolic, and functional abnormalities in diabetic rats. Curr Eye Res 2009; 34(11): 928-38.
[http://dx.doi.org/10.3109/02713680903205238] [PMID: 19958109]

[202] Muriach M, Bosch-Morell F, Alexander G, *et al.* Lutein effect on retina and hippocampus of diabetic mice. Free Radic Biol Med 2006; 41(6): 979-84.
[http://dx.doi.org/10.1016/j.freeradbiomed.2006.06.023] [PMID: 16934681]

[203] Brazionis L, Rowley K, Itsiopoulos C, O'Dea K. Plasma carotenoids and diabetic retinopathy. Br J Nutr 2009; 101(2): 270-7.

[http://dx.doi.org/10.1017/S0007114508006545] [PMID: 18554424]

[204] Hu BJ, Hu YN, Lin S, Ma WJ, Li XR. Application of Lutein and Zeaxanthin in nonproliferative diabetic retinopathy. Int J Ophthalmol 2011; 4(3): 303-6.
[PMID: 22553667]

[205] Neelam K, Goenadi CJ, Lun K, Yip CC, Au Eong K-G. Putative protective role of lutein and zeaxanthin in diabetic retinopathy. Br J Ophthalmol 2017; 101(5): 551-8.
[http://dx.doi.org/10.1136/bjophthalmol-2016-309814] [PMID: 28232380]

[206] Hodge WG, Schachter HM, Barnes D, *et al.* Efficacy of ω-3 fatty acids in preventing age-related macular degeneration: a systematic review. Ophthalmology 2006; 113(7): 1165-72.
[http://dx.doi.org/10.1016/j.ophtha.2006.02.043] [PMID: 16815401]

[207] Hodge WG, Barnes D, Schachter HM, *et al.* Evidence for the effect of ω-3 fatty acids on progression of age-related macular degeneration: a systematic review. Retina 2007; 27(2): 216-21.
[http://dx.doi.org/10.1097/01.iae.0000233322.83713.2d] [PMID: 17290205]

[208] Souied EH, Delcourt C, Querques G, *et al.* Oral docosahexaenoic acid in the prevention of exudative age-related macular degeneration: the Nutritional AMD Treatment 2 study. Ophthalmology 2013; 120(8): 1619-31.
[http://dx.doi.org/10.1016/j.ophtha.2013.01.005] [PMID: 23395546]

[209] Lawrenson JG, Evans JR. Omega 3 fatty acids for preventing or slowing the progression of age-related macular degeneration. Cochrane Database Syst Rev 2015; 4(4)CD010015
[http://dx.doi.org/10.1002/14651858.CD010015.pub3] [PMID: 25856365]

[210] Wu J, Cho E, Giovannucci EL, *et al.* Dietary intakes of eicosapentaenoic acid and docosahexaenoic acid and risk of age-related macular degeneration. Ophthalmology 2017; 124(5): 634-43.
[http://dx.doi.org/10.1016/j.ophtha.2016.12.033] [PMID: 28153441]

[211] Nguyen CTO, Bui BV, Sinclair AJ, Vingrys AJ. Dietary omega 3 fatty acids decrease intraocular pressure with age by increasing aqueous outflow. Invest Ophthalmol Vis Sci 2007; 48(2): 756-62.
[http://dx.doi.org/10.1167/iovs.06-0585] [PMID: 17251475]

[212] Hodge W, Barnes D, Schachter HM, *et al.* Effects of omega-3 fatty acids on eye health. Evid Rep Technol Assess (Summ) 2005; 117(117): 1-6.
[PMID: 16111433]

[213] Lu M, Cho E, Taylor A, Hankinson SE, Willett WC, Jacques PF. Prospective study of dietary fat and risk of cataract extraction among US women. Am J Epidemiol 2005; 161(10): 948-59.
[http://dx.doi.org/10.1093/aje/kwi118] [PMID: 15870159]

[214] Mohammadpour M, Mehrabi S, Hassanpoor N, Mirshahi R. Effects of adjuvant omega-3 fatty acid supplementation on dry eye syndrome following cataract surgery: A randomized clinical trial. J Curr Ophthalmol 2016; 29(1): 33-8.
[http://dx.doi.org/10.1016/j.joco.2016.05.006] [PMID: 28367524]

[215] Hobbs RP, Bernstein PS. Nutrient supplementation for age-related macular degeneration, cataract, and dry eye. J Ophthalmic Vis Res 2014; 9(4): 487-93.
[http://dx.doi.org/10.4103/2008-322X.150829] [PMID: 25709776]

[216] Packer L, Roy S, Sen CK. Alpha-lipoic acid: a metabolic antioxidant and potential redox modulator of transcription. Adv Pharmacol 1997; 38: 79-101.
[http://dx.doi.org/10.1016/S1054-3589(08)60980-1] [PMID: 8895805]

[217] Jia L, Liu Z, Sun L, *et al.* Acrolein, a toxicant in cigarette smoke, causes oxidative damage and mitochondrial dysfunction in RPE cells: protection by (R)-alpha-lipoic acid. Invest Ophthalmol Vis Sci 2007; 48(1): 339-48.
[http://dx.doi.org/10.1167/iovs.06-0248] [PMID: 17197552]

[218] Sun Y-D, Dong Y-D, Fan R, Zhai L-L, Bai Y-L, Jia L-H. Effect of (R)-α-lipoic acid supplementation on serum lipids and antioxidative ability in patients with age-related macular degeneration. Ann Nutr

Metab 2012; 60(4): 293-7.
[http://dx.doi.org/10.1159/000338444] [PMID: 22678104]

[219]   Tao Y, Jiang P, Wei Y, Wang P, Sun X, Wang H. α-lipoic acid treatment improves vision-related quality of life in patients with dry age-related macular degeneration. Tohoku J Exp Med 2016; 240(3): 209-14.
[http://dx.doi.org/10.1620/tjem.240.209] [PMID: 27840374]

[220]   Sarezky D, Raquib AR, Dunaief JL, Kim BJ. Tolerability in the elderly population of high-dose alpha lipoic acid: a potential antioxidant therapy for the eye. Clin Ophthalmol 2016; 10: 1899-903.
[http://dx.doi.org/10.2147/OPTH.S115900] [PMID: 27729766]

[221]   Inman DM, Lambert WS, Calkins DJ, Horner PJ. α-Lipoic acid antioxidant treatment limits glaucoma-related retinal ganglion cell death and dysfunction. PLoS One 2013; 8(6)e65389
[http://dx.doi.org/10.1371/journal.pone.0065389] [PMID: 23755225]

[222]   Ekinci M, Cagatay HH, Ceylan E, *et al.* Reduction of conjunctival fibrosis after trabeculectomy using topical α-lipoic acid in rabbit eyes. J Glaucoma 2014; 23(6): 372-9.
[http://dx.doi.org/10.1097/IJG.0000000000000052] [PMID: 25055213]

[223]   Gomes MB, Negrato CA. Alpha-lipoic acid as a pleiotropic compound with potential therapeutic use in diabetes and other chronic diseases. Diabetol Metab Syndr 2014; 6(1): 80.
[http://dx.doi.org/10.1186/1758-5996-6-80] [PMID: 25104975]

[224]   Maitra I, Serbinova E, Trischler H, Packer L. Alpha-lipoic acid prevents buthionine sulfoximine-induced cataract formation in newborn rats. Free Radic Biol Med 1995; 18(4): 823-9.
[http://dx.doi.org/10.1016/0891-5849(94)00195-P] [PMID: 7750805]

[225]   Kilic F, Handelman GJ, Traber K, Tsang K, Packer L, Trevithick JR. Modelling cortical cataractogenesis XX. *In vitro* effect of alpha-lipoic acid on glutathione concentrations in lens in model diabetic cataractogenesis. Biochem Mol Biol Int 1998; 46(3): 585-95.
[PMID: 9818098]

[226]   Borenshtein D, Ofri R, Werman M, *et al.* Cataract development in diabetic sand rats treated with alpha-lipoic acid and its gamma-linolenic acid conjugate. Diabetes Metab Res Rev 2001; 17(1): 44-50.
[http://dx.doi.org/10.1002/1520-7560(0000)9999:9999<::AID-DMRR153>3.0.CO;2-S]   [PMID: 11241890]

[227]   Kojima M, Sun L, Hata I, Sakamoto Y, Sasaki H, Sasaki K. Efficacy of alpha-lipoic acid against diabetic cataract in rat. Jpn J Ophthalmol 2007; 51(1): 10-3.
[http://dx.doi.org/10.1007/s10384-006-0384-3] [PMID: 17295134]

[228]   Sun L, Zhang J-S. [Effects of DL-alpha-lipoic acid on the experimentally induced diabetic cataract in rats]. Zhonghua Yan Ke Za Zhi 2004; 40(3): 193-6.
[PMID: 15307993]

[229]   Chen Y, Yi L, Yan G, *et al.* alpha-Lipoic acid alters post-translational modifications and protects the chaperone activity of lens alpha-crystallin in naphthalene-induced cataract. Curr Eye Res 2010; 35(7): 620-30.
[http://dx.doi.org/10.3109/02713681003768211] [PMID: 20597648]

[230]   Li Y, Liu Y-Z, Shi J-M, Jia S-B. Alpha lipoic acid protects lens from H_2O_2-induced cataract by inhibiting apoptosis of lens epithelial cells and inducing activation of anti-oxidative enzymes. Asian Pac J Trop Med 2013; 6(7): 548-51.
[http://dx.doi.org/10.1016/S1995-7645(13)60094-2] [PMID: 23768827]

[231]   Kan E, Kiliçkan E, Ayar A, Çolak R. Effects of two antioxidants; α-lipoic acid and fisetin against diabetic cataract in mice. Int Ophthalmol 2015; 35(1): 115-20.
[http://dx.doi.org/10.1007/s10792-014-0029-3] [PMID: 25488016]

[232]   Haritoglou C, Gerss J, Hammes HP, Kampik A, Ulbig MW. Alpha-lipoic acid for the prevention of

diabetic macular edema. Ophthalmologica 2011; 226(3): 127-37.
[http://dx.doi.org/10.1159/000329470] [PMID: 21811051]

[233] Kowluru RA, Odenbach S. Effect of long-term administration of alpha-lipoic acid on retinal capillary cell death and the development of retinopathy in diabetic rats. Diabetes 2004; 53(12): 3233-8.
[http://dx.doi.org/10.2337/diabetes.53.12.3233] [PMID: 15561955]

[234] Roberts R, Luan H, Berkowitz BA. α-lipoic acid corrects late-phase supernormal retinal oxygenation response in experimental diabetic retinopathy. Invest Ophthalmol Vis Sci 2006; 47(9): 4077-82.
[http://dx.doi.org/10.1167/iovs.06-0464] [PMID: 16936127]

[235] Musabayane CT, Bwititi PT, Ojewole JAO. Effects of oral administration of some herbal extracts on food consumption and blood glucose levels in normal and streptozotocin-treated diabetic rats. Methods Find Exp Clin Pharmacol 2006; 28(4): 223-8.
[http://dx.doi.org/10.1358/mf.2006.28.4.990202] [PMID: 16801983]

[236] Shukla S, Dubey KK. CoQ10 a super-vitamin: review on application and biosynthesis. 3 Biotech 2018; 8: 249.

[237] Blasi MA, Bovina C, Carella G, *et al.* Does coenzyme Q10 play a role in opposing oxidative stress in patients with age-related macular degeneration? Ophthalmologica 2001; 215(1): 51-4.
[http://dx.doi.org/10.1159/000050826] [PMID: 11125270]

[238] Qu J, Kaufman Y, Washington I. Coenzyme Q10 in the human retina. Invest Ophthalmol Vis Sci 2009; 50(4): 1814-8.
[http://dx.doi.org/10.1167/iovs.08-2656] [PMID: 19060288]

[239] Zhang X, Tohari AM, Marcheggiani F, *et al.* Therapeutic potential of co-enzyme Q10 in retinal diseases. Curr Med Chem 2017; 24(39): 4329-39.
[http://dx.doi.org/10.2174/0929867324666170801100516] [PMID: 28762311]

[240] Kernt M, Hirneiss C, Neubauer AS, Ulbig MW, Kampik A. Coenzyme Q10 prevents human lens epithelial cells from light-induced apoptotic cell death by reducing oxidative stress and stabilizing BAX / Bcl-2 ratio. Acta Ophthalmol 2010; 88(3): e78-86.
[http://dx.doi.org/10.1111/j.1755-3768.2010.01875.x] [PMID: 20374575]

[241] Shafaa MW, Elshazly AH, Dakrory AZ, Elsyed MR. Interaction of coenzyme Q10 with liposomes and its impact on suppression of selenite - induced experimental cataract. Adv Pharm Bull 2018; 8(1): 1-9.
[http://dx.doi.org/10.15171/apb.2018.001] [PMID: 29670833]

[242] Ozates S, Elgin KU, Yilmaz NS, Demirel OO, Sen E, Yilmazbas P. Evaluation of oxidative stress in pseudo-exfoliative glaucoma patients treated with and without topical coenzyme Q10 and vitamin E. Eur J Ophthalmol 2019; 29(2): 196-201.
[http://dx.doi.org/10.1177/1120672118779486] [PMID: 29869538]

[243] Ates O, Bilen H, Keles S, *et al.* Plasma coenzyme Q10 levels in type 2 diabetic patients with retinopathy. Int J Ophthalmol 2013; 6(5): 675-9.
[PMID: 24195048]

[244] Domanico D, Fragiotta S, Cutini A, Carnevale C, Zompatori L, Vingolo EM. Circulating levels of reactive oxygen species in patients with nonproliferative diabetic retinopathy and the influence of antioxidant supplementation: 6-month follow-up. Indian J Ophthalmol 2015; 63(1): 9-14.
[http://dx.doi.org/10.4103/0301-4738.151455] [PMID: 25686055]

[245] Rodríguez-Carrizalez AD, Castellanos-González JA, Martínez-Romero EC, *et al.* The effect of ubiquinone and combined antioxidant therapy on oxidative stress markers in non-proliferative diabetic retinopathy: A phase IIa, randomized, double-blind, and placebo-controlled study. Redox Rep 2016; 21(4): 155-63.
[http://dx.doi.org/10.1179/1351000215Y.0000000040] [PMID: 26321469]

[246] Fioravanti M, Buckley AE. Citicoline (Cognizin) in the treatment of cognitive impairment. Clin Interv Aging 2006; 1(3): 247-51.

[http://dx.doi.org/10.2147/ciia.2006.1.3.247] [PMID: 18046877]

[247] Parisi V, Manni G, Colacino G, Bucci MG. Cytidine-5'-diphosphocholine (citicoline) improves retinal and cortical responses in patients with glaucoma. Ophthalmology 1999; 106(6): 1126-34.
[http://dx.doi.org/10.1016/S0161-6420(99)90269-5] [PMID: 10366081]

[248] Rejdak R, Toczołowski J, Kurkowski J, *et al.* Oral citicoline treatment improves visual pathway function in glaucoma. Med Sci Monit 2003; 9(3): PI24-8.
[PMID: 12640353]

[249] Parisi V, Coppola G, Centofanti M, *et al.* Evidence of the neuroprotective role of citicoline in glaucoma patients. Prog Brain Res 2008; 173: 541-54.
[http://dx.doi.org/10.1016/S0079-6123(08)01137-0] [PMID: 18929133]

[250] Frolov MA, Gonchar PA, Barashkov VI, *et al.* The effect of parenteral citicoline on visual functions and life quality of patients with primary open-angle glaucoma. Vestn Oftalmol 2011; 127(5): 18-21.
[PMID: 22165093]

[251] Ottobelli L, Manni GL, Centofanti M, Iester M, Allevena F, Rossetti L. Citicoline oral solution in glaucoma: is there a role in slowing disease progression? Ophthalmologica 2013; 229(4): 219-26.
[http://dx.doi.org/10.1159/000350496] [PMID: 23615390]

[252] Parisi V, Centofanti M, Ziccardi L, *et al.* Treatment with citicoline eye drops enhances retinal function and neural conduction along the visual pathways in open angle glaucoma. Graefes Arch Clin Exp Ophthalmol 2015; 253(8): 1327-40.
[http://dx.doi.org/10.1007/s00417-015-3044-9] [PMID: 26004075]

[253] Sahebkar A. A systematic review and meta-analysis of the effects of pycnogenol on plasma lipids. J Cardiovasc Pharmacol Ther 2014; 19(3): 244-55.
[http://dx.doi.org/10.1177/1074248413511691] [PMID: 24346156]

[254] Iravani S, Zolfaghari B. Pharmaceutical and nutraceutical effects of Pinus pinaster bark extract. Res Pharm Sci 2011; 6(1): 1-11.
[PMID: 22049273]

[255] Spadea L, Balestrazzi E. Treatment of vascular retinopathies with Pycnogenol. Phytother Res 2001; 15(3): 219-23.
[http://dx.doi.org/10.1002/ptr.853] [PMID: 11351356]

[256] Schönlau F, Rohdewald P. Pycnogenol for diabetic retinopathy. A review. Int Ophthalmol 2001; 24(3): 161-71.
[http://dx.doi.org/10.1023/A:1021160924583] [PMID: 12498513]

[257] Kamuren ZT, McPeek CG, Sanders RA, Watkins JB III. Effects of low-carbohydrate diet and Pycnogenol treatment on retinal antioxidant enzymes in normal and diabetic rats. J Ocul Pharmacol Ther 2006; 22(1): 10-8.
[http://dx.doi.org/10.1089/jop.2006.22.10] [PMID: 16503770]

[258] Steigerwalt R, Belcaro G, Cesarone MR, *et al.* Pycnogenol improves microcirculation, retinal edema, and visual acuity in early diabetic retinopathy. J Ocul Pharmacol Ther 2009; 25(6): 537-40.
[http://dx.doi.org/10.1089/jop.2009.0023] [PMID: 19916788]

[259] Trevithick JR, Bantseev V, Hirst M, Dzialoszynski TM, Sanford ES. Is pycnogenol a double-edged sword? Cataractogenic *in vitro*, but reduces cataract risk in diabetic rats. Curr Eye Res 2013; 38(7): 751-60.
[http://dx.doi.org/10.3109/02713683.2013.770038] [PMID: 23537316]

[260] De Marino S, Gala F, Borbone N, *et al.* Phenolic glycosides from *Foeniculum vulgare* fruit and evaluation of antioxidative activity. Phytochemistry 2007; 68(13): 1805-12.
[http://dx.doi.org/10.1016/j.phytochem.2007.03.029] [PMID: 17498761]

[261] Keskin I, Gunal Y, Ayla S, *et al.* Effects of *Foeniculum vulgare* essential oil compounds, fenchone and limonene, on experimental wound healing. Biotech Histochem 2017; 92(4): 274-82.

[http://dx.doi.org/10.1080/10520295.2017.1306882] [PMID: 28426256]

[262] Mhaidat NM, Abu-zaiton AS, Alzoubi KH, Alzoubi W, Alazab RS. Antihyperglycemic properties of *Foeniculum vulgare* extract in streptozocin-induced diabetes in rats. Int J Pharmacol 2015; 11(1): 72-5.
[http://dx.doi.org/10.3923/ijp.2015.72.75]

[263] Kronschläger M, Forsman E, Yu Z, *et al.* Pharmacokinetics for topically applied caffeine in the rat. Exp Eye Res 2014; 122: 94-101.
[http://dx.doi.org/10.1016/j.exer.2014.03.009] [PMID: 24704471]

[264] Varma SD. Effect of coffee (caffeine) against human cataract blindness. Clin Ophthalmol 2016; 10: 213-20.
[http://dx.doi.org/10.2147/OPTH.S96394] [PMID: 26869755]

[265] Zhang S, Zhou R, Li B, *et al.* Caffeine preferentially protects against oxygen-induced retinopathy. FASEB J 2017; 31(8): 3334-48.
[http://dx.doi.org/10.1096/fj.201601285R] [PMID: 28420694]

[266] Higgins RD, Sanders RJ, Yan Y, Zasloff M, Williams JI. Squalamine improves retinal neovascularization. Invest Ophthalmol Vis Sci 2000; 41(6): 1507-12.
[PMID: 10798670]

[267] Ciulla TA, Criswell MH, Danis RP, Williams JI, McLane MP, Holroyd KJ. Squalamine lactate reduces choroidal neovascularization in a laser-injury model in the rat. Retina 2003; 23(6): 808-14.
[http://dx.doi.org/10.1097/00006982-200312000-00011] [PMID: 14707832]

[268] Genaidy M, Kazi AA, Peyman GA, *et al.* Effect of squalamine on iris neovascularization in monkeys. Retina 2002; 22(6): 772-8.
[http://dx.doi.org/10.1097/00006982-200212000-00014] [PMID: 12476105]

[269] Wroblewski JJ, Hu AY. Topical squalamine 0.2% and intravitreal ranibizumab 0.5 mg as combination therapy for macular edema due to branch and central retinal vein occlusion: an open-label, randomized study. Ophthalmic Surg Lasers Imaging Retina 2016; 47(10): 914-23.
[http://dx.doi.org/10.3928/23258160-20161004-04] [PMID: 27759857]

[270] Lock JY, Carlson TL, Carrier RL. Mucus models to evaluate the diffusion of drugs and particles. Adv Drug Deliv Rev 2018; 124: 34-49.
[http://dx.doi.org/10.1016/j.addr.2017.11.001] [PMID: 29117512]

[271] Irimia T, Ghica MV, Popa L, Anuţa V, Arsene A-L, Dinu-Pîrvu C-E. Strategies for improving ocular drug bioavailability and corneal wound healing with chitosan-based delivery systems. Polymers (Basel) 2018; 10(11)E1221
[http://dx.doi.org/10.3390/polym10111221] [PMID: 30961146]

[272] Elieh-Ali-Komi D, Hamblin MR. Chitin and chitosan: production and application of versatile biomedical nanomaterials. Int J Adv Res (Indore) 2016; 4(3): 411-27.
[PMID: 27819009]

[273] Rong X, Ji Y, Zhu X, *et al.* Neuroprotective effect of insulin-loaded chitosan nanoparticles/PLGA-PEG-PLGA hydrogel on diabetic retinopathy in rats. Int J Nanomedicine 2018; 14: 45-55.
[http://dx.doi.org/10.2147/IJN.S184574] [PMID: 30587984]

[274] Ochiai T, Soeda S, Ohno S, Tanaka H, Shoyama Y, Shimeno H. Crocin prevents the death of PC-12 cells through sphingomyelinase-ceramide signaling by increasing glutathione synthesis. Neurochem Int 2004; 44(5): 321-30.
[http://dx.doi.org/10.1016/S0197-0186(03)00174-8] [PMID: 14643749]

[275] Maccarone R, Di Marco S, Bisti S. Saffron supplement maintains morphology and function after exposure to damaging light in mammalian retina. Invest Ophthalmol Vis Sci 2008; 49(3): 1254-61.
[http://dx.doi.org/10.1167/iovs.07-0438] [PMID: 18326756]

[276] Falsini B, Piccardi M, Minnella A, *et al.* Influence of saffron supplementation on retinal flicker

sensitivity in early age-related macular degeneration. Invest Ophthalmol Vis Sci 2010; 51(12): 6118-24.
[http://dx.doi.org/10.1167/iovs.09-4995] [PMID: 20688744]

[277]   Makri OE, Ferlemi A-V, Lamari FN, Georgakopoulos CD. Saffron administration prevents selenite-induced cataractogenesis. Mol Vis 2013; 19: 1188-97.
[PMID: 23734088]

[278]   Stellpflug SJ, Cole JB, Isaacson BA, Lintner CP, Bilden EF. Massive atropine eye drop ingestion treated with high-dose physostigmine to avoid intubation. West J Emerg Med 2012; 13(1): 77-9.
[http://dx.doi.org/10.5811/westjem.2011.7.6817] [PMID: 22461927]

[279]   Liesegang TJ. Viscoelastic substances in ophthalmology. Surv Ophthalmol 1990; 34(4): 268-93.
[http://dx.doi.org/10.1016/0039-6257(90)90027-S] [PMID: 2111587]

[280]   Espíndola RF, Castro EF, Santhiago MR, Kara-Junior N. A clinical comparison between DisCoVisc and 2% hydroxypropylmethylcellulose in phacoemulsification: a fellow eye study. Clinics (São Paulo) 2012; 67(9): 1059-62.
[http://dx.doi.org/10.6061/clinics/2012(09)13] [PMID: 23018304]

[281]   Higashide T, Sugiyama K. Use of viscoelastic substance in ophthalmic surgery - focus on sodium hyaluronate. Clin Ophthalmol 2008; 2(1): 21-30.
[http://dx.doi.org/10.2147/OPTH.S1439] [PMID: 19668386]

[282]   Chumbley LC, Morgan AM, Musallam I. Hydroxypropyl methylcellulose in extracapsular cataract surgery with intraocular lens implantation: intraocular pressure and inflammatory response. Eye (Lond) 1990; 4(Pt 1): 121-6.
[http://dx.doi.org/10.1038/eye.1990.15] [PMID: 2323463]

[283]   Salwowska NM, Bebenek KA, Żądło DA, Wcisło-Dziadecka DL. Physiochemical properties and application of hyaluronic acid: a systematic review. J Cosmet Dermatol 2016; 15(4): 520-6.
[http://dx.doi.org/10.1111/jocd.12237] [PMID: 27324942]

[284]   Goa KL, Benfield P. Hyaluronic acid. A review of its pharmacology and use as a surgical aid in ophthalmology, and its therapeutic potential in joint disease and wound healing. Drugs 1994; 47(3): 536-66.
[http://dx.doi.org/10.2165/00003495-199447030-00009] [PMID: 7514978]

[285]   Moreland LW. Intra-articular hyaluronan (hyaluronic acid) and hylans for the treatment of osteoarthritis: mechanisms of action. Arthritis Res Ther 2003; 5(2): 54-67.
[http://dx.doi.org/10.1186/ar623] [PMID: 12718745]

[286]   Barbucci R, Lamponi S, Borzacchiello A, *et al.* Hyaluronic acid hydrogel in the treatment of osteoarthritis. Biomaterials 2002; 23(23): 4503-13.
[http://dx.doi.org/10.1016/S0142-9612(02)00194-1] [PMID: 12322970]

[287]   van Beek M, Weeks A, Jones L, Sheardown H. Immobilized hyaluronic acid containing model silicone hydrogels reduce protein adsorption. J Biomater Sci Polym Ed 2008; 19(11): 1425-36.
[http://dx.doi.org/10.1163/156856208786140364] [PMID: 18973721]

[288]   Fechner PU, Fechner MU. Methylcellulose and lens implantation. Br J Ophthalmol 1983; 67(4): 259-63.
[http://dx.doi.org/10.1136/bjo.67.4.259] [PMID: 6830744]

[289]   Mikami T, Kitagawa H. Biosynthesis and function of chondroitin sulfate. Biochim Biophys Acta 2013; 1830(10): 4719-33.
[http://dx.doi.org/10.1016/j.bbagen.2013.06.006] [PMID: 23774590]

[290]   Moschos MM, Chatziralli IP, Sergentanis TN. Viscoat *versus* Visthesia during phacoemulsification cataract surgery: corneal and foveal changes. BMC Ophthalmol 2011; 11: 9.
[http://dx.doi.org/10.1186/1471-2415-11-9] [PMID: 21529354]

[291]   Oh HN, Kim CE, Lee JH, Yang JW. Effects of quercetin in a mouse model of experimental dry eye.

Cornea 2015; 34(9): 1130-6.
[http://dx.doi.org/10.1097/ICO.0000000000000543] [PMID: 26203745]

[292] Ivanova D, Richer S, Bhandari A. Improved visual acuity and retinal integrity with resveratrol-based supplementation in patients with macular degeneration. Int J Ophthalmol Clin Res 2017; 4: 082.

[293] Unsal AIA, Kocaturk T, Gunel C, *et al*. Effect of Pycnogenol® on an experimental rat model of allergic conjunctivitis. Graefes Arch Clin Exp Ophthalmol 2018; 256(7): 1299-304.
[http://dx.doi.org/10.1007/s00417-018-3988-7] [PMID: 29675725]

[294] Lashay A, Sadough G, Ashrafi E, Lashay M, Movassat M, Akhondzadeh S. Short-term outcomes of saffron supplementation in patients with age-related macular degeneration: a double-blind,p lacebo-controlled, randomized trial. Med Hypothesis Discov Innov Ophthalmol 2016; 5(1): 32-8.
[PMID: 28289690]

[295] Christen WG, Glynn RJ, Chew EY, Albert CM, Manson JE. Folic acid, vitamin B6, and vitamin B12 in combination and age-related cataract in a randomized trial of women. Ophthalmic Epidemiol 2016; 23(1): 32-9.
[http://dx.doi.org/10.3109/09286586.2015.1130845] [PMID: 26786311]

[296] Roberti G, Tanga L, Parisi V, Sampalmieri M, Centofanti M, Manni G. A preliminary study of the neuroprotective role of citicoline eye drops in glaucomatous optic neuropathy. Indian J Ophthalmol 2014; 62(5): 549-53.
[http://dx.doi.org/10.4103/0301-4738.133484] [PMID: 24881599]

[297] Barar J, Aghanejad A, Fathi M, Omidi Y. Advanced drug delivery and targeting technologies for the ocular diseases. Bioimpacts 2016; 6(1): 49-67.
[http://dx.doi.org/10.15171/bi.2016.07] [PMID: 27340624]

[298] Velpandian T, Ed. Pharmacology of ocular therapeutics. Switzerland: Springer International Publishing 2016; pp. 479-83.
[http://dx.doi.org/10.1007/978-3-319-25498-2]

[299] Hornof M, Toropainen E, Urtti A. Cell culture models of the ocular barriers. Eur J Pharm Biopharm 2005; 60(2): 207-25.
[http://dx.doi.org/10.1016/j.ejpb.2005.01.009] [PMID: 15939234]

[300] Urtti A. Challenges and obstacles of ocular pharmacokinetics and drug delivery. Adv Drug Deliv Rev 2006; 58(11): 1131-5.
[http://dx.doi.org/10.1016/j.addr.2006.07.027] [PMID: 17097758]

SUBJECT INDEX